Coronary Artery Spasm and Thrombosis

Cardiovascular Clinics Series

*Not Available

Coronary Artery Spasm and Thrombosis

Sheldon Goldberg, M.D. | Editor

Associate Professor of Medicine
Jefferson Medical College
Director, Cardiac Catheterization Laboratory
Thomas Jefferson University Hospital
Philadelphia, Pennsylvania

CARDIOVASCULAR CLINICS

Albert N. Brest, M.D. | Editor-in-Chief

James C. Wilson Professor of Medicine
Director, Division of Cardiology
Jefferson Medical College
Philadelphia, Pennsylvania

 F. A. DAVIS COMPANY, PHILADELPHIA

Cardiovascular Clinics, 14/1, Coronary Artery Spasm and Thrombosis

Copyright © 1983 by F. A. Davis Company

Printed in the United States of America

Library of Congress Cataloging in Publication Data
Main entry under title:

Coronary artery spasm and thrombosis.

(Cardiovascular clinics ; 14/1)
Includes bibliographical references and index.
1. Coronary vasospasm—Addresses, essays, lectures.   2. Coronary heart disease—Addresses, essays, lectures.   I. Goldberg, Sheldon, 1946-   . II. Brest, Albert N.   III. Series. [DNLM: 1. Coronary vasospasm—Physiopathology. 2. Coronary disease—Physiopathology. 3. Coronary vessels—Physiopathology. W1 CA77N v. 14 no. 1] RC685.C65C67
1983   616.1'23   83-1850
ISBN 0-8036-4161-3

Preface

We are witnessing a time of important advances in the understanding and therapy of ischemic heart disease. Over the last five to ten years, new insights have been formulated regarding the causes of angina and myocardial infarction. Attention has been focused on primary intracoronary events, including coronary artery spasm and thrombosis. The importance of these observations in the elucidation of pathophysiology and in treatment of patients forms the basis of this volume.

This is a time for development of more effective, safe, and elegant therapy for patients with ischemic heart disease. It was not long ago that the idea of performing cardiac catheterization in patients with unstable angina or myocardial infarction was considered contrary to the best interests of patient care. Today, however, transluminal catheter therapy of acute coronary obstruction is widespread and effective. In addition, studies on coronary artery spasm have led to development of potent agents to prevent vasospastic angina.

I thank those who contributed to this book. Also to those colleagues and teachers who encouraged efforts to investigate the areas of spasm and thrombosis I am especially indebted. It is hoped that future efforts will enable us to write improved, important, and timely chapters. Finally, especial thanks to my wife and children who make all these ventures worthwhile.

Sheldon Goldberg, M.D.
Guest Editor

Editor's Commentary

Coronary heart disease continues to be the major cause of mortality in the westernized world and remains our most challenging clinical problem. Two conditions—thrombosis and spasm—have re-emerged during recent years as key contributors to the coronary occlusive process. An essential role for coronary thrombosis has been documented in acute transmural myocardial infarction. Likewise it is evident that coronary artery spasm has fundamental importance in various anginal syndromes, and probably in the evolution of at least some instances of myocardial infarction. The purpose of this issue of *Cardiovascular Clinics* is to examine the interrelated roles and clinical importance of these conditions in coronary artery disease. I am extremely grateful to Sheldon Goldberg, M.D., for his energetic guidance in the formulation of this issue, and both of us are indeed indebted to the contributing authors for their exemplary contributions.

Albert N. Brest, M.D.
Editor-in-Chief

Arnold J. Greenspon, M.D.
Assistant Professor of Medicine, Jefferson Medical College; Assistant Director, Cardiac Catheterization Laboratory, Thomas Jefferson University Hospital, Philadelphia, Pennsylvania

Alden H. Harken, M.D.
Associate Professor of Surgery, University of Pennsylvania School of Medicine, Philadelphia, Pennsylvania

Richard H. Helfant, M.D.
Professor of Clinical Medicine, Chief, Division of Cardiology, Presbyterian-University of Pennsylvania Medical Center; Director, Mid-Atlantic Heart and Vascular Institute, Philadelphia, Pennsylvania

L. David Hillis, M.D.
Assistant Professor of Internal Medicine, University of Texas Health Science Center; Director, Cardiac Catheterization Laboratory, Parkland Memorial Hospital, Dallas, Texas

Paul D. Hirsh, M.D.
Fellow in Cardiology, University of Texas Health Science Center, Dallas, Texas

Joseph S. Janicki, Ph.D.
Associate Professor of Medicine, University of Pennsylvania School of Medicine, Philadelphia, Pennsylvania

Rex MacAlpin, M.D.
Professor of Medicine/Cardiology, UCLA Center for Health Sciences, Los Angeles, California

Peter R. Maroko, M.D.
Adjunct Professor of Physiology and Medicine, Jefferson Medical College, Philadelphia, Pennsylvania; Director, Deborah Cardiovascular Research Institute, Browns Mills, New Jersey

Philip B. Oliva, M.D.
Director, Cardiology Research and Education, Proctor Community Hospital, Peoria, Illinois

Carl J. Pepine, M.D.
Professor of Medicine, University of Florida, Gainesville, Florida

Lair G. T. Ribeiro, M.D.
Adjunct Assistant Professor of Physiology, Jefferson Medical College, Philadelphia, Pennsylvania; Assistant Director, Deborah Cardiovascular Research Institute, Browns Mills, New Jersey

John S. Schroeder, M.D.
Associate Professor of Clinical Medicine and Cardiology, Stanford University Medical Center, Stanford, California

Geoffrey Scott, M.S.
Graduate Student, Cardio-Pulmonary Research Laboratories, University of Pennsylvania School of Medicine, Philadelphia, Pennsylvania

CONTRIBUTORS

Sol Sherry, M.D.
Professor and Chairman, Department of Medicine, Temple University School of Medicine, Philadelphia, Pennsylvania

Sanjeev Shroff, Ph.D.
Research Associate in Medicine, Cardio-Pulmonary Research Laboratories, University of Pennsylvania School of Medicine, Philadelphia, Pennsylvania

Paul Urban, M.D.
Fellow in Cardiology, Jefferson Medical College, Philadelphia, Pennsylvania

David D. Waters, M.D.
Montreal Heart Institute, Montreal, Canada

Karl T. Weber, M.D.
Associate Professor of Medicine, University of Pennsylvania School of Medicine, Philadelphia, Pennsylvania

William S. Weintraub, M.D.
Assistant Professor of Medicine, Division of Cardiology, Presbyterian-University of Pennsylvania Medical Center, Philadelphia, Pennsylvania

Contents

Coronary Artery Spasm: Historic Aspects

William S. Weintraub, M.D., and
Richard H. Helfant, M.D.

The current interest in coronary artery spasm as a potentially important cause of clinical manifestations of coronary heart disease is by no means new. In fact it more accurately represents the resurgence of an historic hypothesis. The history of coronary artery spasm is actually an integral part of the history of coronary artery disease itself. The ancient Greeks recognized that chest pain could be associated with serious diseases, but they failed to provide a detailed clinical description, and they did not have insight into the pathophysiology. The Greeks referred to diseases of the oral pharynx as angina. Galen, in the second century A.D., referred to chest pain as "kardialgia." He recognized that chest pain could come from the heart, and postulated that pain from the heart was probably very serious. Galen is credited with naming the coronary arteries. Aretaeus, a contemporary of Galen, wrote that "cardiac passion" was associated with syncope and sudden death.[1,2]

Little advancement was made thereafter until William Harvey's pathfinding physiologic studies were published in 1628. Vieussens of Montpelier accurately described the coronary arteries in 1706. Ossification of the coronary arteries was referred to by Drelincourt (1633–1697), Bellin (1643–1704), and Thebesius (1708). Lancisi of Rome (1654–1720) noted that calcified coronary arteries could cause cardiac enlargement.[2]

The first major advance clinically was made by the English clinician William Heberden when he delivered his classic paper entitled "Some Account of a Disorder of the Breast" to the Royal College of Physicians in 1768. This discourse was subsequently published in 1772.[3] In this essay Heberden coined the term angina pectoris and described 20 cases. His clinical description remains unparalleled to this day. He recognized and characterized the variations in chest pain symptoms, the variable natural history of patients with these symptoms, and described rest angina and nocturnal angina in addition to classic effort angina. He also recognized that both rest and exertional angina could coexist in one patient, and he appreciated, too, that there was a danger of sudden death from this disease. Interestingly, Heberden proposed that angina was due to "spasm," although he did not clearly state where the spasm was occurring, and in fact did not recognize the cardiac origin of these symptoms.

Late in the 18th century, however, a patient of John Fothergill with a history of Heberden's angina came to autopsy by the great English pathologist John Hunter. He described "many parts of the left ventricle almost white and hard. . . . The two coronary arteries . . . were become one piece of bone." John Hunter himself suffered from angina; at the time of his death in 1793, his student Edward Jenner predicted in advance that Hunter would have coronary disease, which indeed his autopsy revealed.[4]

Curiously, despite these great insights, the 19th century provided little new information on coronary artery disease. Great physicians such as Laennec, Virchow, and Stokes failed to

1

understand the central role of the coronary arteries in angina pectoris. There are several reasons for this lack of progress. The extreme variability of the natural history undoubtedly was confusing. John C. Warren wrote in 1813 of autopsies he had performed in which there was coronary ossification without a prior history of angina.[2] In the 19th century the great advances in the field of medicine related to the major infectious diseases. Immunization became a reality. Antisepsis and later asepsis revolutionized the practice of obstetrics and surgery. The patients who were more well off and more likely to have coronary artery disease were apt to be treated at home rather than in a hospital, and thus the disease was overlooked as a public health issue. Coronary artery disease was in fact considered a medical rarity until the 1920s!

However, one of the medical giants of the 19th century, Peter Mere Latham (1789–1875), appears to be the first to have considered angina to be due to coronary artery spasm. He accurately described the clinical variations of coronary artery disease, but failed to recognize the importance of atherosclerosis, as Jenner and others had done years previously.[5] In 1867 Nothnagel proposed an entity called "angina pectoris vasomotoria," associated with spasm in multiple arterial beds.[6]

Another investigator, Cohnheim, postulated in 1881 that the coronary arteries were end-arteries without anastomoses, and that occlusion (by whatever mechanism) would lead to death within several minutes.[7] This point of view held sway for more than 30 years and prevented the differentiation of angina pectoris from myocardial infarction.

In the early 20th century Sir William Osler defined his concept of angina, its pathophysiology, and the role of coronary artery spasm. Osler's clinical description of angina rivaled Heberden's, and his knowledge of the pathology was more complete than Jenner's. He recognized that most patients with angina had coronary artery disease. He wrote, "A heart the coronary arteries of which are sclerotic or calcified any extra exertion is likely to be followed by a relative ischemia and spasm." Here he was writing of spasm of the myocardium! However, he was among the first to support the notion that coronary artery spasm was a likely explanation for angina in at least some patients.[8] Osler speculated in the Lumleian lectures in 1910 that "there may be a perverted internal secretion that favors spasm of the coronary arteries," and further stated, "I do not know any better explanation for anginal pain."[9]

Perhaps, in retrospect, the stage was being set for one of the major current controversies, when James Herrick first gave a clearcut description of a myocardial infarction in 1912.[10] He called this disorder a coronary thrombosis, and the phrase was to remain popular for 50 years. Initially, coronary thrombosis was considered a medical rarity. Osler's and McCrae's massive five-volume text in 1914 devoted only one paragraph to coronary thrombosis.[11] However, in 1923, Joseph Wearn presented a series of 19 patients with coronary thrombosis.[12] He was the first to state that this syndrome is not rare. He recognized the variable history, course, complications, and prognosis. In 1920 Pardee described the electrocardiographic ST and T wave changes.[13] In 1929, Samuel Levine stressed the importance of Q waves in the diagnosis of coronary thrombosis.[14] It was during this period in the 1920s that coronary artery disease was initially recognized as the primary cause of angina pectoris.

The relationship between fixed and dynamic obstruction was considered in the 1930s. In 1931, Sir Thomas Lewis[15] commented on angina in patients with hypertension and postulated generalized vasospasm, including the coronary arteries, in these patients—as previously proposed by Nothnagel.[6] Paul Dudley White, in his famous 1937 textbook on the heart,[16] recognized the great frequency of coronary artery disease. He described the oxygen supply-demand relationship, with imbalance leading to angina. He considered atherosclerosis to be the overwhelming cause, but believed that coronary artery spasm might lead to angina in some patients with underlying atherosclerosis or other cardiac diseases.

The current era could be said to have been ushered in by Herman Blumgart and his colleagues in a series of classic pathologic studies of more than 450 patients with coronary artery disease.[17,18] Blumgart postulated that angina was due to an oxygen supply-demand imbalance, and, if more severe, the imbalance would lead to myocardial infarction. He recognized that patients with acute myocardial infarction might not exhibit coronary thrombosis at autopsy. He also noted that there could be total coronary occlusion without evidence of infarction, and thus suggested that the term coronary thrombosis was inaccurate, and that the term myocardial infarction should be used instead. He did not, however, speculate on the pathogenesis of myocardial infarction without total occlusion.

The careful delineation of angina and myocardial infarction, as well as methods of accurately diagnosing infarction during life, made it possible to consider the nature of ischemic chest pain at rest without myocardial infarction. In fact, a patient with rest angina and ST segment elevation simulating myocardial infarction was reported in 1941.[19] In the 1950s, Myron Prinzmetal made landmark contributions on classic angina pectoris, and described a new "variant" form.[20-22] Prinzmetal's work delineated and clarified the clinical and pathophysiologic mechanisms in the various anginal syndromes. He and his colleagues clearly described for the first time a syndrome of angina occurring at rest with ST segment elevation, often associated with arrhythmias, and without a change in myocardial oxygen demand. He noted a frequent circadian pattern and observed that the symptoms were relieved by nitroglycerin. He also noted that the syndrome often coexists with typical angina and is associated with atherosclerosis. He postulated that this "variant form of angina pectoris" was associated with "a temporary and often cyclic increase in tonus in a narrowed vessel," and that this spasm was the cardinal point separating variant from Heberden's effort angina.[22]

The 1960s marked the clinical introduction by F. Mason Sones of selective cine coronary arteriography. This advance heralded an era of literally revolutionary changes in our understanding and approach to the diagnostic, prognostic, and therapeutic aspects of coronary heart disease. In retrospect, however, it almost seems as if coronary arteriography initially retarded our appreciation of the pathophysiology, at least where coronary artery spasm is concerned. Paradoxically, it can be appreciated now that the arteriographic procedure was almost designed to prevent coronary artery spasm from manifesting itself. It was routine to administer sedatives and analgesics prior to catheterization, as well as sublingual nitroglycerin just before coronary arteriography. This routine strongly mitigated against spasm occurring during coronary studies. Moreover, the contrast agent itself is a vasodilator, and there was an understandable reluctance to inject dye into the coronary arterial system during a significant episode of ischemic chest pain.

Coronary artery spasm was often observed in the 1960s, but it was iatrogenically produced by the catheter itself in the coronary ostia (usually in the right coronary artery). Clinically, catheter-induced spasm seemed to be of no consequence. Despite reduction of the coronary lumen, no significant reduction in coronary flow was noted, and the patients did not suffer chest pain, nor did the electrocardiogram show changes suggestive of myocardial ischemia. Nonetheless, increasing reports of patients with Prinzmetal's angina appeared in the late 1960s and early 1970s,[23-26] in some cases without obstructive coronary atherosclerosis disease.

During the past decade, spontaneously occurring coronary artery spasm on coronary arteriography has been demonstrated conclusively in variant angina (concomitant with chest pain and ST segment elevation), as well as in patients with other manifestations of coronary heart disease.[27] Decreased myocardial perfusion (as assessed by thallium scan) has also been demonstrated during episodes of variant angina without change in myocardial oxygen demand.[28] Considerable effort has now focused on the underlying pathophysiologic mechanisms. Concomitantly, powerful new antispasmodic agents, the calcium flux inhibitors, have also been developed, and appear to represent a potentially invaluable, new therapeutic approach.

As we have noted, the historical development of our understanding of coronary artery spasm is related in a complex manner to our overall understanding of coronary artery disease. It has only been in the last decade that coronary artery spasm has been widely recognized as a clinically important disorder, and thus as we begin the 1980s, the role of coronary artery spasm has once again been revived. The overall clinical importance of coronary artery spasm is still under active investigation, and the current state of our understanding is detailed in this book. Undoubtedly, we will learn considerably more about this entity in the future as we have (albeit intermittently) in the past. Perhaps one of the most important lessons we should have already learned, however, is that in the future one should not lightly dismiss the contributions of medical giants of the past.

REFERENCES

1. HARRIS, CRS: *The Heart and the Vascular System in Ancient Greek Medicine.* Clarendon Press, Oxford, 1973.

2. HERRICK, JB: *A Short History of Cardiology.* Charles C Thomas, Springfield, Illinois, 1940.

3. HEBERDEN, W: *Some account of a disorder of the breast.* Read before Royal College of Physicians, July 21, 1768, Med Trans Royal College of Physicians, London 2:59, 1772.

4. JENNER, E: In PARRY, CH: *An inquiry into the symptoms and causes of the syncope anginosa, commonly called angina pectoris; illustrated by dissections.* R Cruttwell, Bath, 1799.

5. LATHAM, PM: *Collected Works.* Vol. 1. New Sydenham Society, London, 1876.

6. NOTHNAGEL, H: *Angina pectoris vasomotoria.* Deutsch Arch f klin Med 3:309, 1867.

7. COHNHEIM, S: *Ueber die Folgen der Kranzarterien-verschliessungfur das Herz Virchows.* Arch f path Anal 85:503, 1881.

8. OSLER, W: *The Principles and Practice of Medicine,* ed 7. D Appleton, New York, 1909.

9. OSLER, W: *The Lumleian lectures on angina pectoris.* Lancet 1:697, 1910.

10. HERRICK, JB: *Clinical features of sudden obstruction of the coronary arteries.* JAMA 59:2015, 1912.

11. OSLER, W: In OSLER, W, AND MCCRAE, T (EDS): *Modern Medicine.* Lea & Febiger, Philadelphia and New York, 1914.

12. WEARN, JT: *Thrombosis of the coronary arteries with infarction of the heart.* Am J Med Sci 165:250, 1923.

13. PARDEE, HBB: *An electrocardiographic sign of coronary artery obstruction.* Arch Intern Med 26:244, 1920.

14. LEVINE, SA: *Coronary thrombosis: Its various clinical features.* Medicine 8:245, 1929.

15. LEWIS, T: *Angina pectoris associated with high blood pressure and its relief by amyl nitrite: With a note on Nothnagel's syndrome.* Heart 15:305, 1931.

16. WHITE, PD: *Heart Disease.* Macmillan, New York, 1937.

17. BLUMGART, HL, SCHLESINGER, MJ, AND DAVIS, D: *Studies of the relation of the clinical manifestations of angina pectoris, coronary thrombosis and myocardial infarction to the pathologic findings with particular reference to the significance of the collateral circulation.* Am Heart J 19:1, 1940.

18. BLUMGART, HL, SCHLESINGER, MJ, AND ZOLL, PM: *Angina pectoris, coronary failure, and acute myocardial infarction: Role of coronary occlusion and collateral circulation.* JAMA 16:91, 1941.

19. WILSON, FN, AND JOHNSTON, FD: *The occurrence of angina pectoris with electrocardiographic changes similar in magnitude and in kind to those produced by myocardial infarction.* Am Heart J 22:375, 1941.

20. PRINZMETAL, M, KENNAMER, R, MERLISS, R, ET AL: *Angina pectoris 1. A variant form of angina pectoris.* Am J Med 27:375, 1959.

21. PRINZMETAL, M, ET AL: *Angina pectoris 2. Observations on classic form of angina pectoris (preliminary report).* Am Heart J 57:530, 1959.

22. PRINZMETAL, M, EKMECKI, A, KENNAMER, R, ET AL: *Variant form of angina pectoris: Previously undelineated syndrome.* JAMA 174:102, 1960.

23. BOTTI, RE: *A variant form of angina pectoris with recurrent transient complete heart block.* Am J Cardiol 17:443, 1966.

24. GIANELLY, R, MUGLER, F, AND HARRISON, DC: *Prinzmetal's variant of angina pectoris with only slight coronary atherosclerosis.* Calif Med 108:129, 1968.

25. WHITING, RB, KLEIN, MD, VANDER VEER, J, ET AL: *Variant angina pectoris.* N Engl J Med 282:709, 1970.

26. SILVERMAN, ME, AND FLAMM, MD: *Variant angina pectoris: Anatomic findings and prognostic implications.* Ann Intern Med 75:339, 1971.

27. DHURANDHER, RW, WATT, DL, AND SILVER, MD, ET AL: *Prinzmetal's variant form of angina with arteriographic evidence of coronary arterial spasm.* Am J Cardiol 30:902, 1972.

28. MASERI, A, PARODI, O, SEVERI, S, ET AL: *Transient transmural reduction of myocardial blood flow, demonstrated by thallium 201 scintigraphy as a cause of variant angina.* Circulation 54:280, 1976.

Coronary Thrombosis: Historic Aspects

Albert N. Brest, M.D., and Sheldon Goldberg, M.D.

There can be no doubt that William Harvey's epoch-making contribution, published in 1628, on the anatomy and physiology of the heart and circulation provided the foundation for all subsequent discoveries and advances in this field.[1,2] Not only did Harvey describe the systemic and pulmonary circulations, but he also was the first to recognize the coronary circulation. In 1772, William Heberden published the classic description of angina pectoris.[3] Edward Jenner (1749–1823) and Caleb Hillier Parry (1755–1822) went on to correlate angina pectoris with occlusive disease of the coronary arteries. Subsequently, in 1878, Adam Hammer (a professor of surgery from St. Louis) described the first case of coronary thrombosis with correct diagnosis ante mortem.[4,5] In 1910, the first completed description was published by the Russian physicians Obrastzow and Straschesko.[6] However, it was the Chicago physician James B. Herrick who provided the classic account of this disorder. In his report in the *Journal of the American Medical Association* in 1912, Herrick correlated the clinical and postmortem features of myocardial infarction.[7] He wrote:

> A study of cases of this type shows that nearly all are in men past the middle period of life. Previous attacks of angina have generally been experienced, though, as shown by my first case, the fatal thrombosis may bring on the first seizure. The seizure is described by patients who have had previous experience with angina as of unusual severity, and the pain persists much longer. In some instances there has been no definite radiation of the pain, as to the neck or left arm, though this may have been a feature of other anginal attacks, and the pain, as in these two cases, may be referred to the lower sternal region or definitely to the upper abdomen. Cases with little or no pain have been described.

Prior to Herrick's paper, the view was widely held that obstruction of a coronary artery was almost always suddenly fatal. However, Herrick emphasized that "even large branches of the coronary arteries may be occluded—at times acutely occluded—without resulting death, at least without death in the immediate future." He went on to point out, contrary to prevailing opinion in many quarters, that the "coronaries are not so strictly end-arteries, i.e., with merely capillary anastomoses, as Cohnheim and others thought. By careful dissections, by injection of one artery from another, by skiagraphs of injected arteries and by direct inspection of hearts made translucent by special methods, there is proof of an anatomic anastomosis that is by no means negligible." He stated further that "there is proof not only of anatomic connection between the two coronaries, but that in certain instances, at least, such connection is of functional value. Experiments on lower animals and the clinical experiment of disease of the coronaries with autopsy findings show this." Offering an example, he said,

"I have seen the descending branch completely occluded with an extensive fibrous area in the interventricular septum and at the apex, the latter aneurysmally dilated, where the process was clearly one of long standing." He concluded that "while sudden death often does occur, yet at times it is postponed for several hours or even days, and in some instances a complete, i.e., functionally complete, recovery ensues." With great perspicacity, Herrick reasoned that the clinical manifestations of coronary obstruction will depend on the size, location, and number of vessels occluded; the blood pressure; the condition of the myocardium not immediately affected by the obstruction; and the ability of the remaining vessels to carry on their work, "as determined by their health or disease." In this regard, he suggested that "presumably a sudden overwhelming obstruction, with comparatively normal vessels, would be followed by a profounder shock than the gradual narrowing of a lumen through sclerosis which has accustomed the heart to this pathologic condition and has perhaps caused collateral circulation through neighboring or anastomosing vessels to be compensatorily increased." Although most of Herrick's assumptions regarding the pathophysiology of coronary occlusion have now been confirmed by coronary angiography and other studies, and are widely accepted, his foresight was astonishing, given the state of medical knowledge in his day.

From a therapeutic standpoint, Herrick suggested certain drug remedies (such as digitalis), and he stressed the importance of "absolute rest in bed for several days." However, one other suggestion by Herrick is particularly noteworthy: "The hope for the damaged myocardium lies in the direction of securing a supply of blood through friendly neighboring vessels so as to restore so far as possible its functional integrity." The latter concept was perhaps the forerunner for later ideas regarding vasodilator and thrombolytic therapy.

Herrick's concept of the relationship between coronary thrombosis and myocardial infarction gradually gained general acceptance. Indeed, the terms "coronary occlusion" and "coronary thrombosis" became virtually synonymous with myocardial infarction. However, even while the concept was gaining support, others began to question whether coronary thrombosis was the cause or the effect of the myocardial necrosis. Moreover, in recent years, there has been a spate of reports detailing cases of myocardial infarction in the absence of coronary disease.[8] It is generally agreed, however, that this latter disorder accounts for a relatively small percentage of cases of myocardial infarction.

Pathologists, especially, have been bothered by the concept that coronary thrombosis and myocardial infarction are inevitably linked. In this regard, Spain and Bradess[9] commented, "The relative frequency of coronary thrombi in cases dying from acute myocardial ischemia increases with the duration of survival from the onset of the acute terminal episode." In their study, they noted a 16 percent frequency of coronary thrombi in those cases surviving under one hour, 37 percent in those surviving 24 hours, and 54 percent in those surviving over one day. They said, "This would indicate that for reasons as yet not clearly understood an acute episode of myocardial ischemia is precipitated in individuals with advanced coronary atherosclerosis and that perhaps secondary to the lowering of pressure with slowed and diminished flow in narrowed and damaged coronary arteries, thrombosis occurs as a secondary manifestation. If the formation of thrombi is the primary precipitous event for these episodes of acute myocardial ischemia, then it is difficult to account for the frequency sequence just described." Spain and Bradess[10] reexamined this relationship 10 years later in another autopsy study, and they again reported similar findings and an increase in the frequency of recent coronary thrombi with increasing survival time from the onset of the acute coronary heart attack. However, they cautioned, "Autopsies unfortunately provide only one still picture of a process which during life is rapidly evolving, changing and dynamic. The cause often cannot be distinguished from effect."

Roberts[11] summarized "acute or recent lesions observed in major coronary arteries in patients with fatal ischemic heart disease" as follows: (1) thrombi are infrequent (about 10 percent) in patients dying suddenly and in those in whom the necrosis is limited to the subendocardium; (2) thrombus in a coronary artery is found in about 60 percent of patients with

6

fatal acute transmural myocardial infarction; (3) among patients with transmural myocardial necrosis, the major determinant of the presence of coronary thrombosis seems to be cardiogenic shock; (4) the larger the area of myocardial necrosis, the greater the likelihood of coronary thrombosis; (5) when coronary thrombosis is associated with acute infarction, the thrombus is always located in the artery responsible for perfusing the area of myocardial necrosis; (6) in fatal ischemic heart disease, thrombi occur in coronary arteries that are already severely narrowed by old atherosclerotic plaques; and (7) coronary thrombi in fatal acute myocardial infarction are usually single, occlusive, short, and located entirely in the major trunks. Roberts went on to outline the evidence for and against coronary thrombosis as the usual cause for acute myocardial infarction. He stated: "Two factors implicate coronary thrombosis as the *precipitating cause* of AMI (acute myocardial infarction): (1) the occurrence of coronary arterial thrombi in many patients with fatal AMI and (2) the location of the thrombus in the coronary artery responsible for supplying the area of myocardial necrosis. Five factors, however, tend to indicate that coronary thrombosis is a *consequence* rather than the precipitating cause of AMI: (1) the very low frequency of thrombi in patients dying suddenly with or without previous evidence of cardiac disease; (2) the increasing frequency of thrombi with increasing intervals between onset of symptoms of AMI and death; (3) the absence of thrombi in fatal transmural AMI nearly as often as they are present; (4) the near absence of thrombi in fatal subendocardial AMI; and (5) the occurrence of thrombi in high percentage only in patients with cardiogenic shock, most of whom have large transmural infarcts." Despite these cogent points, it must be noted that autopsies provide a category of patients whose pathology may be different from those individuals with myocardial infarction who survive the acute attack. Furthermore, the final autopsy findings need not necessarily reflect the in vivo sequence of events, that is, early initiation of natural thrombolysis may alter significantly the findings ultimately recognized at death. And, finally, perhaps the patient with coronary disease who dies suddenly may represent still another pathogenetic sequence; for example, in some such patients, coronary spasm may be responsible for death. In these cases, there would be no coronary thrombosis and no acute myocardial infarction. In other instances, cardiac arrhythmias—in the absence of myocardial infarction—may cause sudden death.

There is probably an important difference(s) in the pathogenesis of transmural versus subendocardial infarction. In a study of 500 cases of fatal acute myocardial infarction, it was found that in those having transmural infarction (469 subjects), occlusive thrombosis of the related artery was present in 95 percent. In contrast, only 4 of 31 with subendocardial necrosis had recent coronary occlusion.[12]

Furthermore, much new information has been derived from coronary angiographic studies performed during acute myocardial infarction. DeWood and coworkers[13] found that total occlusion of the infarct-related coronary artery was present in 87 percent of 126 patients studied within 4 hours of the onset of symptoms. The incidence of total occlusion dropped significantly to 65 percent of 57 patients studied 12 to 24 hours after the onset of symptoms. Among 59 patients with angiographic features of coronary thrombosis, the thrombus was retrieved by Fogarty catheter in 52 (88 percent). The authors concluded that total coronary obstruction is frequent during the early hours of transmural infarction and decreases in frequency during the initial 24 hours. Subsequent recanalization of the affected vessel (by the body's intrinsic fibrinolytic system) may explain the variable incidence of thrombosis found in postmortem studies.

Coronary angiographic studies performed in vivo, taken together with observations that coronary thrombolysis can be accomplished safely and with potential myocardial salvage, open a new frontier in the therapy of myocardial infarction.[14,15] These developments also add a new dimension to the history of coronary thrombosis.

Other chapters in this book will dwell on the potential roles of prostaglandins and coronary artery spasm in the initiation of coronary artery thrombosis. In addition, acute and chronic antithrombotic therapy and the physiologic basis of infarct size reduction will be further explored. Physicians have learned a great deal since Adam Hammer's original case report of acute coronary artery thrombosis. We owe much to Herrick and others, who have contributed so brilliantly to our present understanding of the relationship between coronary thrombosis and myocardial infarction. Our patients will be the ultimate beneficiaries of past and present investigations in this area.

REFERENCES

1. HARVEY, W: *Exercitatio Anatomica de Motu Cordis et Sanguinis in Animalibus.* London, 1628.
2. WILLIUS, FA, AND KEYS, TE: *Classics of Cardiology.* Dover, New York, 1961.
3. HEBERDEN, W: *Some account of a disorder of the breast.* Med Tr Roy Coll Phys (London) 2:59, 1772.
4. *A case of thrombotic occlusion of a coronary artery of the heart: Diagnosed clinically and reported by Dr. A. Hammer, Professor of Surgery from St. Louis, currently in Vienna.* Wien med Wchnschr 28:97, 1878.
5. LIE, JT: *Centenary of the first correct antemortem diagnosis of coronary thrombosis by Adam Hammer (1818–1878): English translation of the original report.* Am J Cardiol 42:849, 1978.
6. OBRASTZOW, WP, AND STRASCHESKO, ND: *Zur Kenntnis der Thrombose der Koronar arterien des Herzens.* Ztschr F Klin Med 71:116, 1910.
7. HERRICK, JB: *Clinical features of sudden obstruction of the coronary arteries.* JAMA 59:2015, 1912.
8. BREST, AN: *Myocardial infarction without demonstrable coronary artery disease.* In BREST, AN, WIENER, L, CHUNG, EK, ET AL: *Innovations in the Diagnosis and Management of Acute Myocardial Infarction.* Cardiovascular Clinics 7/2. FA Davis, Philadelphia, 1975, p 291.
9. SPAIN, DM, AND BRADESS, VA: *The relationship of coronary thrombosis to coronary atherosclerosis and ischemic heart disease.* Am J Med Sci 240:701, 1960.
10. SPAIN, DM, AND BRADESS, VA: *Sudden death from coronary heart disease. Survival time, frequency of thrombi, and cigarette smoking.* Chest 58:107, 1970.
11. ROBERTS, WC: *The status of the coronary arteries in fatal ischemic heart disease.* In BREST, AN, WIENER, L, CHUNG, EK, ET AL: *Innovations in the Diagnosis and Management of Acute Myocardial Infarction.* Cardiovascular Clinics 7/2. FA Davis, Philadelphia, 1975, p 1.
12. DAVIES, MJ, WOOLF, N, AND ROBERTSON, WB: *Pathology of acute myocardial infarction with particular reference to occlusive coronary thrombi.* Br Heart J 38:659, 1976.
13. DEWOOD, MA, SPORES, J, NOTSKE, R, ET AL: *Prevalence of total coronary occlusion during the early hours of transmural myocardial infarction.* N Engl J Med 303:897, 1980.
14. RENTROP, P, BLANKE, H, KARSCH, KR, ET AL: *Selective intracoronary thrombolysis in acute myocardial infarction and unstable angina pectoris.* Circulation 63:307, 1981.
15. MATHEY, DG, KUCK, KH, TILSNER, V, ET AL: *Nonsurgical coronary artery recanalization in acute transmural myocardial infarction.* Circulation 63:689, 1981.

The Normal Regulation
of Coronary Blood Flow*

Karl T. Weber, M.D.,† Geoffrey Scott, M.S.,
Joseph S. Janicki, Ph.D.,† and Sanjeev Shroff, Ph.D.

The work of the heart is continuous. It follows, therefore, that the energy requirements of the heart must be continuous. The conversion of chemical energy to mechanical work within the myocardium is highly dependent on oxidative reactions and aerobic conditions. The heart cannot work in the absence of oxygen; without oxygen, energy production falters and cardiac performance rapidly deteriorates. The myocardium, however, is well suited for continuous aerobic work. A rich vascular network provides each muscle fiber with a capillary. Mitochondria, the predominant site of oxidative phosphorylation, are in great abundance in each muscle cell. Moreover, the concentration of oxidative enzymes within the myocardium is the highest of any tissue in the body, and cardiac muscle extracts a large fraction of the oxygen with which it is supplied. Because the myocardium normally extracts 65 to 70 percent of the oxygen delivered to it, even when the body is at rest, any increase in myocardial work requirement and oxygen utilization (for example, exercise) must be met by an increase in coronary blood flow (CBF). Thus, the regulation of CBF is essential to maintaining adequate oxygen delivery to the perpetually working myocardium.

CBF is regulated by the gradient in perfusion pressure across the coronary vascular bed and the resistance to flow offered by the coronary circulation. This simplistic separation, though not precisely true under all circumstances, serves to facilitate our discussion of CBF and its regulation under normal physiologic conditions.

NORMAL CBF REGULATION

Cardiac output, together with the resistance offered by the systemic circulation, establishes a pressure in the aorta. Aortic pressure is the driving, or inflow, pressure for CBF. An outflow pressure which resists this driving pressure is generated at a more distal site within the coronary circulation. Thus, the gradient in perfusion pressure may be expressed as the difference between inflow and outflow pressures. Any increase in the magnitude of this gradient will cause an increase in CBF.

The resistance characteristics of the coronary vessels (CVR) also determine CBF. In accordance with the theorem of Poiseuille, CVR is determined by blood viscosity and by coronary blood vessel length and cross-sectional area. Large changes in fluid flow are produced by relatively small changes in vessel diameter, because CBF is proportional to the fourth power

*This work was supported in part by National Heart, Lung and Blood Institute Grant HL08805.
†Drs. Weber and Janicki are the recipients of NHLBI Research Career Development Awards HL-00187 and HL-00411, respectively.

9

of vessel radius. For example, doubling the radius of the vessel would increase CBF sixteen-fold. Vessel length and blood viscosity do not vary under normal conditions and therefore need not be considered further. For any given perfusion pressure gradient, therefore, a decrease in vessel radius is associated with an increase in CVR and a decrease in CBF. The various factors that influence the gradient to perfusion and that regulate CVR are reviewed below.

Factors Influencing the Gradient in Coronary Perfusion Pressure

The perfusion pressure gradient has traditionally been calculated as the difference between aortic pressure and coronary venous pressure, where right atrial pressure has been used to reflect venous pressure. This approach would hold true if the coronary vessels were rigid or were located entirely on the epicardium. However, because the collapsible coronary vasculature traverses the myocardium, the vessels are rhythmically compressed by an extravascular pressure (Fig. 1). This extravascular, or tissue, pressure normally exceeds coronary venous pressure and therefore is more representative of the outflow pressure which opposes the driving pressure.[1] Consequently, the perfusion pressure gradient is most accurately represented as the difference between aortic pressure and intramyocardial tissue pressure.

Conceptually, this gradient to perfusion in the coronary circulation is analogous to a waterfall, where the pressure or height of the water level downstream from the falls does not influence the flow of water over the brink of the falls.[1] In applying the waterfall concept to the coronary circulation, vascular resistance, or the extent of vessel collapse, will also be influenced by the dynamic interplay between the inlet and extravascular pressures.

The rhythmic contraction of the myocardium determines phasic left coronary artery flow, as shown in Figure 2. CBF falls during systole, confining the bulk of flow to the diastolic portion of the cardiac cycle. Hence, the very process of contraction, which not only establishes the driving pressure to coronary perfusion and accounts for most of the oxygen consumed by the myocardium, tends to impede myocardial perfusion. This impediment to CBF during systole has been attributed to two mechanical factors which determine the extravascular pressure on the coronary vessels: (1) the contracting muscle fibers create a direct compression of intramyocardial vessels, and (2) the transmission of ventricular chamber pressure to the myocardium creates an indirect compression of the vessels.

Extravascular or Tissue Pressure

Muscle shortening is thought to create a uniform shearing strain on all vessels, irrespective of their location within the myocardium. The extent of this strain would be related to the direction of the vessel (that is, perpendicular or parallel) relative to the muscle fibers. A vessel aligned parallel to muscle is less likely to be "kinked" during systole. On the other hand, the intramyocardial pressure transmitted from the ventricle would be greatest adjacent to the

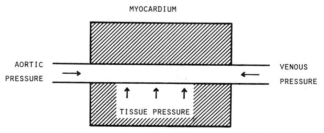

Figure 1. The perfusion pressure gradient to coronary flow is determined by the difference between the inflow, aortic pressure and a downstream, outflow pressure. An intramyocardial tissue pressure compresses the collapsible coronary vessel. Because this extravascular pressure exceeds venous pressure, it is the more appropriate outflow pressure.

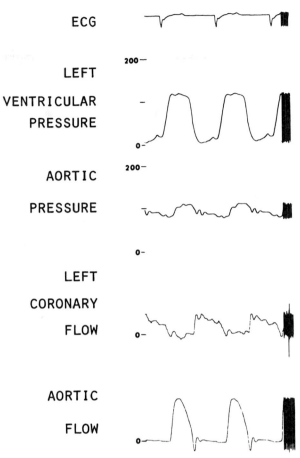

Figure 2. Phasic left main coronary artery flow measured in a calf by an electromagnetic flow probe. Note that commencing with isovolumic relaxation in the left ventricle, coronary flow increases significantly, reaching its peak in early diastole and then declining gradually. During systole, epicardial coronary flow is impeded by the increased intramyocardial tissue pressure.

chamber and least within the subepicardium, where intrapericardial pressure equals intrapleural pressure. Therefore, a nonuniform shearing of the vessels would be operative across the myocardium. Several recent studies have clarified the relative importance of these mechanical factors in regulating systolic CBF.

Borg and Caulfield[2] have demonstrated that capillaries run parallel to their respective myocytes and that each capillary is tethered to the myocytes by collagenous struts measuring 120 to 150 nm in diameter. These struts are inserted tangentially on each myocyte and perpendicularly to the capillary (Fig. 3). With the contraction of the myocytes and the increase in their respective diameters, the collagenous struts are drawn taut. The resultant tension exerted on the capillary wall preserves the patency of the capillary and prevents its translocation relative to the myocyte. These anatomic findings suggest that the shearing forces created by muscle fiber shortening play only a minor role in the throttling of CBF during systole. Physiologic data to support this conclusion have been provided by Downey and coworkers.[3] Thus, it would appear that the intramyocardial pressure created by the transmission of ventricular pressure is the dominant mechanical factor that impedes systolic CBF.

The measurement of intramyocardial pressures has both intrigued and baffled the physiologist. A variety of techniques have been utilized, but each method has its own limitations. Nevertheless, subendocardial tissue pressure has been found to exceed subepicardial pressure

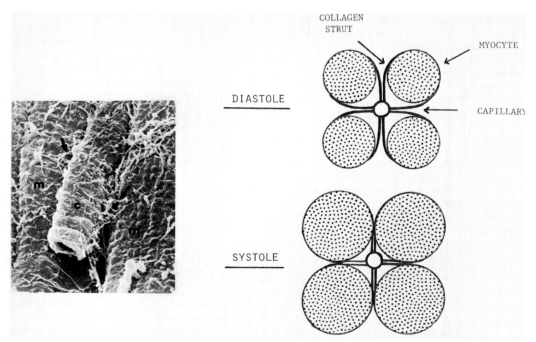

Figure 3. The collagenous network connecting myocytes and capillaries are shown. On the left, the collagen struts, which interconnect a capillary (c) and two myocytes (m), are shown. On the right, the angle of insertion of these struts and the tension created on the capillary during myocyte contraction serves to preserve the patency of the capillary during systole. Adapted from Borg and Caulfield.[2]

during systole. Accordingly, subendocardial perfusion is restricted during systole to a greater extent than is subepicardial flow.[4] These observations draw attention to the fact that a series of vascular waterfalls must exist across the myocardium.

Further evidence in support of the dominant role of this transmitted tissue pressure in throttling systolic CBF relates to the difference in phasic right and left coronary artery flows. In the left coronary artery, CBF is greatest during diastole (see Fig. 2) when the difference between aortic and tissue pressures is greatest. During the isovolumic phase of left ventricular contraction, when chamber pressure rises to the level of aortic pressure, CBF is markedly reduced and remains low throughout ejection; this is particularly true in the subendocardium. On the other hand, right ventricular systolic pressure is much less than aortic pressure. Consequently, systolic right coronary artery flow equals or exceeds diastolic flow; and, hence, CBF here is more continuous, resembling the time course of aortic pressure.[5]

Diastolic CBF is principally regulated by the vasomotor activity of the coronary resistance vessels which, in turn, is closely linked to myocardial oxygen utilization.

Factors Influencing Coronary Vascular Resistance

The heart cannot work in the absence of oxygen for any significant period of time. Accordingly, the heart is considered to be an obligatory aerobic organ. The consumption of oxygen by the heart ($M\dot{V}O_2$) may therefore be used to monitor its energy requirements. Because the heart extracts a large portion of the oxygen delivered to it, increments in $M\dot{V}O_2$ require increased oxygen delivery (that is, CBF · arterial oxygen content). CBF follows myocardial oxygen requirements and preserves oxygen availability by the autoregulatory vasodilation of the coronary resistance vessels. Therefore, increments in myocardial work and $M\dot{V}O_2$ are accompanied by a reduction in coronary vascular resistance. Before discussing coronary autoregulation, however, the concept of myocardial work should be reviewed.

Myocardial Work

In physical terms, work is performed when a force is exerted in moving an object over a given distance. The hemodynamic work of the heart has traditionally been expressed as the integral of the pressure and volume events of the ventricle. The recognition that the work of this muscular pump is more accurately reflected in the force generated and sustained by the contracting muscle fibers has provided a more detailed and quantitative assessment of work, and thereby the determinants of $M\dot{V}O_2$.

The net wall force created by the contracting muscle fibers is related to the pressure created inside the ventricular chamber and to the size and shape of the chamber (that is, its cross-sectional area). As shown in Figure 4, wall force rises during early systole; the magnitude of this developed force is determined by the pressure required to initiate ejection and by the size of the ventricle (for example, in the enlarged heart, a greater force is generated for any given aortic valve opening pressure). The rate with which force is developed is determined by the volume of the ventricle and the contractile state of the myocardium. In the normal heart, the greater the diastolic volume, the more rapid the rate of force development. Similarly, an increment in myocardial contractility (for example, during exercise) will augment the rate of force development. During ejection, wall force must be sustained. The magnitude of this ejection force is related to the level of ejection pressure and the rate and extent of ventricular emptying. Hence the integral of systolic wall force, which includes the magnitude of the force developed and sustained from onset contraction to aortic valve closure, is a major determinant of $M\dot{V}O_2$.[6] The rate of force development and the frequency with which force is developed per unit of time represent the other two major determinants of $M\dot{V}O_2$.[7] The importance of ventricular pressure and volume, myocardial contractile state, and heart rate in regulating $M\dot{V}O_2$ are apparent when considered in light of their influence on these various components of wall force. For a more detailed discussion of these issues, the interested reader is referred

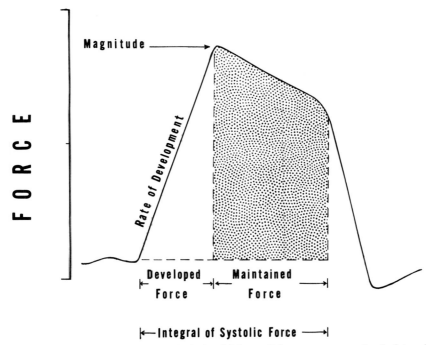

Figure 4. The time course of systolic wall force is depicted. Myocardial oxygen consumption is determined by the integral of systolic force (per beat), the frequency with which systolic force is generated per unit time, and the rate of force development. See text for details.

elsewhere.[8] Normally, major adjustments in CBF are confined to periods of exercise[9] (for example, CBF is increased three- to fourfold) when the pumping requirements of the ventricle and energy expenditure of the myocardium are significantly increased.

Autoregulation

The vasomotor activity of the coronary resistance vessels determines the level of diastolic CBF. The concept of autoregulation suggests that the coronary circulation adjusts its vasomotor tone in accordance with the oxygen requirements of the myocardium. Therefore, a link exists between the heart's mechanical activity and its CVR. An increase in oxygen utilization is accompanied by coronary vasodilation and increased oxygen delivery. On the other hand, steady state CBF changes little over a wide range of perfusion pressure when the level of oxygen utilization remains constant. This behavior of the coronary circulation is demonstrated in Figure 5, where its pressure-flow relations are plotted for several constant levels of oxygen utilization. Isopleths of oxygen utilization were obtained in our isolated heart preparation by manipulating ventricular filling volume, ejection pressure, heart rate, and myocardial contractility. For any constant level of oxygen utilization (for example, 20 to 40 μl oxygen consumed per beat per 100 g of myocardium), it is apparent that CBF does not vary for perfusion pressures ranging between 60 and 110 mm Hg. When $M\dot{V}O_2$ is raised to 40 to 60 μl per beat, CBF is greater for any given perfusion pressure, although the autoregulatory behavior remains intact. Adenosine, a potent coronary vasodilator, will abolish vasomotor activity. As a result, CVR remains constant as CBF becomes a linear function of perfusion pressure.

The vasomotor-dependent activity of the coronary circulation differs in various segments of the myocardium to preserve uniform transmural perfusion throughout the cardiac cycle. For example, subendocardial flow during diastole exceeds subepicardial flow,[4,10] thus restoring

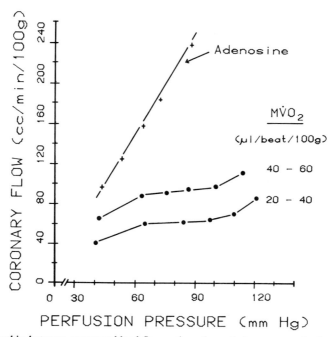

Figure 5. The relationship between coronary blood flow and aortic perfusion pressure is shown for the isolated canine heart performing at two different levels of myocardial work. Each work load is defined according to a constant range of oxygen utilization. The linear pressure-flow relation following coronary vasodilation with adenosine is also shown.

the imbalance in perfusion created during systole. The greater vascular density of the sub-endocardium may also contribute to its preferential perfusion in diastole.[11] Nevertheless, autoregulatory adjustments of the coronary circulation serve to maintain myocardial perfusion in a manner that is consonant with both its global and regional perfusion requirements. These phenomena are most convincingly demonstrated during the increased $M\dot{V}O_2$ attendant with exercise.[12] However, a limit to oxygen delivery does exist in the myocardium, beyond which anaerobic metabolism and a depression in cardiac performance do occur.[13] Additionally, the work load placed on the myocardium to achieve this aerobic limit is substantial. If present over a prolonged period of time, these excessive oxygen requirements might exhaust available energy stores and result in myocardial necrosis. As a case in point, acute myocardial infarction has been reported in a marathon runner without coronary artery disease.[14]

The control mechanism(s) whereby CBF and oxygen utilization are coupled has received much attention. The current prevailing concept of coronary autoregulation has been attributed to a work-dependent local release of a metabolite from the myocardial cell into the interstitium. The principal site of action of this vasodilating metabolite is at the terminal arteriole or precapillary sphincter, or both. Various substances have been incriminated in mediating this response.[15] Adenosine has received the greatest attention in recent years. According to the adenosine hypothesis, adenosine triphosphate is degraded during oxidative metabolism to adenosine, which freely diffuses out of the cell to dilate vascular smooth muscle. The release of this potent coronary vasodilator is related to the level of aerobic metabolism and ATP degradation. Thus, the release of adenosine is closely coupled to oxygen utilization to preserve oxygen availability on a beat-to-beat basis, and thereby provides the link between myocardial work and coronary vasomotion.

Neural Control

Anatomic studies have failed to identify the sympathetic or parasympathetic innervation of coronary vascular smooth muscle. For example, the extent to which postganglionic fibers innervate the coronary vessels remains to be elucidated. The results of physiologic studies dealing with neural control of the coronary circulation are often difficult to evaluate because of concomitant changes in myocardial contractility, heart rate, and arterial pressure, which accompany stimulation of either the sympathetic or the parasympathetic nervous system. These extravascular effects will independently alter $M\dot{V}O_2$ and CBF, quite apart from any primary effect on coronary vasomotor control. However, a mounting body of evidence does suggest that stimulation of the alpha-adrenergic receptor will promote vasoconstriction of the large epicardial coronary arteries as well as the remainder of the coronary vasculature.[16-18] These issues are discussed elsewhere in this book.

REFERENCES

1. DOWNEY, JM, AND KIRK, ES: *Inhibition of coronary blood flow by a vascular waterfall mechanism.* Circ Res 36:753, 1975.
2. BORG, TK, AND CAULFIELD, JB: *The collagen matrix of the heart.* In WEBER, KT, AND HAWTHORNE, EW: *Symposium on Cardiac Shape and Structure.* Fed Proc 40:2037, 1981.
3. DOWNEY, JM, DOWNEY, HF, AND KIRK, ES: *Effects of myocardial strains on coronary blood flow.* Circ Res 34:286, 1974.
4. HESS, DS, AND BACHE, RJ: *Transmural distribution of myocardial blood flow during systole in the awake dog.* Circ Res 38:5, 1976.
5. GREGG, DE, AND SHIPLEY, RE: *Changes in right and left coronary artery inflow with cardiac nerve stimulation.* Am J Physiol 141:382, 1944.
6. WEBER, KT, AND JANICKI, JS: *Myocardial oxygen consumption: The role of wall force and shortening.* Am J Physiol 233:H421, 1977.

7. WEBER, KT, AND JANICKI, JS: *Interdependence of cardiac function, coronary flow and oxygen extraction.* Am J Physiol 236:H784, 1978.

8. WEBER, KT, AND JANICKI, JS: *The metabolic demand and oxygen supply of the heart: Physiologic and clinical considerations.* Am J Cardiol 44:722, 1979.

9. LOMBARDO, TA, ROSE, L, TAESCHLER, M, ET AL: *The effect of exercise on coronary blood flow, myocardial oxygen consumption and cardiac efficiency in man.* Circulation 7:71, 1953.

10. MOIR, TW: *Subendocardial distribution of myocardial blood flow and the effect of antianginal drugs.* Circ Res 30:621, 1972.

11. DOWNEY, HF, BASHOUR, FA, BOATWRIGHT, RB, ET AL: *Uniformity of transmural perfusion in anesthetized dogs with maximally dilated coronary circulations.* Circ Res 37:111, 1975.

12. BALL, RM, BACHE, RJ, COBB, FR, ET AL: *Regional myocardial blood flow during graded treadmill exercise in the dog.* J Clin Invest 55:43, 1975.

13. WEBER, KT, JANICKI, JS, AND FISHMAN, AP: *Aerobic limit of the heart perfused at constant pressure.* Am J Physiol 238:H118, 1980.

14. GREEN, LH, COHEN, SI, AND KURLAND, G: *Fatal myocardial infarction in marathon racing.* Ann Intern Med 84:704, 1976.

15. RUBIO, R, AND BERNE, RM: *Regulation of coronary blood flow.* Prog Cardiovasc Dis 18:105, 1975.

16. MOHRMAN, DE, AND FEIGL, EO: *Competition between sympathetic vasoconstriction and metabolic vasodilation in the canine coronary circulation.* Circ Res 42:79, 1978.

17. KELLY, KD, AND FEIGL, EO: *Segmental α-receptor mediated vasoconstriction in the canine coronary circulation.* Circ Res 43:908, 1978.

18. MURRAY, PA, AND VATNER, SF: *α-Adrenoceptor attenuation of the coronary vascular response to severe exercise in the conscious dog.* Circ Res 45:654, 1979.

Pathophysiology of Angina Pectoris due to Coronary Artery Spasm

Arnold J. Greenspon, M.D., and Sheldon Goldberg, M.D.

Angina pectoris is now known to occur by two broad mechanisms: there may be a primary increase in myocardial oxygen consumption or an abrupt reduction in myocardial oxygen supply.

Myocardial demand for oxygen must be met by a sufficient myocardial oxygen supply in order for there to be metabolic stability (Fig. 1). If there is an imbalance between myocardial oxygen supply and myocardial oxygen demand, myocardial ischemia will ensue. The predominant symptom of myocardial ischemia is angina pectoris. As first described by William Heberden in 1772, the symptom complex of angina pectoris is usually precipitated by activities such as walking or eating and relieved by rest: "They who are afflicted with it, are seized while they are walking, (more especially if it be up hill, and soon after eating) with a painful and most disagreeable sensation in the breast, which seems as if it would extinguish life, if it were to increase or to continue; but the moment they stand still, all this uneasiness vanishes."[1] Later it was recognized that most patients with angina pectoris had fixed obstructive disease of the coronary arteries.[2-4] At rest, their myocardial oxygen supply is sufficient to meet the myocardial needs for oxygen. During the stress of activity, myocardial ischemia develops when myocardial oxygen supply cannot increase sufficiently to meet the increased myocardial oxygen demand.[5] In the latter circumstance, ischemia results because demand exceeds supply. The mechanism of ischemia in most patients with classic angina pectoris is that of an increase in myocardial oxygen demand in the setting of a restricted myocardial oxygen supply.

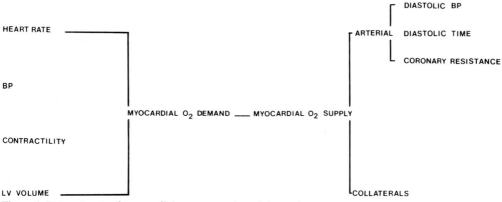

Figure 1. Determinants of myocardial oxygen supply and demand.

ISCHEMIA DUE TO INCREASE IN DEMAND

In coronary artery disease, an atherosclerotic plaque in an epicardial vessel introduces a fixed obstruction to coronary flow. This fixed resistance in a capacitance vessel is met by a reflex decrease in resistance of the smaller vessels. At rest, flow is adequate because the resistance vessels can dilate sufficiently. However, with a sudden increase in myocardial oxygen demand, ischemia develops because myocardial oxygen supply is fixed. The resistance vessels are already maximally dilated and cannot meet the increased metabolic needs of the myocardium. Therefore, in fixed obstructive coronary disease, ischemia develops owing to an increase in the determinants of myocardial oxygen demand.

Episodes of ischemia in patients with fixed obstructive coronary disease are usually preceded by increases in the heart rate and blood pressure—two determinants of myocardial oxygen demand. Such episodes can be provoked by atrial pacing or exercise.[26-30] The value of the exercise electrocardiogram in the diagnosis of coronary artery disease is based on the concept that an increase in myocardial oxygen demand due to the increased heart rate and blood pressure of exercise will precipitate ischemia if myocardial oxygen supply is already significantly restricted (Fig. 2). A positive exercise test is marked by signs and symptoms of myocardial ischemia at a time when myocardial oxygen demand is increased. These signs resolve as the patient rests and the heart rate and blood pressure return to normal.

Signs of myocardial ischemia develop when myocardial oxygen demand exceeds supply. ST segment depression appears on the electrocardiogram during episodes of ischemia.[26] Anaerobic metabolism is documented by lactate production rather than lactate extraction in coronary arteriovenous lactate measurements.[27] Associated hemodynamic abnormalities reflect left ventricular dysfunction during the stress of ischemia. The left ventricular end-diastolic pressure rises as the result of abnormal ventricular compliance.[28] An elevation in pulmonary capillary wedge pressure may also follow. Left ventricular contraction abnormalities may also be seen on radionuclide gated scans (MUGA) and contrast ventriculography.[31] Consequently, exercise MUGA scans may be a sensitive indicator of significant fixed obstructive coronary disease. Regional myocardial perfusion is also abnormal during ischemia, as reflected by perfusion defects on exercise scintigraphy with thallium-201 or other potassium analogs.[32]

In summary (Table 1), angina pectoris due to an increase in myocardial oxygen demand is marked by an increase in the heart rate and blood pressure prior to the ischemic episode. Ischemia is precipitated by exercise, emotion, or other factors that increase the determinants of myocardial oxygen demand, that is, heart rate, blood pressure, left ventricular volume, and myocardial contractility. There is evidence of fixed obstructive coronary disease on coronary angiography. Ischemia occurs reproducibly at a specific level of myocardial oxygen consumption. Therefore, ischemia is frequently documented by exercise ECG or thallium scintigraphy post-exercise. Finally, treatment of angina pectoris due to an increase in myocardial oxygen demand is directed at decreasing the energy requirements of the myocardium. Drug treatment with nitrates and beta-adrenergic blockade is often effective in decreasing anginal episodes. Nitrates are effective because they produce venodilation and also systemic vasodilation, which reduces left ventricular wall tension secondary to decreased ventricular volume and lowered blood pressure.[33] Beta blockade is effective because it decreases the heart rate

Table 1. Features of angina secondary to increased demand

1. Preceded by increased heart rate and blood pressure
2. Precipitated by exertion, emotion, and other factors that increase oxygen demand
3. Evidence of fixed obstructive coronary disease on coronary angiography
4. Ischemia occurs reproducibly at a specific level of myocardial oxygen consumption
5. Evidence of ischemia on exercise ECG or exercise thallium-201 scintigraphy
6. Treatment directed at decreasing myocardial oxygen demand with beta-blockade and nitrates

and the contractility of the myocardium.[34,35] By decreasing the determinants of myocardial oxygen consumption, the threshold for ischemia secondary to an increased demand is improved.

ISCHEMIA DUE TO DECREASE IN SUPPLY

In 1959, Prinzmetal and associates described a "variant" form of angina pectoris in which angina pectoris was associated with ST segment elevation rather than ST segment depression.[36] In contrast to the typical patient with angina pectoris who developed angina with effort, these patients developed angina at rest. Though coronary spasm was inferred to be the cause of this type of angina, Oliva and coworkers in 1973 were the first to document angiographically that myocardial ischemia in these patients was due to spasm of a large epicardial conductance vessel.[25] Thus it was shown that patients with "variant angina" develop ischemia on the basis of a primary reduction in myocardial oxygen supply.

The initial observations of reversible coronary obstruction during an episode of spontaneous "variant" angina were made by the chance occurrence of a spontaneous attack in the cardiac catheterization laboratory. Later, in studies of patients with angina at rest, Maseri[37] and others[38,39] demonstrated angiographic evidence of reversible coronary spasm during spontaneous episodes of angina, associated with ST segment elevation. Angiographic evidence for

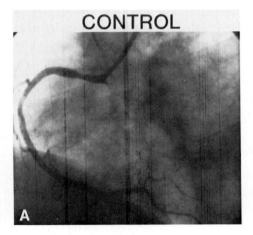

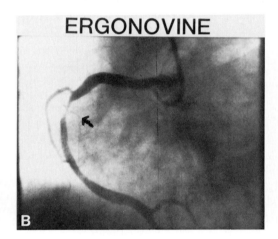

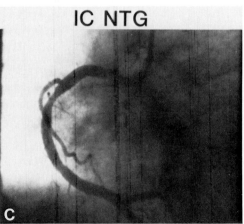

Figure 3. A 44-year-old man with variant angina underwent provocative testing with ergonovine maleate in the cardiac catheterization laboratory. *A,* Initially, an angiogram of the right coronary artery showed no evidence of obstructive coronary disease. Following the administration of ergonovine maleate the patient developed angina associated with ST segment elevation in lead 2. *B,* Severe spasm developed in the right coronary artery. *C,* After the administration of the intracoronary nitroglycerin the area of spasm resolved, and the right coronary angiogram returned to normal.

coronary spasm during episodes of angina at rest has also been documented by provocative drug testing in the cardiac catheterization laboratory. The administration of ergonovine maleate, an ergot alkaloid and alpha-adrenergic agonist, has been used to induce coronary spasm in patients with "variant" angina[40] (Fig. 3). Electrocardiographic changes during ergonovine-induced spasm are identical to those encountered during spontaneous episodes of "variant" angina. Methacholine[41] as well as epinephrine and propranolol in combination[42] have also been used to provoke coronary spasm. Coronary angiography during spontaneous and provoked episodes of rest angina has conclusively shown that these episodes of angina at rest are associated with a primary reduction in the caliber of a large capacitance vessel.

Cardiac Hemodynamics

Guazzi and Maseri and their associates studied patients with spontaneous episodes of variant angina using constant electrocardiographic and hemodynamic monitoring.[37,43-45] Hemodynamic observations during angina showed that these episodes were not preceded by an increased demand for oxygen. Therefore, there must have been a primary reduction in myocardial oxygen supply.

Maseri and coworkers extended these observations to patients with spontaneous angina at rest.[10,45] Patients with frequent episodes of angina at rest were studied using constant electrocardiographic and hemodynamic monitoring. Right ventricular and left ventricular pressures or aortic and pulmonary artery pressures were recorded continuously to determine if angina was preceded by an increase in oxygen demand. Ischemic episodes at rest were characterized by either ST segment depression or elevation. More than 60 percent of these episodes were asymptomatic. No increases in heart rate, blood pressure, or first derivative of left ventricular pressure (dp/dt) were noted before the onset of angina.

Berndt and colleagues studied the hemodynamic changes during angina in patients with unstable angina and coronary artery disease.[46] They found that the double product (heart rate $\times$ arterial pressure) and triple product (heart rate $\times$ arterial pressure $\times$ systolic ejection time) were smaller during spontaneous angina than pacing-induced angina. Therefore, the determinants of myocardial oxygen demand were less in patients with spontaneous angina. They concluded that there had to be a primary reduction in coronary blood flow to account for the angina.

Several conclusions may be drawn from these studies. First, the direction of ST segment change during spontaneous angina does not determine the mechanism of ischemia. Both ST segment depression and ST segment elevation may be encountered. The direction of ST segment change is determined by the degree of ischemia. If there is a decrease in myocardial oxygen supply sufficient to cause transmural ischemia, ST segment elevation will result. Less of a decrease in supply will cause ST segment depression or pseudonormalization of the T wave. Any or all of these changes may be encountered in the same patient. Second, pain is a late finding in relation to the development of ischemia on the ECG. Some episodes of ischemia may be asymptomatic. Third, angina at rest is due to decreased myocardial oxygen supply because the determinants of myocardial oxygen demand do not precede spontaneous angina.

Changes in left ventricular performance are encountered during episodes of rest angina.[18,41,43] These changes reflect ischemia in the area of myocardium supplied by the involved coronary artery. There is a decreased rate of pressure rise during systole and pressure fall during diastole. Increases in left ventricular end-diastolic pressure reflect abnormal left ventricular compliance. The left ventricular systolic pressure falls along with the cardiac output. With more advanced ischemia, segmental wall motion abnormalities occur. Many of these changes in left ventricular mechanical performance are also encountered in ischemia secondary to an increase in myocardial oxygen demand. The left ventricle will not perform normally whenever there is ischemia, whether it is due to an increase in myocardial oxygen demand or a decrease in myocardial oxygen supply.

Regional Myocardial Perfusion

Radionuclide studies during spontaneous angina are characterized by perfusion defects corresponding to the electrocardiographic changes and the involved artery demonstrated angiographically. Myocardial scintigraphy with thallium-201[45,46−48] or intracoronary macroaggregated albumin labeled with ^{99}Tc and ^{131}I has demonstrated transmural perfusion defects during spontaneous or provoked episodes of angina associated with ST segment elevation.[49] Episodes of angina with ST segment elevation are associated with transmural reduction in coronary blood flow.

Coronary Hemodynamics and Myocardial Metabolic Alterations

The pathophysiology of angina occurring without an increase in myocardial oxygen demand has been further clarified by studying the coronary hemodynamic and metabolic changes accompanying coronary spasm. Goldberg and associates studied patients with atypical chest pain and those with variant angina to detect changes in arterial pressure, coronary sinus blood flow, and calculated coronary vascular resistance after the administration of ergonovine maleate[50] (Fig. 4). Patients with atypical chest pain showed diffuse narrowing of the coronary arteries without ST segment changes on the ECG after the administration of ergonovine. Arterial pressure rose along with a concomitant increase in coronary sinus blood flow. Coronary vascular resistance was not significantly changed. Coronary sinus lactate concentrations were also not significantly changed after ergonovine. By contrast, their patients with variant angina demonstrated focal spasm of the left anterior descending coronary artery associated with ST segment elevation after ergonovine. During provoked coronary spasm, arterial pressure fell rather than increased in three of six patients, reflecting poor left ventricular mechanical performance during transmural ischemia. A dramatic decrease in coronary sinus blood flow was associated with a marked increase in coronary vascular resistance. These findings suggested a marked reduction in myocardial oxygen supply secondary to a decrease in coronary blood flow. Myocardial metabolism was also altered during provoked spasm. Arteriovenous oxygen difference and lactate production increased considerably owing to the ischemia produced by coronary spasm.

Ricci and coworkers studied four patients with either spontaneous or provoked spasm of the left anterior descending coronary artery.[51] During episodes of coronary spasm, coronary sinus blood flow fell and calculated coronary vascular resistance rose. Further evidence for a marked reduction in coronary blood flow was an increased myocardial arteriovenous oxygen difference and anterior perfusion defects on thallium-201 scintigraphy during spontaneous spasm in one of their patients.

Further evidence for ischemia secondary to a primary reduction in myocardial oxygen supply was provided by Curry and associates. They evaluated left ventricular hemodynamics and myocardial lactate metabolism in patients with atypical chest pain and those with variant angina after administration of ergonovine maleate.[52] In patients with variant angina, chest pain and ST segment elevation following ergonovine were associated with angiographic evidence of marked focal reduction in the caliber of a coronary artery. During the time of coronary spasm, lactate extraction markedly declined and the coronary sinus lactate/pyruvate ratio increased. The left ventricular systolic pressure fell while the left ventricular end-diastolic pressure rose. Patients with atypical chest pain showed neither angiographic evidence of coronary spasm nor metabolic evidence of myocardial ischemia following ergonovine.

These studies performed during episodes of angina at rest associated with ST segment elevation indicate the following: (1) there is angiographic evidence of dynamic coronary obstruction of a major epicardial vessel, (2) angina is associated with a marked reduction in coronary sinus blood flow and an increase in coronary vascular resistance, and (3) myocardial ischemia is demonstrated by a change from lactate extraction to lactate production and an increase in

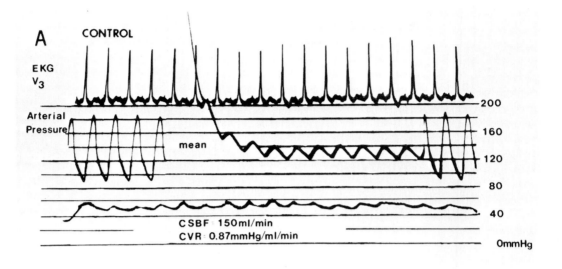

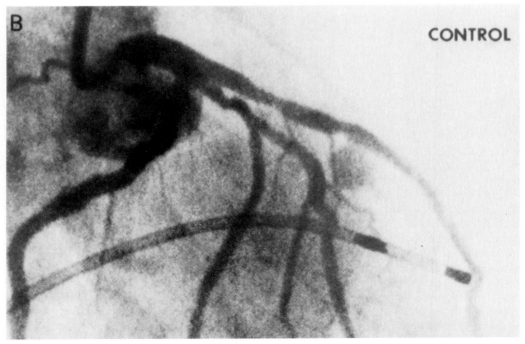

Figure 4. A 47-year-old woman with variant angina had the following electrocardiographic and hemodynamic findings at rest: the heart rate was kept constant by coronary sinus pacing. *A,* The ECG, arterial pressure, and coronary sinus blood flow (CSBF) in the control state. *B,* A coronary angiogram performed seconds after these measurements showed only luminal irregularities of the left coronary artery. (From Am J Cardiol 43:481, 1979, with permission.)

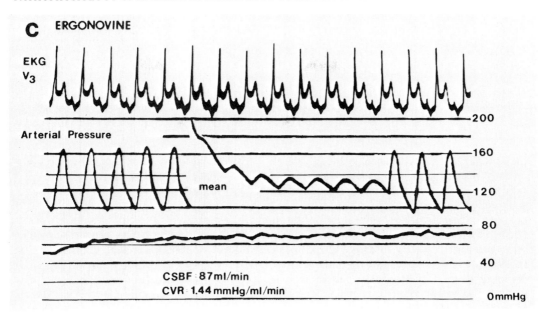

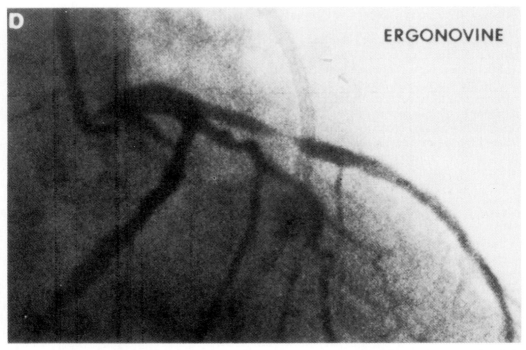

Figure 4. *Continued.* Following the administration of ergonovine maleate the patient's angina was reproduced. *C,* With heart rate constant, ST segment elevation developed and blood pressure fell slightly. CSBF dropped substantially to 87 ml per minute. *D,* The repeat coronary angiogram showed focal spasm of the left anterior descending coronary artery. These findings indicate that this patient's angina was not caused by a primary increase in myocardial oxygen consumption (heart rate constant, blood pressure fell) but, rather, a primary decrease in supply (CSBF fell) owing to coronary spasm.

Table 2. Features of angina secondary to decreased supply

1. Not preceded by increased heart rate and blood pressure
2. Usually occurs at rest
3. Coronary arteriography may be normal or show fixed disease
4. ST segment shifts during ischemia depend on extent of decrease in supply
5. Associated with decreased coronary blood flow and increased coronary vascular resistance
6. Treatment directed at reducing coronary vasoconstriction with nitrates or calcium channel blockade

the coronary arteriovenous oxygen difference. Thus, the etiology of the angina at rest is a primary reduction in myocardial oxygen supply due to focal coronary spasm.

In summary (Table 2), the features of angina secondary to a reduction in myocardial oxygen supply include: (1) myocardial ischemia which is not preceded by an increase in blood pressure or heart rate, (2) most episodes occur at rest even though exercise-induced coronary spasm has been reported,[53] (3) coronary arteriography may be normal or show evidence of atherosclerotic coronary disease, (4) ST segment shifts during ischemia depend on the extent that supply is decreased and the area of myocardium involved, (5) during angina there is a decrease in coronary blood flow and an increase in coronary vascular resistance, and (6) treatment is directed at reducing coronary vasoconstriction. Coronary vasodilators such as nitrates or calcium channel blockers (nifedipine, verapamil, diltiazem) are often effective in preventing repeated episodes of variant angina.[54,55] The role of calcium channel blockade in the setting of unstable angina remains to be determined.

Etiology of Primary Increase in Coronary Resistance

In the basal state the epicardial capacitance vessels contribute very little to total coronary resistance. However, because these vessels carry a high flow, even a small change in this resistance will have a profound effect on myocardial oxygen supply. There is evidence that neural and biochemical factors play a role in the regulation of coronary resistance.

Experimental evidence suggests that the normal coronary circulation vasoconstricts in response to alpha-adrenergic stimulation.[19-24,56-58] Sympathetic stimulation of the unanesthetized dog causes coronary vasoconstriction in the presence of beta-adrenergic blockade. When alpha-adrenergic blockade is substituted, coronary vasoconstriction does not occur.[56] Carotid sinus stimulation in conscious dogs reduces tonic alpha-adrenergic tone, causing a decrease in coronary resistance.[57] Furthermore, heart transplant patients have less of a rise in coronary vascular resistance after alpha-adrenergic blockade than normal patients.[58] These findings suggest that there is a tonic level of alpha-adrenergic stimulation causing coronary vasoconstriction in the intact heart.

Patients with coronary artery disease respond to alpha-adrenergic stimulation with an increase in coronary vascular resistance. In a series of experiments, Mudge and coworkers studied the effects of the cold pressor test,[59,60] a known alpha-adrenergic stimulus, on coronary vascular resistance. Arterial pressure and coronary sinus flow were measured in normal individuals and in patients with coronary artery disease. Coronary vascular resistance was calculated from these two values. The cold pressor stimulus was applied for one minute, and the studies were repeated. The cold pressor test produced a hypertensive response in both the normal subjects and the coronary artery disease group. Coronary resistance was unchanged in normal subjects but rose significantly in patients with coronary disease.

In another study, patients were evaluated during atrial pacing and the cold pressor test. Three of fourteen patients with coronary disease developed angina during both atrial pacing and the cold pressor test. Myocardial oxygen demand was estimated by calculating the double product (heart rate $\times$ blood pressure). The double product during angina induced by cold was lower than that induced by atrial pacing. Therefore, under the vasoconstrictor influence of cold, ischemia was produced at a lower level of oxygen demand. This suggests that alpha-adrenergic stimulation induces coronary vasoconstriction and causes angina on the basis of a decrease in myocardial oxygen supply.

Pharmacologic agents are also known to cause an increase in coronary resistance.[40-42] Ergonovine maleate, methacholine, and the combination of epinephrine and propranolol have been shown to provoke coronary spasm in susceptible individuals. The action of these drugs appears to be mediated via the alpha-adrenergic system. Coronary spasm has also been implicated in the sudden deaths of munitions workers suddenly withdrawn from chronic nitroglycerin exposure.[61] The sudden withdrawal of nitroglycerin, a known coronary vasodilator, in these workers may cause excessive coronary vasoconstriction.

Finally, circulating prostaglandins such as thromboxane A_2 may be important in influencing coronary vascular resistance. Thromboxane A_2 has been shown to have potent coronary vasoconstrictor and platelet aggregating properties.[62-65] Elevated levels of its inactive metabolite, thromboxane B_2, have been found in patients with Prinzmetal's variant angina[64] and during pacing-induced angina.[65] By increasing coronary vascular resistance, thromboxane A_2 may be an important determinant in decreasing myocardial oxygen supply in patients with fixed coronary disease and rest angina.

CONCLUSIONS

The concept that angina pectoris is always due to increased metabolic needs of the myocardium in the setting of fixed obstructive coronary disease is not sufficient to explain the varied clinical presentations of ischemic heart disease. It will not explain the presentation of myocardial infarction with normal coronary arteries, Prinzmetal's variant angina, or rest angina without antecedent changes in blood pressure or heart rate. Inasmuch as myocardial ischemia develops whenever there is an imbalance between myocardial oxygen demand and supply, recent investigations have focused on primary alterations in myocardial oxygen supply to account for ischemia. Primary changes in oxygen supply may be important in the genesis of unstable angina and myocardial infarction. Understanding the pathophysiology of the various clinical manifestations of ischemic heart disease should lead to more direct and effective therapy.

REFERENCES

1. HEBERDEN, W: *Some account of a disorder of the breast.* Med Trans Coll Physicians (London) 2:59, 1772.
2. HERRICK, JB, AND NUZUM, FR: *Angina pectoris: Clinical experience with 200 cases.* JAMA 70:67, 1918.
3. ZOLL, PM, WESSLER, S, AND BLUMGART, HL: *Angina pectoris: Clinical and pathological correlation.* Am J Med 11:331, 1951.
4. REEVES, TJ, OBERMAN, A, JONES, WB, ET AL: *Natural history of angina pectoris,* Am J Cardiol 33:423, 1974.
5. MACALPIN, RN, KATTUS, AA, AND ALVARO, AB: *Angina pectoris at rest with preservation of exercise capacity: Prinzmetal's variant angina.* Circulation 47:946, 1973.
6. HERMAN, MV: *The clinical picture of ischemic heart disease.* Prog Cardiovasc Dis 14:321, 1971.
7. FOWLER, NO: *Angina pectoris: Clinical diagnosis.* Circulation 46:1079, 1972.
8. KEMP, HG, VOKONAS, PS, COHN, PF, ET AL: *The original syndrome associated with normal coronary arteriograms. Report of a six year experience.* Am J Med 54:735, 1973.
9. HILLIS, LD, AND BRAUNWALD, E: *Coronary artery spasm.* N Engl J Med 299:695, 1978.
10. MASERI, A, L'ABBATE, AL, BAROLD, G, ET AL: *Coronary vasospasm as a possible cause of myocardial infarction, a conclusion derived from the study of "pre-infarction" angina.* N Engl J Med 299:1271, 1978.
11. FISCHL, S, GORLIN, R, AND HERMAN, MV: *The intermediate coronary syndrome: Clinical, angiographic, and therapeutic aspects.* N Engl J Med 288:1193, 1973.
12. FOWLER, NO: *Pre-infarction angina.* Circulation 44:755, 1971.
13. BERNE, RM: *Regulation of coronary blood flow.* Physiol Rev 44:1, 1964.
14. GORLIN, R: *Regulation of coronary blood flow.* Br Heart J 33(Suppl):9, 1971.

15. McKeever, WP, Gregg, DE, and Carrey, PC: *Oxygen uptake of the non-working left ventricle.* Circ Res 6:612, 1958.
16. Sarnoff, SJ, Braunwald, E, Welch, GH, et al: *Hemodynamic determinants of oxygen consumption of the heart with special reference to the tension-time index.* Am J Physiol 192:148, 1958.
17. Braunwald, E, Sarnoff, SJ, Case, RB, et al: *Hemodynamic determinants of coronary flow: Effect of changes in aortic pressure and cardiac output on the relationship between oxygen consumption and coronary flow.* Am J Physiol 192:157, 1958.
18. Luchi, RJ, Chahine, RA, and Raizner, AE: *Coronary artery spasm.* Ann Intern Med 91:441, 1979.
19. Ross, G: *Adrenergic responses of the coronary vessels.* Circ Res 39:461, 1976.
20. Feigl, EO: *Control of myocardial oxygen tension by sympathetic coronary vasoconstriction in the dog.* Circ Res 37:88, 1975.
21. Feigl, EO: *Reflex parasympathetic coronary vasodilatation elicited from cardiac receptors in dog.* Circ Res 37:175, 1975.
22. Berne, RM: *Effect of epinephrine and norepinephrine on coronary circulation.* Circ Res 6:644, 1958.
23. Berne, RM, DeGeest, H, and Levy, MN: *Influence of the cardiac nerves on coronary resistance.* Am J Physiol 208:763, 1965.
24. McRaven, DR, Mark, AL, Abboud, FM, et al: *Responses of coronary vessels to adrenergic stimuli.* J Clin Invest 50:773, 1971.
25. Oliva, PB, Potts, DE, and Pluss, RG: *Coronary arterial spasm in Prinzmetal's angina: Documentation by coronary arteriography.* N Engl J Med 288:745, 1973.
26. Helfant, RH, Forrester, JS, Hampton, JR, et al: *Coronary heart disease: Differential hemodynamic, metabolic, and electrocardiographic effects in subjects with and without angina pectoris during atrial pacing.* Circulation 42:601, 1970.
27. Parker, JO, Chiang, MA, West, RO, et al: *Sequential alterations in myocardial lactate metabolism, ST segments, and left ventricular function during angina induced by atrial pacing.* Circulation 40:113, 1969.
28. Parker, JO, Ledwich, JR, West, RO, et al: *Reversible cardiac failure during angina pectoris: Hemodynamic effects of atrial pacing in coronary artery disease.* Circulation 39:745, 1969.
29. Faris, JV, McHenry, PL, and Morris, SN: *Concepts and application of treadmill exercise testing and the exercise electrocardiogram.* Am Heart J 95:102, 1978.
30. Goldschlager, N, Selzer, A, and Cohn, K: *Treadmill tests as indicators of presence and severity of coronary artery disease.* Ann Intern Med 85:277, 1976.
31. Borer, JS, Bacharach, SL, Green, MV, et al: *Real-time radionuclide-cineangiography in the non-invasive evaluation of global and regional left ventricular function at rest and during exercise in patients with coronary artery disease.* N Engl J Med 296:839, 1977.
32. Pitt, B, and Strauss, HW: *Myocardial imaging in the non-invasive evaluation of patients with suspected ischemic heart disease.* Am J Cardiol 37:797, 1976.
33. Cohn, PF, and Gorlin, R: *Physiologic and clinical actions of nitroglycerin.* Med Clin N Am 58:407, 1974.
34. Epstein, SE, and Braunwald, E: *Beta adrenergic receptor blockade: Mechanisms of action and clinical application.* N Engl J Med 275:1106, 1966.
35. Wolfson, S, and Gorlin, R: *Cardiovascular pharmacology of propranolol in man.* Circulation 40:501, 1969.
36. Prinzmetal, M, Kennaner, R, Merliss, R, et al: *Angina Pectoris. I. A variant form of angina pectoris.* Am J Med 27:375, 1969.
37. Maseri, A, Mimmo, R, Chierchia, S, et al: *Coronary spasm as a cause of acute myocardial ischemia in man.* Chest 68:625, 1975.
38. Gaasch, WH, Adyanthaya, A, Wang, V, et al: *Prinzmetal's variant angina: Hemodynamic and angiographic observations during pain.* Am J Cardiol 35:683, 1975.
39. Higgins, CG, Wexler, L, Silverman, JF, et al: *Clinical and arteriographic features of Prinzmetal's variant angina: Documentation of etiologic factors.* Am J Cardiol 37:831, 1976.
40. Schroeder, JS, Bolen, JL, Quint, RA, et al: *Provocation of coronary spasm with ergonovine maleate: A new test with results in 57 patients undergoing coronary arteriography.* Am J Cardiol 40:487, 1977.
41. Endo, M, Hirosawa, K, Kaneko, N, et al: *Prinzmetal's variant angina: Coronary arteriogram and left ventriculogram during anginal attack induced by methacholine.* N Engl J Med 294:252, 1976.
42. Yasue, H, Touyama, M, Kato, H, et al: *Prinzmetal's variant form of angina as a manifestation of alpha-adrenergic receptor mediated coronary artery spasm: Documentation by coronary arteriography.* Am Heart J 91:148, 1976.
43. Guazzi, M, Polese, A, Fiorentini, P, et al: *Left ventricular performance and related hemodynamic changes in Prinzmetal's variant angina pectoris.* Br Heart J 33:84, 1971.

28

44. GUAZZI, M, POLESE, A, FIORENTINI, P, ET AL: *Left and right heart hemodynamics during spontaneous angina pectoris: Comparison between angina with ST segment depression and angina with ST segment elevation.* Br Heart J 37:401, 1975.

45. MASERI, A, SEVERI, S, DENES, M, ET AL: *"Variant angina": One aspect of a continuous spectrum of vasospastic myocardial ischemia.* Am J Cardiol 42:1019, 1978.

46. BERNDT, TB, FITZGERALD, J, HARRISON, DC, ET AL: *Hemodynamic changes at the onset of spontaneous versus pacing induced angina.* Am J Cardiol 39:784, 1977.

47. MCLAUGHLIN, PR, DOHERTY, PW, MARTIN, RP, ET AL: *Myocardial imaging in a patient with reproducible variant angina.* Am J Cardiol 39:126, 1977.

48. RICCI, DR, ORLICK, AE, DOHERTY, PW, ET AL: *Reduction of coronary blood flow during coronary artery spasm occurring spontaneously and after provocation with ergonovine maleate.* Circulation 57:392, 1978.

49. BERMAN, ND, MCLAUGHLIN, PR, HUCKELL, VF, ET AL: *Prinzmetal's angina with coronary artery spasm: Angiographic, pharmacologic, metabolic and radionuclide perfusion studies.* Am J Med 60:727, 1976.

50. GOLDBERG, S, LAM, W, AND MUDGE, G: *Coronary hemodynamic and metabolic alterations accompanying coronary spasm.* Am J Cardiol 43:481, 1979.

51. RICCI, DR, ORLICK, AE, CIPRIANO, P, ET AL: *Altered adrenergic activity in coronary artery spasm: Insight into mechanism based on study of coronary hemodynamics and the electrocardiogram.* Am J Cardiol 43:1073, 1979.

52. CURRY, RC, PEPINE, CJ, SABOUR, MB, ET AL: *Hemodynamic and myocardial metabolic effects of ergonovine in patients with chest pain.* Circulation 58:648, 1978.

53. SPECCHIA, G, DESERVI, S, FALCONE, C, ET AL: *Coronary arterial spasm as a cause of exercise induced ST segment elevation in patients with variant angina.* Circulation 59:948, 1979.

54. ANTMAN, EA, MULLER, J, GOLDBERG, S, ET AL: *Nifedipine therapy for coronary artery spasm. Experience in 127 patients.* N Engl J Med 302:1269, 1980.

55. JOHNSON, SM, MAURHSON, DR, WILLERSON, JT, ET AL: *A controlled trial of verapamil for Prinzmetal's variant angina.* N Engl J Med 304:862, 1981.

56. PITT, B, ELLIOT, EC, AND GREGG, DE: *Adrenergic receptor activity in the coronary arteries of the unanesthesized dog.* Circ Res 21:75, 1967.

57. VATNER, SG, FRANKLIN, D, VAN CITTERS, RL, ET AL: *Effects of carotid sinus nerve stimulation on the coronary circulation of the conscious dog.* Circ Res 27:11, 1970.

58. ORLICK, AE, RICCI, DE, ALDERMAN, EL, ET AL: *Effects of alpha-adrenergic blockade upon coronary hemodynamics.* J Clin Invest 62:459, 1978.

59. MUDGE, GH, JR, GROSSMAN, W, MILLS, RM, JR, ET AL: *Reflex increase in coronary vascular resistance in patients with ischemic heart disease.* N Engl J Med 295:1333, 1976.

60. MUDGE, GH, JR, GOLDBERG, S, GUNTHER, S, ET AL: *Comparison of metabolic and vasoconstrictor stimuli on coronary vascular resistance in man.* Circulation 59:544, 1979.

61. LANGE, R, REID, M, TRESCH, D, ET AL: *Non-atheromatous ischemic heart disease following withdrawal from chronic nitroglycerin exposure.* Circulation 46:666, 1972.

62. NEEDLEMAN, P, KALKARNI, PS, AND RAZ, A: *Coronary tone modulation: Formation and actions of prostaglandins, endoperoxides and thromboxanes.* Science 195:409, 1977.

63. HAMBERG, M, SVENSSON, J, AND SAMUELSSON, B: *Thromboxanes: A new group of biologically active compounds derived from prostaglandin endoperoxides.* Proc Nat Acad Sci USA 72:2294, 1975.

64. LEVY, RI, SMITH, JB, SILVER, MJ, ET AL: *Detection of thromboxane B_2 in the peripheral blood of patients with Prinzmetal's angina.* Prostaglandins Med 2:243, 1979.

65. LEVY, RI, WIENER, L, WALINSKY, P, ET AL: *Thromboxane release during pacing induced angina pectoris: Possible vasoconstrictor influence on the coronary vasculature.* Circulation 61:1165, 1980.

Interactions of the Arterial Wall, Plaque, and Platelets in Myocardial Ischemia and Infarction

L. David Hillis, M.D., Paul D. Hirsh, M.D.,
William B. Campbell, Ph.D.,
and Brian G. Firth, M.D., Ph.D.

During the past 10 years there has been considerable interest in the role of platelets and certain vasoactive compounds both in the initiation and progression of the atherosclerotic process and in the occurrence of the various clinical syndromes of ischemic heart disease. Numerous studies have suggested that enhanced platelet aggregation may play a role in the formation of the atherosclerotic plaque, and other studies have demonstrated a strong association between the various risk factors for atherosclerosis and an imbalance between circulating thromboxane and prostacyclin. Once the atherosclerotic process is established, platelet hyperaggregability and a continued thromboxane:prostacyclin imbalance may be of pathophysiologic importance in the occurrence of certain clinical syndromes in patients with ischemic heart disease, such as unstable angina pectoris, acute myocardial infarction, and sudden death. Thus, platelet function abnormalities as well as alterations in thromboxane and prostacyclin concentrations may be of importance in patients with myocardial ischemia and infarction.

THE INITIATION AND PROGRESSION OF ATHEROSCLEROSIS

The Role of Platelets

Extensive investigations have been performed in an attempt to elucidate the pathophysiologic events leading to the atherosclerotic process. One theory of atherogenesis, the so-called "response-to-injury" hypothesis,[1-4] contends that atherosclerosis is a pathologic response to repetitive vascular endothelial cell injury. In response to endothelial cell disruption, platelets adhere to exposed subendothelial collagen, aggregate, synthesize thromboxane, and release the contents of their granules.[5,6] This platelet response to exposed collagen can be observed for up to 48 hours after injury and may occur for a much longer period.[7-12] Subsequent to this platelet aggregation and within 5 to 7 days of the initial injury, smooth muscle cell proliferation and migration occur, connective tissue matrix is laid down, and there is deposition of lipids both within the cells and in their surrounding connective tissue matrix.[4,7,8] Within 1 to 3 months, the intima contains 5 to 15 layers of newly-proliferated smooth muscle cells, which, in turn, are surrounded by newly-formed collagen fibrils and elastic fibers.[13] Such intimal smooth muscle proliferation has been observed after all forms of endothelial injury examined thus far, including mechanical injury,[1,7,8,14-17] homocystinemia,[18] hypercholesterolemia,[19-26] and immunologic injury.[27,28]

According to the theory, if both the endothelial injury and the ensuing tissue response are limited, restoration of the endothelial barrier eventually occurs. However, if such injury is repetitive, platelet adherence and activation also occur repetitively, leading to an eventual pathologic accumulation of connective tissue and lipid, which, in turn, forms the nidus of an atherosclerotic plaque. Recent studies in experimental animals have demonstrated that repeated platelet aggregation plays an integral part in this process and, furthermore, that the proliferation of smooth muscle cells at the site of repetitive endothelial injury can be prevented by aspirin[29] (an inhibitor of platelet aggregation and prostanoid synthesis) and antiplatelet serum.[30]

In short, the "response-to-injury" hypothesis of atherogenesis states that the initiation and possibly even the progression of the atherosclerotic process are intimately linked with repetitive platelet adherence and activation at the site of endothelial cell disruption. As a result, if platelet activation is inhibited pharmacologically, the development of an atherosclerotic plaque may be impeded.

The Role of Thromboxane and Prostacyclin

Prostanoids (thromboxanes and prostaglandins) are not stored anywhere in the body. Rather, they are synthesized in response to a variety of mechanical and humoral stimuli, act

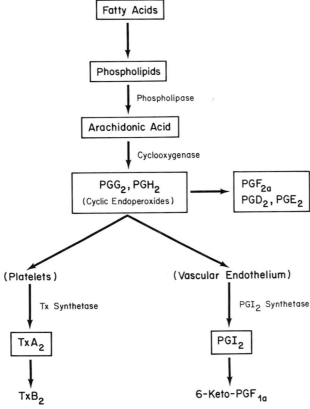

Figure 1. The pathway by which arachidonic acid is formed and then metabolized to the various prostanoids. In response to a variety of stimuli, a series of phospholipases is activated, which enzymatically cleaves arachidonic acid. Subsequently, arachidonic acid is converted by the enzyme cyclooxygenase to PGG_2 and PGH_2, which are known collectively as cyclic endoperoxides. In turn, these substances are converted to a series of prostaglandins ($PGF_{2\alpha}$, PGD_2, PGE_2) as well as to thromboxane $A_2(TxA_2)$ and prostacyclin (PGI_2). Specifically, PGG_2 and PGH_2 are converted in platelets by thromboxane synthetase to TxA_2, a powerful vasoconstrictor and aggregator of platelets. Alternatively, the cyclic endoperoxides are converted in vascular endothelium by prostacyclin synthetase to PGI_2, a powerful vasodilator and inhibitor of platelet aggregation. Finally, both TxA_2 and PGI_2 are unstable and are quickly converted to inactive metabolites, TxB_2 and 6-keto $PGF_{1\alpha}$, respectively.

locally, and are then degraded. The major precursor of thromboxane A_2 and prostacyclin is arachidonic acid, a polyunsaturated fatty acid that is obtained from the essential fatty acid, linoleic acid, which is present in dietary meat and vegetable oils.[31] Arachidonic acid is converted by the enzyme cyclooxygenase to prostaglandins G_2 (PGG_2) and H_2 (PGH_2) (the cyclic endoperoxides),[32] which, in turn, are converted to thromboxane A_2 and various prostaglandins, including prostacyclin (Fig. 1). The particular end-product of arachidonic acid metabolism is determined by the cell type in which the cyclic endoperoxides become available. In platelets, they are converted by thromboxane synthetase to thromboxane A_2 (TxA_2); in vascular endothelium, they are converted by prostacyclin synthetase to prostacyclin (PGI_2).

Thromboxane A_2, a powerful endogenous constrictor of arteries and promoter of platelet aggregation,[33] is synthesized and released by aggregating platelets. At body temperature and pH, it is unstable, with a half-life of only about 30 seconds in aqueous media; it is spontaneously hydrolyzed to thromboxane B_2, an inactive compound with sufficient stability to allow its quantitation. Prostacyclin has actions diametrically opposite to those of thromboxane A_2:

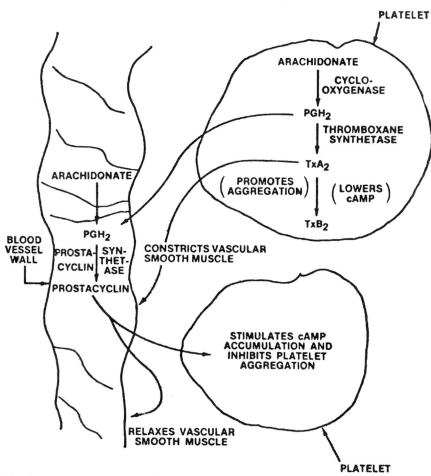

Figure 2. A schematic representation of thromboxane:prostacyclin balance within the circulation. On the left, the blood vessel wall; on the right, the lumen of the vessel, within which there are two platelets. In the blood vessel wall, arachidonic acid (arachidonate) is converted to PGH_2 (a cyclic endoperoxide) and then to prostacyclin, which (1) relaxes vascular smooth muscle and (2) stimulates cAMP accumulation in platelets and, therefore, inhibits platelet aggregation. In contrast, in the platelet, arachidonate is converted to PGH_2 and then to TxA_2, which (1) constricts vascular smooth muscle and (2) lowers cAMP accumulation in platelets, thus promoting aggregation. (From Gorman, RR, Bunting, S, and Miller, OV: *Modulation of human platelet adenylate cyclase by prostacyclin (PGX)*. Prostaglandins 13:377, 1977, with permission.)

it causes relaxation of vascular smooth muscle and is a potent inhibitor of platelet aggregation.[32,34] It is produced within vascular endothelial cells. The ability to synthesize prostacyclin is greatest nearest the vessel lumen and progressively diminishes toward the adventitial surface. Like thromboxane A_2, prostacyclin is unstable at physiologic temperature and pH and has a half-life of only 2 to 3 minutes in aqueous media. It spontaneously degrades to 6-keto-$PGF_{1\alpha}$.

Thus, although thromboxane A_2 and prostacyclin are synthesized from the same parent compound (arachidonic acid), they have opposite physiologic properties. Numerous investigators have postulated that normal vascular function depends on a balance between thromboxane A_2 and prostacyclin (Fig. 2). Furthermore, recent studies have suggested that many of the so-called risk factors for the development of atherosclerosis exert their effects, at least in part, by adversely influencing the thromboxane:prostacyclin balance.

We will briefly review some of the data that suggest an association between these "risk factors" and a thromboxane:prostacyclin imbalance (Fig. 3).

1. Hyperlipidemia, specifically hypercholesterolemia, has been shown to enhance platelet sensitivity and aggregability[35,36] and to increase thromboxane production.[37] At the same time, human atherosclerotic tissue has a reduced ability to synthesize and to release prostacyclin.[38–40]

2. Several studies have demonstrated that diabetes mellitus is associated with alterations in prostaglandin production and platelet function. For example, rats with both spontaneous[41] and streptozotocin-induced[42] diabetes as well as diabetic humans[43–46] have hyperactive platelets with enhanced platelet thromboxane generation in response to adenosine diphosphate, epinephrine, collagen, and arachidonic acid. Simultaneously, diabetes mellitus is associated with reduced vascular prostacyclin synthesis.[42,47–49]

3. There is some evidence that smoking causes a thromboxane:prostacyclin imbalance. It increases platelet activity[50] and proaggregatory prostaglandin production,[51] and it potentiates the effects of hyperlipidemia on platelet aggregability.[52] Nicotine inhibits the ability of the coronary arteries to synthesize prostacyclin-like substances in vitro,[53] and this effect is more pronounced in vascular tissue from individuals who smoke than from nonsmoking controls.[54,55]

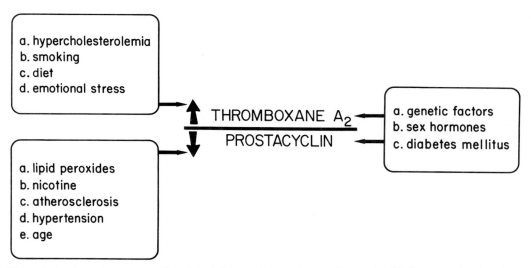

Figure 3. A schematic representation of the influence of the various cardiovascular risk factors on the thromboxane:prostacyclin balance. Certain genetic factors, sex hormones, and diabetes mellitus induce an excess of thromboxane relative to prostacyclin by adversely affecting the levels of both substances. The other risk factors either increase thromboxane *(upper left)* or reduce prostacyclin *(lower left)*.

4. Recent reports have suggested that patients with essential hypertension have a reduced urinary excretion of prostaglandin E_2 and 6-keto-$PGF_{1\alpha}$ with a normal excretion of thromboxane B_2,[56] leading to an increased ratio of vasoconstrictive:vasodilatory prostanoids.

5. Some of the effects of sex hormones and age on cardiovascular risk may be related to alterations in thromboxane and prostacyclin. Several studies have suggested that continuously elevated estrogen concentrations are associated with heightened cardiovascular risk. For example, such risk is increased in men[57] and postmenopausal women[58] given estrogenic hormones, as well as in young women on oral contraceptives.[59] Although the exact mechanism whereby estrogens increase cardiovascular risk is not understood, estrogen administration has been shown to enhance platelet aggregability and to reduce vascular production of prostacyclin-like material in both experimental animals[60] and man.[61] In addition, spontaneous platelet aggregation occurs in vitro in blood from young women on oral contraceptives but not in men or young women on no therapy, and such aggregation is abolished by aspirin.[62] In experimental animals, aging is accompanied by reduced vascular prostacyclin production.[63]

6. It is well established that individuals with a family history of premature coronary artery disease are at increased risk for the early development of such disease. A recent report of a family with an inherited thromboxane synthetase deficiency[64] suggests that the presence and activity of prostaglandin regulatory enzymes may be genetically controlled. Thus, it is possible that the familial occurrence of premature vascular events may be causally related to abnormalities of these enzymes.

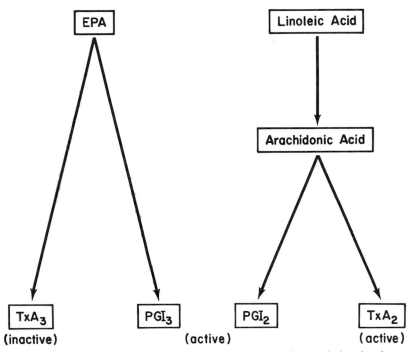

Figure 4. A schematic representation of how dietary manipulation may lead to a relative abundance of prostacyclin. The normal American diet contains an abundance of arachidonic acid precursors, such as linoleic acid. Arachidonic acid is metabolized to PGI_2 and TxA_2, both active compounds. In contrast, mackerel and cod contain a large quantity of eicosapentaenoic acid (EPA), which is metabolized to prostaglandins and thromboxanes of the "3" series. Although PGI_3 is similar in activity to PGI_2, TxA_3 is physiologically inactive and, in fact, may block platelet TxA_2 receptors. Thus, by serving as the parent compound of different prostaglandin end-products, EPA promotes vascular dilatation and inhibits platelet aggregation. (From Hirsh, Campbell, Willerson, et al,[55] with permission.)

7. Some cardiovascular events appear to be associated with emotional stress, and these events may be mediated by catecholamine-induced activation of platelets and stimulation of thromboxane production.[65]

8. Diet may affect the occurrence of cardiovascular events independent of its influence on hyperlipidemia. Greenland eskimos, who have a high dietary intake of cold-water fish (mackerel and cod), have a diminished incidence of vascular disease as well as a prolonged bleeding time.[66] Cold-water fish contain large amounts of eicosapentaenoic acid, and, as a result, the plasma of these eskimos contains a predominance of eicosapentaenoic acid rather than arachidonic acid (eicosatetraenoic acid). Eicosapentaenoic acid is metabolized to thromboxane A_3 and PGI_3. Although PGI_3 is physiologically as active as PGI_2, TxA_3 is inactive[67] and, in fact, may even block platelet TxA_2 receptors (Fig. 4). In short, a diet containing an abundance of eicosapentaenoic acid leads to a predominance of substances that promote vascular dilatation and inhibit platelet aggregation. This mechanism may account for the low incidence of cardiovascular events in Greenland eskimos.[68] In support of this hypothesis, Caucasian men fed a diet rich in eicosapentaenoic acid develop similar alterations in prostaglandins with concomitant hemostatic alterations to those seen in the eskimos.[69,70] However, it is unknown if this rather drastic dietary alteration would reduce the incidence of cardiovascular events in Caucasian men.

In summary, there is an abundance of evidence suggesting that both platelets and a thromboxane:prostacyclin imbalance may be involved in the development and progression of atherosclerosis. Platelets appear to play an integral part in the initiation and possibly the progression of the atherosclerotic process. A thromboxane:prostacyclin imbalance—that is, excessive thromboxane compared to the available prostacyclin—may be the pathway whereby the numerous risk factors for atherosclerotic vascular disease become manifest. If a prostanoid imbalance is indeed important in the pathogenesis of atherosclerosis, attention should be directed toward its physiologic and pharmacologic correction.

THE CLINICAL MANIFESTATIONS OF ISCHEMIC HEART DISEASE

The Role of Platelets

Both experimental and clinical data have suggested that platelets may contribute to the adverse clinical events associated with atherosclerotic coronary artery disease.[71,72] For example, fluctuations in coronary flow after experimental coronary arterial narrowing in the dog have been shown to be related to the formation of platelet aggregates and, in turn, to be abolished by the administration of cyclooxygenase inhibitors, such as aspirin, ibuprofen, and sulfinpyrazone.[73,74] In man, autopsy studies of individuals dying suddenly have shown platelet aggregates in the coronary microcirculation,[75] and more recent clinical investigations have suggested that sulfinpyrazone may reduce the incidence of sudden death during the year after myocardial infarction.[76] Thus, increasing evidence suggests that heightened platelet aggregation may be of pathophysiologic importance in patients with several different clinical forms of ischemic heart disease.

Stable (Exertional) Angina Pectoris

Several studies have suggested that there may be an important interrelationship among atherosclerotic coronary artery disease, platelet function, and stress-induced myocardial ischemia. Patients with underlying coronary artery disease—unlike those without such disease—have diminished platelet aggregation in coronary venous blood,[77,78] probably a result of the removal of hyperaggregable platelets by the atherosclerotic coronary vasculature. Experimental endothelial injury in the coronary and other vascular beds has been shown to promote formation of platelet aggregates.[79-82] Morphologic studies have demonstrated that platelets are trapped in the ischemic myocardium,[80,81] and others[83–85] (using indium-111-tagged platelets) have shown that hyperaggregable platelets are indeed sequestered in damaged vessels.

In response to stress, induced by either rapid cardiac pacing or exercise, platelet reactivity within the coronary vasculature increases.[86] With treadmill exercise, the concentration of peripheral venous platelet factor IV, a platelet-specific protein liberated during the platelet release reaction,[72] may increase in patients with coronary artery disease and exercise-induced myocardial ischemia but not in those in whom the exercise tolerance test is negative.[87] However, other investigators have been unable to confirm these observations.[88] Despite this variance in published results, it seems plausible that platelet activation occurs within the coronary vasculature in patients with coronary artery disease who develop angina pectoris.

Unstable Angina Pectoris

Several recent studies[89–92] have demonstrated that many episodes of angina pectoris at rest are caused by a primary reduction in coronary artery flow, due to either increased coronary artery tone (that is, coronary artery spasm) or transient platelet aggregation. That enhanced

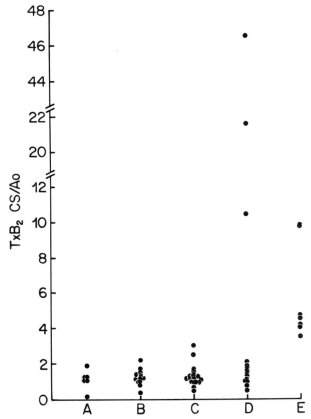

Figure 5. The resting thromboxane B_2 coronary sinus/ascending aortic (TxB$_2$ CS/Ao) ratios for five groups of patients with various kinds of cardiac disease. Each point represents the data from one patient. In Groups A (valvular and congenital non-ischemic heart disease), B (chest pain syndrome without ischemic heart disease), and C (ischemic heart disease without chest pain for at least 96 hours), all patients had TxB$_2$ CS/Ao ratios less than 3.1. Group D (ischemic heart disease with chest pain 24–96 hours prior to study) had a bimodal distribution: 12 individuals had low TxB$_2$ CS/Ao ratios, whereas three had very high ratios. Group E (ischemic heart disease and chest pain within 24 hours of study) had TxB$_2$ CS/Ao ratios ranging from 3.5 to 9.9, higher ($p < 0.05$) than Groups A, B, and C.

platelet aggregability may be of pathophysiologic importance in individuals with unstable angina is suggested by the following observations. First, some patients with unstable angina pectoris have elevated peripheral venous concentrations of platelet factor IV, whereas those with stable (exertional) angina do not.[93-95] Second, elevated levels of beta-thromboglobulin (another platelet-specific protein released during platelet degranulation) have been observed in patients hospitalized with unstable angina pectoris but not in those with stable angina.[94,96,97] Sobel and coworkers[94] have demonstrated an especially strong association between platelet activation/secretion and myocardial ischemia: In their study, plasma levels of platelet-specific proteins (platelet factor IV and beta-thromboglobulin) increased and decreased in direct relation to episodes of angina pectoris. Third, Hirsh and associates[98] reported that the transcardiac ratios of thromboxane B_2 (that is, coronary sinus TxB_2/aortic TxB_2) are elevated in patients with unstable angina pectoris but not in those with stable ischemic heart disease or non-ischemic chest pain syndromes (Fig. 5). Thus, in individuals with unstable angina pectoris, there is evidence of enhanced platelet aggregability and metabolic activity.

In theory, platelets could participate in the development of myocardial ischemia in at least two ways. First, platelet adhesion on an atherosclerotic plaque could produce a flow-limiting platelet plug, as has been demonstrated in the dog with coronary arterial narrowing.[73,74] Second, aggregating platelets release thromboxane A_2, a powerful coronary artery constrictor that, upon its release, might induce enough constriction to limit blood flow. In conjunction with this pathophysiologic hypothesis, Maseri and coworkers[89] have suggested that large-caliber coronary arteries can undergo spontaneous and transient vasoconstriction at the site of an atherosclerotic plaque.

Acute Myocardial Infarction

Individuals with recent acute myocardial infarction, like patients with unstable angina pectoris, have been shown to have enhanced platelet aggregability. Specifically, several studies have demonstrated that peripheral venous concentrations of both beta-thromboglobulin[96,99,100] and platelet factor IV[93,95] are elevated in patients with recent myocardial infarction. Detailed postmortem studies of patients dying of acute myocardial infarction have shown that thrombosis of a large epicardial coronary artery is a frequent finding,[101] although there is continued debate over whether such thrombus formation is a cause or consequence of the infarction. Nevertheless, recent attempts to dissolve the thrombus (with the intracoronary infusion of a thrombolytic agent, such as streptokinase) have, in large part, been successful, especially during the early hours after the onset of chest pain.[102,103] The frequency with which thrombolytic therapy is successful shortly after the onset of infarction (73 percent in the study of Mathey and associates[103]) may offer a clue as to the incidence with which coronary artery thrombosis is of pathophysiologic importance in patients with acute myocardial infarction.

Sudden Cardiac Death

Patients dying suddenly of coronary artery disease have been shown to have more intramyocardial arteries occluded by platelet aggregates than those with chronic coronary artery disease who die of noncardiac causes,[75] but the mechanism of formation of these microcirculatory aggregates is unclear. One explanation is that these represent downstream embolization from proximal platelet aggregates formed on atherosclerotic plaques,[104] a phenomenon that has been shown to occur in experimental animals.[105] Alternatively, the aggregates may represent thrombi formed in the microcirculation in situ, as a consequence of a generalized enhancement of platelet reactivity, induced by excessive stimulation by catecholamines[106] or other humoral agents.[107] Thus, as in those with unstable angina pectoris and acute myocardial infarction, individuals with sudden cardiac death demonstrate evidence of platelet hyperaggregability within the coronary macrocirculation and/or microcirculation.

The Role of Thromboxane and Prostacyclin

Because of the powerful influence of thromboxane A_2 as a vasoconstrictor and promoter of platelet aggregation, a thromboxane:prostacyclin imbalance offers an attractive pathophysiologic explanation for many of the clinical manifestations of ischemic heart disease.

Prinzmetal's "Variant" Angina Pectoris

Prinzmetal's angina is caused by coronary artery spasm.[108] Several studies have attempted to delineate the possible role of thromboxane A_2 as the instigator and/or perpetuator of episodes of spasm. Early reports noted detectable levels of thromboxane B_2 in peripheral venous blood of patients with variant angina, whereas it was undetectable in healthy volunteers.[109] However, subsequent studies have demonstrated that thromboxane B_2 concentrations rise only *after* the onset of coronary vasospasm and that the syndrome of variant angina is in no way affected by the administration of cyclooxygenase inhibitors, even though such drugs effectively prevent thromboxane A_2 generation.[110–112] Thus, thromboxane A_2 *alone* is probably not the mediator of variant angina. To date, however, the thromboxane:prostacyclin transcardiac balance has not been examined in these patients. It is conceivable that a transient excess of thromboxane A_2 relative to prostacyclin induces coronary vasospasm. Alternatively, coronary artery spasm may be sustained, but not initiated, by an increase in thromboxane A_2.

Stable (Exertional) Angina Pectoris

Few studies have attempted to examine the possible contribution of a thromboxane:prostacyclin imbalance in patients with stable angina pectoris. Hirsh and colleagues noted, first, that the resting coronary sinus/aortic ratio of thromboxane B_2 is not abnormally elevated in patients with stable angina and, second, that this ratio does not change during myocardial ischemia provoked by rapid cardiac pacing, isometric exercise, or exposure to cold.[98,113] Although several studies have demonstrated increased platelet reactivity during effort-induced angina, others have shown that inhibition of this exercise-induced hyperaggregability with aspirin does not improve exercise tolerance.[114] Thus, although coronary artery spasm or transient platelet "plugging" may occur in some patients with stable angina, most individuals develop exertional myocardial ischemia because of excessive oxygen demand in the setting of limited oxygen supply; neither platelets nor a thromboxane:prostacyclin imbalance appears to be of pathophysiologic importance.

Unstable Angina Pectoris

A recent study[98] has shown that individuals with unstable angina and continuing chest pain have elevated transcardiac ratios of thromboxane B_2 compared with patients without coronary artery disease or those with stable angina (see Fig. 5). Furthermore, we demonstrated that some patients with recent myocardial infarction or unstable angina develop an increase in transcardiac thromboxane B_2 in response to provocation with rapid cardiac pacing, exposure to cold, or isometric exercise; in contrast, individuals with stable angina and those without ischemic heart disease have no such increase.[113] Thus, unstable angina appears to result from a primary fall in myocardial oxygen availability, caused by coronary artery spasm or transient platelet "plugging," both of which may be induced by and result in thromboxane release into the coronary circulation. The fact that prostacyclin (a physiologic thromboxane antagonist) can alleviate unstable angina without exerting a demonstrable effect in those with stable angina[115] supports the hypothesis that thromboxane and platelet aggregation are involved in the pathophysiology of unstable angina.

Acute Myocardial Infarction and Sudden Cardiac Death

Although previous studies in experimental animals have shown a generalized prostaglandin release into the coronary circulation during myocardial ischemia, the significance of such a release is unknown. Some reports have noted no alteration in coronary blood flow when ischemia-induced prostaglandin release is blocked pharmacologically,[116] but others have reported a reduction in reactive hyperemia during such intervention.[117-119] Presently, no studies are available in which the contributory role of a thromboxane:prostacyclin imbalance in patients with myocardial infarction or sudden cardiac death is examined.

CONCLUSIONS

Enhanced platelet reactivity, with the release of thromboxane A_2 and the development of a thromboxane:prostacyclin imbalance, may play an important role, first, in the initiation and progression of atherosclerosis and, second, in at least some of the clinical manifestations of ischemic heart disease.[120] Repetitive endothelial cell injury from any cause induces recurrent platelet aggregation, which, in turn, may serve as the "framework" around which collagen and smooth muscle cells proliferate, eventually forming the nidus of an atherosclerotic plaque. An excess of thromboxane A_2 (relative to available prostacyclin) may stimulate repetitive platelet aggregation and, in addition, may induce such intense vasoconstriction that further "low-flow" aggregation occurs. Once the atherosclerotic plaque is formed, its progression may be accelerated by a chronic thromboxane:prostacyclin imbalance, to which the various risk factors for atherosclerotic vascular disease may contribute.

Subsequent to the development of coronary atherosclerosis, continued platelet hyperaggregability as well as a thromboxane:prostacyclin imbalance may trigger some of the clinical sequelae of ischemic heart disease. Preliminary experimental evidence suggests that intermittent platelet "plugging" at the site of an atherosclerotic coronary stenosis may be the pathophysiologic mechanism underlying the conversion of stable to unstable angina pectoris. Similarly, enhanced platelet reactivity may be operative in many patients with acute myocardial infarction and sudden cardiac death. If, indeed, platelets are of such importance in atherosclerosis and ischemic heart disease, major therapeutic efforts in the future should be directed toward platelet inhibition as well as the correction of a thromboxane A_2 excess or a prostacyclin deficiency.

REFERENCES

1. BJÖRKERUD, S, AND BONDJERS, G: *Arterial repair and atherosclerosis after mechanical injury. II. Tissue response after induction of a total local necrosis (deep longitudinal injury).* Atherosclerosis 14:259, 1971.

2. HARKER, LA, SLICHTER, SJ, SCOTT, CR, ET AL: *Homocystinemia: Vascular injury and arterial thrombosis.* N Engl J Med 291:537, 1974.

3. BJÖRDKERUD, S: *Reaction of the aortic wall of the rabbit after superficial, longitudinal, mechanical trauma.* Virchows Arch (Pathol Anat) 347:197, 1969.

4. ROSS, R, AND GLOMSET, JA: *The pathogenesis of atherosclerosis.* N Engl J Med 295:369, 420, 1976.

5. MUSTARD, JF, AND PACKHAM, MA: *Factors influencing platelet function: adhesion, release, and aggregation.* Pharmacol Rev 22:97, 1970.

6. WEISS, HJ: *Platelet physiology and abnormalities of platelet function.* N Engl J Med 293:531, 580, 1975.

7. ROSS, R, AND GLOMSET, JA: *Atherosclerosis and the arterial smooth muscle cell.* Science 180:1332, 1973.

8. STEMERMAN, MB, AND ROSS, R: *Experimental arteriosclerosis. I. Fibrous plaque formation in primates, an electron microscope study.* J Exp Med 136:769, 1972.

9. STEMERMAN, MB: *Thrombogenesis of the rabbit arterial plaque: An electron microscopic study.* Am J Pathol 73:7, 1973.

10. SHEPPARD, BL, AND FRENCH, JE: *Platelet adhesion in the rabbit abdominal aorta following the removal of the endothelium: A scanning and transmission electron microscopical study.* Proc R Soc Lond (Biol) 176:427, 1971.

11. Moore, S: *Thromboatherosclerosis in normolipemic rabbits: A result of continued endothelial damage.* Lab Invest 29:478, 1973.

12. Friedman, RJ, Moore, S, and Singal, DP: *Repeated endothelial injury and induction of atherosclerosis in normolipemic rabbits by human serum.* Lab Invest 32:404, 1975.

13. Helin, P, Lorenzen, I, Garbarsch, C, et al: *Arteriosclerosis in rabbit aorta induced by mechanical dilatation: Biochemical and morphological studies.* Atherosclerosis 13:319, 1971.

14. Webster, WS, Bishop, SP, and Geer, JC: *Experimental aortic intimal thickening. I. Morphology and source of intimal cells.* Am J Pathol 76:245, 1974.

15. Fishman, JA, Ryan, GB, and Karnovsky, MJ: *Endothelial regeneration in the rat carotid artery and the significance of endothelial denudation in the pathogenesis of myointimal thickening.* Lab Invest 32:339, 1975.

16. Imparato, AM, Baumann, FG, Pearson, J, et al: *Electron microscopic studies of experimentally produced fibromuscular arterial lesions.* Surg Gynecol Obstet 139:497, 1974.

17. Poole, JCF, Cromwell, SB, and Benditt, EP: *Behavior of smooth muscle cells and formation of extracellular structures in the reaction of arterial walls to injury.* Am J Pathol 62:391, 1971.

18. Harker, LA, Ross, R, Slichter, SJ, et al: *Homocystine-induced arteriosclerosis: The role of endothelial cell injury and platelet response in its genesis.* J Clin Invest 58:731, 1976.

19. Manning, PJ, and Clarkson, TB: *Development, distribution, and lipid content of diet-induced atherosclerotic lesions of Rhesus monkeys.* Exp Mol Pathol 17:38, 1972.

20. Scott, PJ, and Harley, PJ: *The distribution of radio-iodinated serum albumin and low-density lipoprotein in tissues and the arterial wall.* Atherosclerosis 11:77, 1970.

21. Armstrong, ML, Megan, MB, and Warner, ED: *Intimal thickening in normocholesterolemic Rhesus monkeys fed low supplements of dietary cholesterol.* Circ Res 34:447, 1974.

22. Wissler, RW; *Recent progress in studies of experimental primate atherosclerosis.* Prog Biochem Pharmacol 4:378, 1968.

23. Florentin, RA, and Nam, SC: *Dietary-induced atherosclerosis in miniature swine. I. Gross and light microscopy observations: Time of development and morphologic characteristics of lesions.* Exp Mol Pathol 8:263, 1968.

24. Wolinsky, H, Goldfischer, S, Daly, M, et al: *Arterial lysosomes and connective tissue in primate atherosclerosis and hypertension.* Circ Res 36:553, 1975.

25. Vesselinovitch, D, Getz, GS, Hughes, RH, et al: *Atherosclerosis in the Rhesus monkey fed three food fats.* Atherosclerosis 20:303, 1974.

26. Kritchevsky, D, Tepper, SA, Vesselinovitch, D, et al: *Cholesterol vehicle in experimental atherosclerosis XI. Peanut oil.* Atherosclerosis 14:53, 1971.

27. Minick, CR, Murphy, GE, and Campbell, WG, Jr: *Experimental induction of atheroarteriosclerosis by the synergy of allergic injury to arteries and lipid-rich diet. I. Effect of repeated injections of horse serum in rabbits fed a dietary cholesterol supplement.* J Exp Med 124:635, 1966.

28. Hardin, NJ, Minick, CR, and Murphy, GE: *Experimental induction of athero-arteriosclerosis by the synergy of allergic injury to arteries and lipid-rich diet. III. The role of earlier acquired fibromuscular intimal thickening in the pathogenesis of later developing atherosclerosis.* Am J Pathol 73:301, 1973.

29. Pick, R, Chediak, J, and Glick, G: *Aspirin inhibits development of coronary atherosclerosis in cynomolgus monkeys (Macaca Fascicularis) fed an atherogenic diet.* J Clin Invest 63:158, 1979.

30. Moore, S, Friedman, RJ, Singal, DP, et al: *Inhibition of injury induced thromboatherosclerotic lesions by antiplatelet serum in rabbits.* Thromb Haemostas 35:70, 1976.

31. Moncada, S, and Vane, JR: *Pharmacology and endogenous roles of prostaglandin endoperoxides, thromboxane A_2, and prostacyclin.* Pharmacol Rev 30:293, 1978.

32. Moncada, S, Gryglewski, R, Bunting, S, et al: *An enzyme isolated from arteries transforms prostaglandin endoperoxides to an unstable substance that inhibits platelet aggregation.* Nature 263:663, 1976.

33. Gorman, RR: *Biochemical and pharmacological evaluation of thromboxane synthetase inhibitors.* Adv Prost Thromb Res 6:417, 1980.

34. Gryglewski, RJ, Bunting, S, Moncada, S, et al: *Arterial walls are protected against deposition of platelet thrombi by a substance (prostaglandin X) which they make from prostaglandin endoperoxides.* Prostaglandins 12:685, 1976.

35. Carvalho, ACA, Colman, RW, and Lees, RS: *Platelet function in hyperlipoproteinemia.* N Engl J Med 290:434, 1974.

36. Shattil, SJ, Anaya-Galindo, R, Bennett, J, et al: *Platelet hypersensitivity induced by cholesterol incorporation.* J Clin Invest 55:636, 1975.

37. Stuart, MJ, Gerrard, JM, and White, JG: *Effect of cholesterol on production of thromboxane B_2 by platelets in vitro.* N Engl J Med 302:6, 1980.

41

38. MONCADA, S, GRYGLEWSKI, RJ, BUNTING, S, ET AL: *A lipid peroxide inhibits the enzyme in blood vessel microsomes that generates from prostaglandin endoperoxides the substance (prostaglandin X) which prevents platelet aggregation.* Prostaglandins 12:715, 1976.

39. D'ANGELO, V, VILLA, S, MYSLIWIEC, M, ET AL: *Defective fibrinolytic and prostacyclin-like activity in human atheromatous plaques.* Thromb Haemostas 39:535, 1978.

40. SINZINGER, H, FEIGL, W, AND SILBERBAUER, K: *Prostacyclin generation in atherosclerotic arteries.* Lancet 2:469, 1979.

41. SUBBIAH, MTR, AND DEITEMEYER, D: *Altered synthesis of prostaglandins in platelet and aorta from spontaneously diabetic Wistar rats.* Biochem Med 23:231, 1980.

42. GERRARD, JM, STUART, MJ, RAO, GHR, ET AL: *Alteration in the balance of prostaglandin and thromboxane synthesis in diabetic rats.* J Lab Clin Med 95:950, 1980.

43. HALUSHKA, PV, ROGERS, RC, LOADHOLT, CB, ET AL: *Increased platelet thromboxane synthesis in diabetes mellitus.* J Lab Clin Med 97:87, 1981.

44. CHASE, HP, WILLIAMS, RL, AND DUPONT, J: *Increased prostaglandin synthesis in childhood diabetes mellitus.* J Pediatr 94:185, 1979.

45. ZIBOH, VA, MARUTA, H, LORD, J, ET AL: *Increased biosynthesis of thromboxane A_2 by diabetic platelets.* Eur J Clin Invest 9:223, 1979.

46. BUTKUS, A, SHRINSKA, VA, AND SCHUMACHER, OP: *Thromboxane production and platelet aggregation in diabetic subjects with clinical complications.* Thromb Res 19:211, 1980.

47. SILBERBAUER, K, SCHERNTHANER, G, SINZINGER, H, ET AL: *Decreased vascular prostacyclin in juvenile-onset diabetes.* N Engl J Med 300:366, 1979.

48. HARRISON, HE, REECE, AH, AND JOHNSON, M: *Decreased vascular prostacyclin in experimental diabetes.* Life Sci 23:351, 1978.

49. DOLLERY, CT, FRIEDMAN, LA, HENSBY, CN, ET AL: *Circulating prostacyclin may be reduced in diabetes.* Lancet 2:1365, 1979.

50. LEVINE, PH: *An acute effect of cigarette smoking on platelet function.* Circulation 48:619, 1973.

51. HORNS, DJ, GERRARD, JM, RAO, GHR, ET AL: *Smoking and platelet labile aggregation stimulating substance (LASS) synthesizing activity.* Thromb Res 9:661, 1976.

52. RENAUD, S, DUMONT, E, BAUDIER, F, ET AL: *Influence of cigarette smoking and saturated fats on platelet function in farmers from east and west Scotland.* Circulation 62 (Suppl 3):97, 1980.

53. WENNMALM, A: *Nicotine inhibits hypoxia and arachidonate-induced release of prostacyclin-like activity in rabbit hearts.* Br J Pharmacol 69:545, 1980.

54. STOEL, I, VAN DER GIESSEN, WJ, ZWOLSMAN, E, ET AL: *Effect of nicotine on prostacyclin production in human umbilical arteries.* Circulation 62 (Suppl 3):97, 1980.

55. HIRSH, PD, CAMPBELL, WB, WILLERSON, JT, ET AL: *Prostaglandins and ischemic heart disease.* Am J Med 71:1009, 1981.

56. GROSE, JH, LEBEL, M, AND GBEASSOR, FM: *Variations in urinary metabolites of prostacyclin and thromboxane A_2 in essential hypertension.* Clin Res 28:685A, 1980.

57. BAILAR, JC III, AND BYAR, DP: *Estrogen treatment for cancer of the prostate: Early results with 3 doses of diethylstilbestrol and placebo.* Cancer 26:257, 1970.

58. GOW, S, AND MACGILLIVRAY, I: *Metabolic, hormonal, and vascular changes after synthetic oestrogen therapy in oophorectomized women.* Br Med J 2:73, 1971.

59. MANN, JI, VESSEY, MP, THOROGOOD, M, ET AL: *Myocardial infarction in young women with special reference to oral contraceptive practice.* Br Med J 2:241, 1975.

60. ELAM, MB, LIPSCOMB, GE, CHESNEY, CM, ET AL: *Effect of synthetic estrogen on platelet aggregation and vascular release of PGI_2-like material in the rabbit.* Prostaglandins 20:1039, 1980.

61. ELKELES, RS, HAMPTON, JR, AND MITCHELL, JRA: *Effect of oestrogens on human platelet behavior.* Lancet 2:315, 1968.

62. NORDOY, A, SVENSSON, B, HAYCRAFT, D, ET AL: *The influence of age, sex, and the use of oral contraceptives on the inhibitory effects of endothelial cells and PGI_2 (prostacyclin) on platelet function.* Scand J Haematol 21:177, 1978.

63. KENT, RS, KITCHELL, BB, SHAND, DG, ET AL: *The ability of vascular tissue to produce prostacyclin decreases with age.* Prostaglandins 21:483, 1981.

64. MACHIN, SJ, CARRERAS, LO, CHAMONE, DAF, ET AL: *Familial deficiency of thromboxane synthetase.* Acta Therapeutica 6:34, 1980.

65. ARKEL, YS, HAFT, JI, KREUTNER, W, ET AL: *Alteration in second phase platelet aggregation associated with an emotionally stressful activity.* Thromb Haemostas 38:552, 1977.

66. DYERBERG, J, AND BANG, HO: *Hemostatic function and platelet polyunsaturated fatty acids in eskimos.* Lancet 2:433, 1979.

67. NEEDLEMAN, P, RAZ, A, MINKES, MS, ET AL: *Triene prostaglandins: Prostacyclin and thromboxane biosynthesis and unique biological properties.* Proc Nat Acad Sci USA 76:944, 1979.

68. DYERBERG, JO, AND BANG, HO: *Lipid metabolism, atherogenesis, and hemostasis in eskimos: The role of the prostaglandin-3-family.* Haemostas 8:227, 1979.

69. SEISS, W, SCHERER, B, BOHLIG, B, ET AL: *Platelet-membrane fatty acids, platelet aggregation, and thromboxane formation during a mackerel diet.* Lancet 1:441, 1980.

70. SANDERS, TAB, NAISMITH, DJ, HAINES, AP, ET AL: *Cod-liver oil, platelet fatty acids, and bleeding time.* Lancet 1:1189, 1980.

71. MUSTARD, JF: *Platelets and thrombosis in acute myocardial infarction.* Hosp Prac 7:115, 1972.

72. SCHAFER, AI, AND HANDIN, RI: *The role of platelets in thrombotic and vascular disease.* Prog Cardiovasc Dis 22:31, 1979.

73. FOLTS, JD, CROWELL, EB Jr AND ROWE, GG: *Platelet aggregation in partially obstructed vessels and its elimination with aspirin.* Circulation 54:365, 1976.

74. FOLTS, JD, AND BECK, RA: *Platelet aggregation in stenosed dog coronary arteries and their inhibition with ibuprofen.* Fed Proc 38:1308, 1979.

75. HAEREM, JW: *Platelet aggregates in intramyocardial vessels of patients dying suddenly and unexpectedly of coronary artery disease.* Atherosclerosis 15:199, 1972.

76. THE ANTURANE REINFARCTION TRIAL RESEARCH GROUP: *Sulfinpyrazone in the prevention of cardiac death after myocardial infarction: The Anturane reinfarction trial.* N Engl J Med 298:289, 1978.

77. MEHTA, P, MEHTA, J, PEPINE, CJ, ET AL: *Platelet aggregation across the myocardial vascular bed in man. I. Normal versus diseased coronary arteries.* Thromb Res 14:423, 1979.

78. MEHTA, J, MEHTA, P, AND PEPINE, CJ; *Platelet aggregation in aortic and coronary venous blood in patients with and without coronary disease. III. Role of tachycardia stress and propranolol.* Circulation 58:881, 1978.

79. ROSENBLUM, WI, AND EL-SABBAN, F: *Platelet aggregation in the cerebral microcirculation. Effect of aspirin and other agents.* Circ Res 40: 320, 1977.

80. MOSCHOS, CB, LAHIRI, K, MANSKOPF, G, ET AL: *Effect of experimental coronary thrombosis upon platelet kinetics.* Thromb Diath Haem 30:339, 1973.

81. MOSCHOS, CB, LAHIRI, K, LYONS, M, ET AL: *Relation of microcirculatory thrombosis to thrombus in the proximal coronary artery: Effect of aspirin, dipyridamole, and thrombolysis.* Am Heart J 86:61, 1973.

82. VIK-MO, H: *Effects of acute myocardial ischemia on platelet aggregation in the coronary sinus and aorta in dogs.* Scand J Haematol 19:68, 1977.

83. THAKUR, ML, WELCH, MJ, JOIST, JH, ET AL: *Indium-111 labeled platelets: Studies on preparation and evaluation of in vitro and in vivo functions.* Thromb Res 9:345, 1976.

84. DEWANJEE, MK, FUSTER, V, KAYE, MP, ET AL: *Imaging platelet deposition with ^{111}In-labeled platelets in coronary artery bypass grafts in dogs.* Mayo Clin Proc 53:327, 1978.

85. DAVIS, HH, SIEGEL, BA, JOIST, JH, ET AL: *Scintigraphic detection of atherosclerotic lesions and venous thrombi in man by indium-111-labeled autologous platelets.* Lancet 1:1185, 1978.

86. MEHTA, J, MEHTA, P, PEPINE, CJ, ET AL: *Platelet function studies in coronary artery disease. VII. Effect of aspirin and tachycardia stress on aortic and coronary venous blood.* Am J Cardiol 45:945, 1980.

87. GREEN, LH, SEROPPIAN, E, AND HANDIN, RI: *Platelet activation during exercise-induced myocardial ischemia.* N Engl J Med 302:193, 1980.

88. MATHIS, PC, WOHL, H, WALLACH, SR, ET AL: *Lack of release of platelet factor 4 during exercise-induced myocardial ischemia.* N Engl J Med 304:1275, 1981.

89. MASERI, A, L'ABBATE, A, BAROLDI, G, ET AL: *Coronary vasospasm as a possible cause of myocardial infarction: A conclusion derived from the study of "preinfarction" angina.* N Engl J Med 299:1271, 1978.

90. CHIERCHIA, S, BRUNELLI, C, SIMONETTI, I, ET AL: *Sequence of events in angina at rest: Primary reduction in coronary flow.* Circulation 61:759, 1980.

91. AIKEN, JW, GORMAN, RR, AND SHEBUSKI, RJ: *Prevention of blockage of partially obstructed coronary arteries with prostacyclin correlates with inhibition of platelet aggregation.* Prostaglandins 17:483, 1979.

92. NEILL, WA, WHARTON, TP, Jr, FLURI-LUNDEEN, J, ET AL: *Acute coronary insufficiency—coronary occlusion after intermittent ischemic attacks.* N Engl J Med 302:1157, 1980.

93. HANDIN, RI, McDONOUGH, M, AND LESCH, M: *Elevation of platelet factor four in acute myocardial infarction: Measurement by radioimmunoassay.* J Lab Clin Med 91:340, 1978.

94. SOBEL, M, SALZMAN, EW, DAVIES, GC, ET AL: *Circulating platelet products in unstable angina pectoris.* Circulation 63:300, 1981.

95. ELLIS, JB, KRENTZ, LS, AND LEVINE, SP: *Increased plasma platelet factor 4(PF4) in patients with coronary artery disease.* Circulation 58 (Suppl 2):116, 1978.

96. SMITHERMAN, TC, MILAM, M, WOO, J, ET AL: *Elevated beta-thromboglobulin in peripheral venous blood of patients with acute myocardial ischemia: Direct evidence for enhanced platelet reactivity in vivo.* Am J Cardiol 48:395, 1981.

97. NERI SERNERI, GG, GENSINI, GF, ABBATE, R, ET AL: *Increased fibrinopeptide A formation and thromboxane A_2 production in patients with ischemic heart disease: Relationships to coronary pathoanatomy, risk factors, and clinical manifestations.* Am Heart J 101:185, 1981.

98. HIRSH, PD, HILLIS, LD, CAMPBELL, WB, ET AL: *Release of prostaglandins and thromboxane into the coronary circulation in patients with ischemic heart disease.* N Engl J Med 304:685, 1981.

99. O'BRIEN, JR, ETHERINGTON, MD, AND SHUTTLEWORTH, R: *Beta-thromboglobulin and heparin-neutralising activity test in clinical conditions.* Lancet 1:1153, 1977.

100. DENHAM, MJ, FISHER, M, JAMES, G, ET AL: *Beta-thromboglobulin and myocardial infarction.* Lancet 1:1154, 1977.

101. CHANDLER, AB, CHAPMAN, I, ERHARDT, LR, ET AL: *Coronary thrombosis in myocardial infarction. Report of a workshop on the role of coronary thrombosis in the pathogenesis of acute myocardial infarction.* Am J Cardiol 34:823, 1974.

102. RENTROP, P, BLANKE, H, KARSCH, KR, ET AL: *Selective intracoronary thrombolysis in acute myocardial infarction and unstable angina pectoris.* Circulation 63:307, 1981.

103. MATHEY, DG, KUCK, KH, TILSNER, V, ET AL: *Nonsurgical coronary artery recanalization in acute transmural myocardial infarction.* Circulation 63:489, 1981.

104. EL-MARAGHI, N, AND GENTON, E: *The relevance of platelet and fibrin thromboembolism of the coronary microcirculation, with special reference to sudden cardiac death.* Circulation 62:936, 1980.

105. JORGENSEN, L: *Experimental platelet and coagulation thrombi.* Acta Pathol Microbiol Scand 62:189, 1964.

106. HAFT, JI, KRANZ, PD, ALBERT, FJ, ET AL: *Intravascular platelet aggregation in the heart induced by norepinephrine. Microscopic studies.* Circulation 46:698, 1972.

107. CORDAY, E, KAPLAN, L, MEERBAUM, S, ET AL: *Consequences of coronary arterial occlusion on remote myocardium: Effects of occlusion and reperfusion.* Am J Cardiol 36:385, 1975.

108. HILLIS, LD, AND BRAUNWALD, E: *Coronary artery spasm.* N Engl J Med 299:695, 1978.

109. LEWY, RI, SMITH, JB, SILVER, MJ, ET AL: *Detection of thromboxane B_2 in peripheral blood of patients with Prinzmetal's angina.* Prostaglandins Med 3:243, 1979.

110. LEWY, RI, WIENER, L, SMITH, JB, ET AL: *Comparison of plasma concentrations of thromboxane B_2 in Prinzmetal's variant angina and classical angina pectoris.* Clin Cardiol 2:404, 1979.

111. ROBERTSON, RM, ROBERTSON, D, ROBERTS, LJ, ET AL: *Thromboxane A_2 in vasotonic angina pectoris: Evidence from direct measurements and inhibitor trials.* N Engl J Med 304:998, 1981.

112. CHIERCHIA, S, DECATERINA, R, BRUNELLI, C, ET AL: *Low dose aspirin prevents thromboxane A_2 synthesis by platelets but not attacks of Prinzmetal's angina.* Circulation 62(Suppl 3):215, 1980.

113. HIRSH, PD, FIRTH, BG, CAMPBELL, WB, ET AL: *Effects of provocation on transcardiac thromboxane and prostacyclin in patients with coronary artery disease.* Submitted for publication.

114. FRISHMAN, WH, CHRISTODOULOU, J, WEKSLER, B, ET AL: *Aspirin therapy in angina pectoris: Effects on platelet aggregation, exercise tolerance, and electrocardiographic manifestations of ischemia.* Am Heart J 92:3, 1976.

115. SZCZEKLIK, A, SZCZEKLIK, J, NIZANKOWSKI, R, ET AL: *Prostacyclin for acute coronary insufficiency.* Artery 8:7, 1980.

116. HINTZE, TH, AND KALEY, G: *Prostaglandins and the control of blood flow in the canine myocardium.* Circ Res 40:313, 1977.

117. KRAEMER, RJ, PHERNETTON, TM, AND FOLTS, JD: *Prostaglandin-like substances in coronary venous blood following myocardial ischemia.* J Pharm Exp Ther 199:611, 1976.

118. OGAWA, K, ITO, T, ENOMOTO, I, ET AL: *Increase of coronary flow and levels of PGE_1 and $PGF_{2\alpha}$ from the ischemic area of experimental myocardial infarction.* Adv Prost Thromb Res 7:665, 1980.

119. AFONSO, S, BANDOW, GT, AND ROWE, GG: *Indomethacin and the prostaglandin hypothesis of coronary blood flow regulation.* J Physiol 241:299, 1974.

120. MEHTA, J, AND MEHTA, P: *Role of blood platelets and prostaglandins in coronary artery disease.* Am J Cardiol 48:366, 1981.

The Role of Coronary Artery Spasm in Acute Myocardial Infarction

Philip B. Oliva, M.D.

For many years, coronary thrombosis was deemed the sole and immediate cause of myocardial infarction. This understandable conclusion was reached because of the high prevalence of coronary thrombi encountered in fatal acute infarction when death occurred more than 6 hours after the onset of symptoms. It was assumed that the thrombus was present at the moment of infarction and initiated the event. In fact, however, the pathologist is hindered in attempts to understand the initiation of infarction because myocardial necrosis cannot be detected by conventional hematoxylin-eosin stain and light microscopy until 6 or more hours have elapsed.[1] Electron microscopy and dehydrogenase stains allow earlier detection of infarction,[2,3] but, nevertheless, it is not possible to confidently diagnose acute infarction during the critical early hours. Consequently, the presence and prevalence of coronary thrombosis at the time of infarction is unknown. It is also unknown how many patients who die within 6 hours from the onset of symptoms, and who lack both histologic evidence of infarction and a thrombus, actually sustained an acute infarction. Death is usually ascribed to "sudden cardiac death," presumably due to a ventricular arrhythmia, under these circumstances. Undoubtedly this is often the case, but it seems intuitively clear that in some instances an acute myocardial infarction leads to sudden death—perhaps by eliciting a ventricular arrhythmia. In two patients who died suddenly after the occurrence of chest pain, and in one instance exhibited ST segment elevation as well, a ruptured plaque with platelet aggregates adhering to subintimal collagen was present, but no occlusive thrombus was present at the time of death.[4] This suggests that some factor other than thrombosis caused the acute plaque changes, and, pari passu, myocardial infarction.

Recently, platelet aggregability has been shown to be increased in patients with an acute myocardial infarction, and coronary artery spasm has been documented by arteriography performed just before and during the onset of infarction. These clinical observations have been complemented by the discovery of two potent substances—thromboxane A_2 and prostacyclin—which affect platelet aggregability and coronary artery tone. In this chapter, these recent observations and discoveries are blended with the older pathologic information in order to attain a more comprehensive understanding of the pathophysiology of acute myocardial infarction.

PATHOLOGIC OBSERVATIONS IN ACUTE MYOCARDIAL INFARCTION

Acute myocardial infarctions are customarily classified as transmural (which involve at least one-half to two-thirds of the left ventricular wall thickness) or subendocardial (which are limited to less than the inner half of the ventricular wall).[5] Transmural infarcts are seg-

45

mental—at least 2 to 3 cm long in one axis—and include a central zone of necrosis surrounded by myocardial cells in varying stages of ischemia. The number of normal, ischemic, and necrotic cells differs in different areas of the region at risk during the early critical hours of infarction. In the canine heart, virtually all cells are potentially viable after only 20 minutes of coronary occlusion, but after 6 hours necrosis is nearly complete.[6,7] The time frame of reversible ischemia in humans is not precisely known and may vary among individuals, depending upon the extent of collaterals nourishing the ischemic border zone. Moreover, it appears that because of collateral flow into the occluded coronary bed, only a central zone with critically reduced flow initially becomes ischemic after occlusion.[8] Over the next few hours, factors that influence the supply and demand of oxygen determine the ultimate amount of myocardium that becomes necrotic. Thus, the ischemic border zone is dynamic and may change during the initial hours of infarction. Platelet trapping,[9] lysomal release,[10] cell swelling,[11] microcirculatory damage,[12] prostaglandin release,[13] and vasospasm[14] are some of the factors influencing the viability of ischemic myocardium.

Subendocardial infarcts are usually not associated with coronary thrombosis, and, conversely, transmural infarcts 6 hours or more old have a thrombus superimposed on an atherosclerotic plaque in the vessel subtending the infarcted region in 90 percent or more of instances (Table 1).[5,15-26] For nonapparent reasons, a few studies have found a lower incidence of thrombi.[27-31] The plaque surface is often ruptured, allowing luminal blood to accumulate beneath an intimal defect and to form a subintimal hemorrhage.[32,33] A plaque rupture usually occurs through a thin layer of intima separating a softened plaque from luminal blood, or at the margin of the plaque at its junction with the vessel wall. The length of the defect is

Table 1. Frequency of coronary thrombosis in acute transmural myocardial infarction

First author, year (reference)	Cases	Age of infarction	% with coronary thrombus
Miller, 1951 (5)	93	<4 weeks	90
Mitchell, 1956, 1963 (15, 16)	26	<4 weeks	96
Ehrlich, 1964 (17)	18	Recent	94
Harland, 1966 (18)	46	Recent	93
Chapman, 1968 (19)	292	<1 month	91
Page, 1971 (20)	34	Recent	91
Sinapius, 1972 (21)	170	4 weeks	96
Davies, 1976 (22)	469	>1 day	95
Bulkley, 1977 (23)	102	<1 month	95
Ridolfi, 1977 (24)	49	<2 weeks	99
Horie, 1978 (25)	185	<1 month	92
Buja, 1981 (26)	55	Recent	90

about 500 to 2,000 μ.[25,34] The defect may be transverse[35] or longitudinal,[36] and the torn ends of the defect usually point toward the lumen.[25,32,33]

The tunica media is variable in thickness in atherosclerotic coronary arteries. In advanced cases, the media is atrophic and there is extensive calcification.[15,37,38] On the other hand, in patients with less advanced disease, the media may be normal or nearly so beneath concentric plaques.[38,39] In addition, many plaques are eccentric, and abundant media is present in the uninvolved wall opposite the plaque.[15,40] Finally, vasa vasora, which are normally confined to the adventitia and outermost portion of the media, are more plentiful and penetrate through the media in atherosclerotic vessels.[35,37,41,42]

PLATELET AGGREGATES

A "hypercoagulable" state due to either accelerated coagulation or depressed fibrinolytic activity, or both, has been known for many years to exist in some patients with an acute myocardial infarction. Recently, attention has shifted from coagulation changes to the role of platelet aggregates in acute myocardial infarction and coronary thrombosis. The sequence of adhesion, release, and aggregation before arterial thrombus formation is now established.[43,44] Platelets initially adhere to exposed intimal collagenous structures or, perhaps, to endothelial cells with deficient prostacyclin production.[45,46] Areas of disturbed flow, created by an atherosclerotic narrowing, may also enhance platelet accumulation.[47-49] After adhesion to the vessel wall, platelets undergo degranulation, the morphologic equivalent of the "release reaction." The release reaction can also be induced by adenosine diphosphate (ADP), thrombin, or epinephrine. These release inducers stimulate the synthesis of thromboxane A_2 from arachidonic acid.[44,45,50,51] Thromboxane A_2 and ADP then initiate platelet aggregation. Both substances cause irreversible aggregation, but the relative importance of each substance during in vivo aggregation is uncertain. Regardless of their relative importance, both ADP and thromboxane A_2 stimulate an increase of intracellular calcium concentration needed for aggregation to occur.[50,52,53]

Platelet aggregates do not form in normal arteries because of the high velocity of blood flow and the strong antiaggregatory effect of prostacyclin synthesized by endothelial cells[54,55] and the lung.[56,57] However, reduced prostacyclin synthesis by atherosclerotic arteries[46,58,59] may impair their ability to resist platelet aggregation. In addition, platelets from animals with diet-induced atherosclerosis and from patients with an acute myocardial infarction synthesize increased amounts of thromboxane A_2.[60,61] Aggregation may be further augmented by transient increases in circulating catecholamines related to stress, smoking, and rapid eye movement sleep.

Platelet aggregation is often enhanced soon after an acute myocardial infarction.[62-66] Moreover, an increased number of circulating peripheral venous platelet aggregates in vivo are present within the first few hours to days following an acute infarction.[67-71] Unfortunately, it is not clear if this altered platelet aggregability is a cause or an effect of the infarction. All studies in man pertaining to platelet aggregability have been conducted on peripheral venous blood—rather than coronary sinus blood—after the onset of infarction. In the dog, platelet aggregates appear in the coronary sinus blood within 15 minutes following ligation of a coronary artery, indicating that the aggregates may form in response to tissue injury.[72] Release of free fatty acids, ADP, or catecholamines from ischemic myocardium may promote platelet aggregation. Thus, it is not yet clear whether the altered platelet aggregability in man with acute myocardial infarction precedes and contributes to the initiation of coronary occlusion or whether it results from the infarction process.

THROMBOXANE A₂ AND PROSTACYCLIN

Thromboxane A_2, discovered in 1975,[51] is synthesized by platelets from arachidonic acid liberated from membrane phospholipids by phospholipase A_2. After arachidonic acid is converted by cyclooxygenase to the prostaglandin endoperoxides, PGG_2 and PGH_2, the latter are acted on by thromboxane synthetase to form thromboxane A_2. Thromboxane A_2 is a more potent platelet aggregator than its endoperoxide precursors; moreover, in contrast to the endoperoxides, it is a powerful vasoconstrictor.[73]

Prostacyclin, discovered in 1976,[74] is the major prostaglandin synthesized by the coronary arteries. It, too, is generated from membrane arachidonic acid via cyclic endoperoxides. Prostacyclin appears to be primarily synthesized by coronary endothelial cells,[74-76] but smooth muscle also is capable of synthesizing this prostaglandin.[77] In addition, the lung is another source that continuously releases prostacyclin into the arterial circulation.[56]

In contrast to thromboxane A_2, prostacyclin is a strong vasodilator. In vitro, prostacyclin relaxes coronary arteries.[78] Intravenous infusion in man causes flushing and, at high concentration, a fall of blood pressure.[79] Prostacyclin also hinders platelet aggregation and can even cause platelet disaggregation.[80,81] Much higher concentrations of prostacyclin are necessary to prevent platelet adhesion than to prevent aggregation.[82,83] Hence, it has been proposed that platelets may normally adhere to or come in close proximity to the endothelium but are prevented from aggregating by local prostacyclin production.[45] Interestingly, human atherosclerotic plaques[59] and rabbit atherosclerotic coronary arteries[46,84] have an impaired ability to synthesize prostacyclin. Thus, impaired prostacyclin production by vascular endothelium and increased thromboxane A_2 synthesis by platelets from patients with an acute myocardial infarction may work in concert to enhance platelet aggregation and, subsequently, thrombosis.

CORONARY ARTERY SPASM

The earliest clinical observations regarding coronary spasm in acute infarction indicate that spasm exists in some patients. Spasm has been demonstrated by coronary arteriography in 7 of 10 patients with an acute inferior infarction studied within 6 hours from the onset of symptoms.[85] After more than 6 hours have elapsed, spasm is infrequently demonstrable, perhaps because an occlusive thrombus forms. Spasm is also infrequently detected in patients with an anterior infarction.[85,86] This could be due to a reduced tendency of the left anterior descending coronary artery to develop spasm for a variety of anatomic or physiologic reasons, or to inability of intracoronary nitroglycerin to reach the point of obstruction in sufficient concentration to relieve spasm. Spasm may be refractory to intracoronary nitroglycerin,[87,88] and occasionally massive doses relieve spasm when usual doses fail.[89] In one instance, spasm was unresponsive to nifedipine and intravenous nitroglycerin, but a continuous intracoronary infusion of nitroglycerin achieved patency.[90]

These studies performed within a few hours after the onset of infarction are complemented by the demonstration of spasm shortly *before* infarction. Four patients with coronary artery disease and spontaneous angina with ST segment elevation had transient spasm at the site of a severe atherosclerotic narrowing 1 hour to 5 days before an acute transmural infarction.[88] In one case, spasm involved the circumflex artery and was associated with transient inferior-lateral myocardial ischemia. Minutes after reversible spasm was demonstrated, an acute inferior-lateral infarction occurred. The circumflex artery had reoccluded and could not be opened by intracoronary nitroglycerin. At autopsy 6 hours later, the circumflex artery was severely narrowed and a small platelet-fibrin thrombus was located at the site of narrowing, but no occlusive thrombus had formed by the time of death. Thus, in this instance, spasm unresponsive to intracoronary nitroglycerin superimposed on a severe atherosclerotic narrowing led to complete occlusion of the vessel and an acute myocardial infarction, but at autopsy the vessel was patent. Three other patients had transient spasm of the left anterior descending artery several days before an acute transmural anterior infarction. These observations suggest, and in one instance prove, that spasm can act in concert with a fixed atherosclerotic lesion to produce infarction. However, because all these patients had antecedent rest angina with ST segment elevation characteristic of Prinzmetal's angina—a subset of patients well known to have a proclivity to develop spasm—the relevance of this information to unselected patients with acute myocardial infarction is unclear.

A patent vessel supplying the infarcted region is found by coronary arteriography in about 35 percent of patients investigated within 6 months after a transmural infarction[91-94] (Table 2). Interestingly, about 20 percent of these patients have only a 50 to 75 percent narrowing. Moreover, several patients who had a coronary arteriogram done before and after an acute anterior infarction had virtually unchanged 75 percent obstruction of the left anterior descending artery and new akinesis of the anterior wall after the infarction.[91-95] These observations suggest that spasm, platelet aggregates, or a thrombus transiently occluded the lumen long enough to produce infarction, and then resolved in a substantial number of cases.

Because the media of an atherosclerotic vessel is often of normal thickness, except in very advanced cases, and atherosclerotic coronary arteries retain the property of spontaneous rhythmic contractions,[96] it is possible that acute infarctions occur during a phase of enhanced coronary vascular reactivity in the course of ischemic heart disease. Among patients with unstable angina, one-third of coronary arteries initially obstructed by an 80 to 95 percent atherosclerotic narrowing became totally occluded over a four-month interval; whereas in patients with stable effort angina, no detectable change in the severity of stenosis occurred over a comparable period.[97] Moreover, more than half of the patients with unstable angina and new occlusions sustained an acute myocardial infarction. These findings suggest that transient spasm causes unstable angina and that more prolonged spasm leads to acute myocardial infarction. In accord with this hypothesis, patients with an acute subendocardial infarction and incomplete coronary occlusion often sustain a recurrent infarction with ST segment elevation in the same region as the initial subendocardial infarction. The coronary artery remains patent after the recurrent infarction, indicating that a transient process, such as spasm, caused both ischemic events.[98] Following an acute transmural infarction, spasm can be provoked by ergot derivatives in 20 percent of cases; also, 37 percent of patients with rest angina but only 2 percent of patients with stable effort angina have provocable spasm.[99,100] Thus, a phase of enhanced vasomotion may punctuate the course of coronary disease, giving rise to unstable angina, a subendocardial infarction, or a transmural infarction.

Most acute myocardial infarctions occur at rest or during low levels of physical activity.[101-103] A similar level of activity exists at the onset of ischemia in patients with Prinzmetal's angina and in those with unstable rest angina. Spasm has been proven to be the cause of ischemia in Prinzmetal's angina,[104,105] and spasm has been observed in patients with unstable rest angina.[106] Arterial pressure and heart rate do not rise before the onset of ischemic ECG changes in either Prinzmetal's angina or unstable rest angina.[107-109] Moreover, despite methoxamine-induced increases of blood pressure and double product exceeding the levels

Table 2. Frequency of totally occluded coronary artery supplying infarced myocardium in transmural infarction

First author, year (reference)	No. patients	No. with total occlusion	% with total occlusion
Haft, 1977 (91)	132	58	44
Bertrand, 1979 (92)	106	56	53
DeWood, 1980 (93)	322	256	80
Hamby, 1981 (94)	140	88	63
Total	700	458	65

19. CHAPMAN, I: *Relationships of recent coronary artery occlusion and acute myocardial infarction.* J Mt Sinai Hosp 35:149, 1968.

20. PAGE, DL, CAULFIELD, JB, AND KASTOR, JA: *Myocardial changes associated with cardiogenic shock.* N Engl J Med 285:133, 1971.

21. SINAPIUS, D: *Beziehungen zwischen koronarthrombosen and myokardinfarkten.* Stsh Med Wochenschr 97:443, 1972.

22. DAVIES, MJ, WOOLF, N, AND ROBERTSON, WB: *Pathology of acute myocardial infarction with particular reference to occlusive coronary thrombi.* Br Heart J 38:659, 1976.

23. BULKLEY, BH, AND HUTCHINS, GM: *Coronary thrombosis: The major cause of acute myocardial infarction in atherosclerotic coronary artery disease.* Circulation 55,56 (Suppl 3):64, 1977.

24. RIDOLFI, RL, AND HUTCHINS, GM: *The relationship between coronary artery lesions and myocardial infarcts: Ulceration of atherosclerotic plaques precipitating coronary thrombosis.* Am Heart J 93:468, 1977.

25. HORIE, T, SEKIGUCHI, M, AND HIROSAWA, K: *Coronary thrombosis in pathogenesis of acute myocardial infarction: Histopathological study of coronary arteries in 108 necropsied cases using serial section.* Br Heart J 40:153, 1978.

26. BUJA, LM, AND WILLERSON, JT: *Cliniocopathologic correlates of acute ischemic heart disease syndromes.* Am J Med 47:343, 1981.

27. BAROLDI, G: *Acute coronary occlusion as a cause of myocardial infarct and sudden coronary heart death.* Am J Cardiol 16:859, 1964.

28. WALSTON, A, HACKEL, DB, AND ESTES, EH: *Acute coronary occlusion and the "power failure" syndrome.* Am Heart J 79:613, 1970.

29. ROBERTS, WC, AND BUJA, LM: *The frequency and significance of coronary arterial thrombi and other observations in fatal acute myocardial infarction: A study of 107 necropsy patients.* Am J Med 52:425, 1972.

30. BAROLDI, G, RADICE, F, SCHMID, G, ET AL: *Morphology of acute myocardial infarction in relation to coronary thrombosis.* Am Heart J 87:65, 1978.

31. BRANWOOD, AW: *The development of coronary thrombosis following myocardial infarction.* Lipids 13:378, 1978.

32. CHAPMAN, I; *Morphogenesis of occluding coronary artery thrombosis.* Arch Pathol 80:256, 1965.

33. FRIEDMAN, M, AND VAN DEN BOVENKAMP, GJ: *The pathogenesis of a coronary thrombus.* Am J Pathol 48:19, 1966.

34. BLUMGART, HL, SCHLESINGER, MJ, AND DAVIS, D: *Studies on the relation of the clinical manifestations of angina pectoris, coronary thrombosis and myocardial infarction to the pathologic findings.* Am Heart J 19:1, 1940.

35. HORN, H, AND FINKELSTEIN, LE: *Arteriosclerosis of the coronary arteries and the mechanism of their occlusion.* Am Heart J 19:655, 1940.

36. CONSTANTINIDES, P: *Plaque fissures in human coronary thrombosis.* J Atheroscler Res 6:1, 1966.

37. CHAPMAN, I: *The initiating cause of coronary artery thrombosis.* J Mt Sinai Hosp 36:361, 1969.

38. LEARY, T: *Coronary spasm as a possible factor in producing sudden death.* Am Heart J 10:338, 1935.

39. LEARY, T: *Experimental atherosclerosis in the rabbit compared with human atherosclerosis.* Arch Pathol 17:453, 1934.

40. FULTON, WFM: *The Coronary Arteries.* Charles C Thomas, Springfield, IL, 1965.

41. RAMSEY, EM: *Nutrition of the blood vessel wall: Review of the literature.* Yale J Biol Med 9:14, 1936–1937.

42. MORGAN, AD: *The Pathogenesis of Coronary Occlusion.* Charles C Thomas, Springfield, IL, 1956.

43. MUSTARD, JF, KINLOUGH-RATHBONE, RL, AND PACKHAM, MA: *Recent status of research in the pathogenesis of thrombosis.* Throm Diath Haemorrh 59(Suppl):157, 1974.

44. WEISS, HJ: *Platelet physiology and abnormalities of platelet function.* N Engl J Med 293:531, 1975.

45. MONCADA, S, AND VANE, JR: *Arachidonic acid metabilities and the interactions between platelets and blood vessel walls.* N Engl J Med 300:1142, 1979.

46. DEMBINSKA-KIEC, A, GRYGLEWSKI, RJ, ZUMUDA, A, ET AL: *The generation of prostacyclin by arteries and by the coronary vascular bed is reduced in experimental atherosclerosis in rabbits.* Prostaglandins 14:1025, 1977.

47. MURPHY, EA, ROWSELL, HC, DOWNIE, HG, ET AL: *Encrustation and atherosclerosis: The analogy between early in vivo lesions and deposits which occur in extracorporeal circulations.* Can Med Assoc J 87:259, 1962.

48. STEIN, PD, AND SABBAH, HN: *Turbulent blood flow and thrombosis.* Circulation 49,50 (Suppl 3):295, 1974.

49. AZUMA, T, AND FUKUSHIMA, T: *Disturbance of blood flow as a factor of thrombosis formation.* Thromb Res 8:375, 1976.

50. GERRARD, JM, AND WHITE, JG: *Prostaglandins and thromboxanes: "Middlemen" modulating platelet function in hemostasis and thrombosis.* Prog Hemost Thromb 4:87, 1978.

51. HAMBERG, M, SVENSSON, J, AND SAMUELSSON, B: *Thromboxanes: A new group of biologically active compounds derived from prostaglandin endoperoxides.* Proc Natl Acad Sci USA 72:2994, 1975.

52. ROBLEE, LS, SHEPRO, D, AND BELAMARICH, FA: *Platelet calcium flux and the release reaction.* Ser Haematol 6:311, 1973.

53. LEBRETON, GC, AND DINERSTEIN, RJ; *Effect of the calcium antagonist TMB-6 on intracellular calcium redistribution associated with platelet shape change.* Thromb Res 10:521, 1977.

54. MONCADA, S, HERMAN, AG, HIGGS, EA, ET AL: *Differential formation of prostacyclin (PGX or PGI$_2$) by layers of the arterial wall: An explanation for the anti-thrombotic properties of vascular endothelium.* Thromb Res 11:323, 1977.

55. MACINTYRE, DE, PEARSON, JD, AND GORDON, JL: *Localization and stimulation of prostacyclin production in vascular cells.* Nature 271:549, 1978.

56. GRYGLEWSKI, RJ, KORBUT, R, AND OCTKIEWICZ, A: *Generation of prostacyclin by lungs in vivo and its release into the arterial circulation.* Nature 273:765, 1978.

57. DOLLERY, CT, AND HENSBY, CN: *Is prostacyclin a circulation anticoagulant?* Nature 273:706, 1978.

58. GRYGLEWSKI, RHJ, DEMBINSKA-KIEC, A, ZUMUDA, A, ET AL: *Prostacyclin and thromboxane A$_2$ biosynthesis capacities of heart arteries and platelets at various stages of experimental atherosclerosis in rabbits.* Atherosclerosis 31:385, 1978.

59. D'ANGELO, V, VILLE, S, MYSLIEIEC, M, ET AL: *Defective fibrinolytic and prostacyclin-like activity in human atheromatous plaques.* Thromb Haemost 39:535, 1978.

60. ZUMUDA, A, DEMBINSKA-KIEC, A, CHYTKOWSKI, A, ET AL: *Experimental atherosclerosis in rabbits: Platelet aggregation, thromboxane A$_2$ generation and anti-aggregatory potency of prostacyclin.* Prostaglandins 14:1035, 1977.

61. SZCZEKLIK, A, GRYGLEWSKI, RJ, MUSIAL, J, ET AL: *Thromboxane generation and platelet aggregation in survivors of myocardial infarction.* Thromb Haemost 40:66, 1978.

62. O'BRIEN, JR, HEYWOOD, JB, AND HEADY, JA: *The quantitation of platelet aggregation induced by four compounds: A study in relation to myocardial infarction.* Thromb Diath Haemorrh 16:752, 1966.

63. ZAHAVI, J, AND DREYFUSS, F: *An abnormal pattern of adenosine diphosphate-induced platelet aggregation in acute myocardial infarction.* Thromb Diath Daemorrh 21:76, 1969.

64. SANO, T, BOXER, MGJ, BOXER, LA, ET AL: *Platelet sensitivity to aggregation in normal and diseased groups: A method for assessment of platelet aggregability.* Thromb Diath Haemorrh 25:524, 1981.

65. DREYFUSS, F, AND ZAHAVI, J: *Adenosine diphosphate induced platelet aggregation in myocardial infarction and ischemic heart disease.* Atherosclerosis 17:107, 1973.

66. YAMAZAKI, H, TAKAHASHI, T, AND SANO, T: *Hyperaggregability of platelets in thromboembolic disorders.* Thromb Diath Haemorrh 34:94, 1975.

67. WU, KK, AND HOAK, JC: *A new method for the quantitative detection of platelet aggregates in patients with arterial insufficiency.* Lancet 2:924, 1974.

68. DOUGHERTY, J, MCINTYRE, N, AND WEKSLER, BB: *Assessment of platelet activation in relation to acute thrombotic events.* Blood 46:1021, 1975.

69. GJESDAL, K: *Platelet function and plasma free fatty acids during acute myocardial infarction and severe angina pectoris.* Scand J Haematol 17:205, 1976.

70. GUYTON, JR, AND WILLERSON, JT: *Peripheral venous platelet aggregates in patients with unstable angina pectoris and acute myocardial infarction.* Angiology 28:695, 1977.

71. MEHTA, P, AND MEHTA, J: *Platelet function studies in coronary artery disease: V. Evidence for enhanced platelet microthrombus formation activity in acute myocardial infarction.* Am J Cardiol 43:757, 1979.

72. VIK-MO, H: *Effects of acute myocardial ischemia on platelet aggregation in the coronary sinus and aorta in dogs.* Scand J Haematol 19:68, 1977.

73. NEEDLEMAN, P, KULKERNI, PS, RAZ, A, ET AL: *Coronary tone modulation: Formation and actions of prostaglandins, endoperoxides and thromboxanes.* Science 195:409, 1977.

74. MONCADA, S, GRYGLEWSKI, R, BUNTING, S, ET AL: *An enzyme isolated from arteries transforms prostaglandin endoperoxides to an unstable substance that inhibits platelet aggregation.* Nature 263:663, 1976.

75. WEKSLER, BB, MARCUS, AJ, AND JAFFE, EA: *Synthesis of prostaglandin I$_2$ (prostacyclin) by cultured human and bovine endothelial cells.* Proc Natl Acad Sci USA 74:3922, 1977.

76. MACINTYRE, DE, PEARSON, JC, AND GORDON, JL: *Localization and stimulation of prostacyclin production in vascular cells.* Nature 274:549, 1978.

77. BAENZIGER, NL, DILLENDER, MJ, AND MAJERUS, PW: *Cultured human skin fibroblasts and arterial cells produce a labile-platelet inhibiting prostaglandin.* Brochem et Biophys Res Comm 78:294, 1977.

134. PACKHAM, MA, NISHIZAQA, EE, AND MUSTARD, JF: *Response of platelets to tissue injury.* Biochem Pharmacol Suppl 17:171, 1968.
135. NACHMAN, Rl, WEKSLER, B, AND FERRIS, B: *Increased vascular permeability produced by human platelet granule cationic extract.* J Clin Invest 49:274, 1970.
136. POMERANCE, A: *Peri-arterial mast cells in coronary atheroma and thrombosis.* J Pathol Bacteriol 76:55, 1958.
137. FRY, DL: *Acute vascular endothelial changes associated with increased blood velocity gradients.* Circ Res 22:165, 1968.

The Clinical Syndrome of Variant Angina

*C. Richard Conti, M.D., Robert L. Feldman, M.D.,
and Carl J. Pepine, M.D.*

In 1959, Prinzmetal and colleagues described a group of 32 patients with angina pectoris that was different from angina of effort.[1] A quote from this report is appropriate because numerous references have been made to this remarkable and original work. "In this variant type of angina, the pain comes on with the subject at rest or during light activity during the day or night. It is not brought on by effort. During an attack ST segments are transiently often markedly elevated and there are reciprocal ST depressions in the opposing leads. The attacks almost always terminate spontaneously but if long continued they may lead to death."

Thus, the diagnosis of variant angina is suspected from the history and confirmed by demonstrating transient ST segment elevation on the electrocardiogram during chest pain. Prinzmetal and colleagues speculated about the pathophysiology of this syndrome and suggested that variant type of angina pectoris "results from temporary occlusion of a large diseased artery with a narrow lumen, due to a normal increase in tonus of the vessel wall."

In 1772, Herberden[2] included along with his original description of classic effort angina pectoris the following statement: "Some have been seized while they are standing still, or sitting, also upon first waking out of sleep." Heberden also describes a patient "who set himself a task sawing wood for ½ hour every day, and was nearly cured." This is perhaps the earliest description of patients whose chest pain was not precipitated or aggravated by effort.

CLINICAL FEATURES OF VARIANT ANGINA

Some confusion exists because the term "coronary artery spasm" has been used interchangably with the specific clinical syndrome of "variant angina or Prinzmetal's angina pectoris." The term "variant angina" should be used only to describe a group of patients with chest pain at rest associated with transient ST segment elevation on the electrocardiogram. The attacks of "variant angina" are usually prolonged and severe, with pain generally located in the same area as in other forms of angina pectoris and often associated with sweating. The chest pain attack is unrelated to exertion, primarily occurs at rest, may often be associated with syncope, and usually occurs at the same time every day—often early in the morning or during sleep. In the usual case, chest pain cannot be provoked by either exercise or emotional stress. In an occasional patient with variant angina, an additional component of exertional angina with accompanying ST segment elevation or depression has been observed. Generally the individual attacks of chest pain are responsive to sublingual nitroglycerin. However, it is not unusual for patients to require more than one dose of sublingual nitroglycerin to relieve chest discomfort and to return the electrocardiogram to its baseline configuration.

During an attack of variant angina, observations at the bedside often provide useful information. For example, during chest pain, heart rate usually does not change significantly; but at the height of the episode, an examination may detect irregularities of pulse, suggesting PVCs, ventricular tachycardia, or heart block in some instances. Blood pressure generally remains constant at the onset of chest pain. Later it may fall owing to left ventricular dysfunction secondary to myocardial ischemia or, in some instances, may rise owing to a sympathetic response to pain. As in myocardial ischemia of any etiology, some degree of ventricular dysfunction occurs, and in many instances a fourth heart sound is audible, and in a few cases a ventricular gallop and/or mitral regurgitation due to transient papillary muscle dysfunction is heard. In this same patient with the aforementioned physical findings, the physical examination may be entirely normal during a pain-free interval.

The electrocardiographic abnormalities during chest pain compared with those during a pain-free interval establish the diagnosis of variant angina. Patients often have a normal electrocardiogram between episodes of chest pain, but during chest discomfort there is marked ST segment elevation with reciprocal ST segment depression in opposing leads. The electrocardiogram of variant angina taken during an episode of chest pain is indistinguishable from the ECG of an acute evolving myocardial infarction (Fig. 1). However, spontaneous relief of pain or relief of pain by nitroglycerin produces a dramatic change in the electrocardiogram toward its control state. During chest pain or following the relief of chest pain, the patient may develop premature ventricular beats, ventricular tachycardia, or heart block (Fig. 2). Ventricular fibrillation has also been documented during spontaneous episodes of variant angina.

Prior to Prinzmetal's report, Wilson and Johnston[3] in 1941 reported on the "occurrence in angina pectoris, of electrocardiographic changes similar in magnitude and kind to those pro-

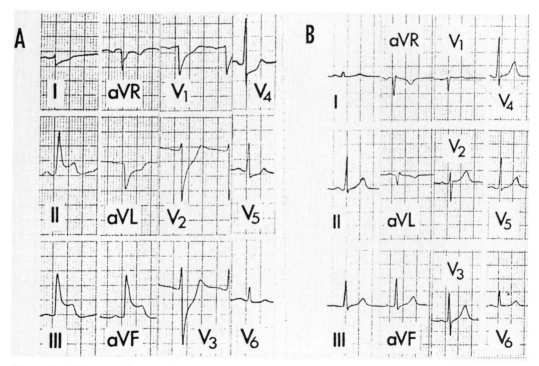

Figure 1. *A,* Electrocardiogram of a patient with variant angina during pain simulates the electrocardiogram of an evolving myocardial infarction. *B,* During a pain-free interval, the ST segments return to their isoelectric baseline, and the electrocardiogram is normal.

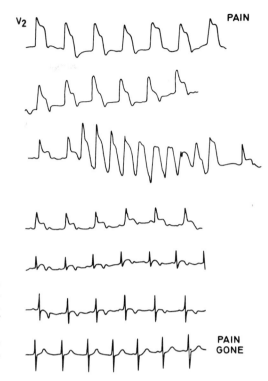

Figure 2. Precordial lead V_2 of a patient during an episode of spontaneous angina. Note marked ST segment elevation (lines 1 and 2), ventricular tachycardia (line 3), heart block (line 4), and normalization of electrocardiogram after pain was relieved. (From Conti, CR, Pepine, CJ, and Feldman, RL: *Coronary artery spasm.* In McIntosh, HD(ed): *Baylor Cardiology Series,* 4(2):9, 1981, with permission.)

duced by myocardial infarction." They postulated that "attacks of angina pain may occur which are accompanied by profound alterations of the electrocardiogram, under circumstances which make it necessary to assume that the attendant myocardial ischemia is due to a change in caliber of the coronary arteries rather than to increase in the work of the heart alone."

PATHOPHYSIOLOGIC STUDIES IN PATIENTS WITH VARIANT ANGINA

The exact sequence of events leading to recurrent episodes of spontaneous variant angina is incompletely understood. However, several investigators have observed the following sequence of events. The first hemodynamic event is a decline in relaxation and/or contraction of left ventricular dP/dT. This is followed by ST segment elevation on the electrocardiogram. Pain, if present, occurs several minutes later. These events are probably preceded by a change in caliber of an epicardial coronary artery. Preceding the ischemic episode there is little change in heart rate or systolic arterial pressure, but once ischemia develops there is a consistent rise in left ventricular end-diastolic pressure. Chierchia and colleagues,[4] by continuous monitoring of coronary sinus oxygen saturation, demonstrated a marked decrease in blood oxygen saturation preceding the impairment of ventricular contraction, ST segment shifts, and chest pain. These latter observations suggest that a reduction in regional coronary blood flow occurred prior to the development of angina pectoris.

In our laboratory several patients with variant angina were studied during unprovoked rest angina associated with ST segment elevation.[5] In a typical patient, chest pain and ST segment elevation occur along with a marked elevation of left ventricular end-diastolic pressure, no significant change in heart rate, and slight elevation or depression of systolic pressure. Figure 3 is a coronary angiogram of a typical patient. The characteristic hemodynamic changes are associated with a decrease in great cardiac vein flow (continuous thermodilution) when isch-

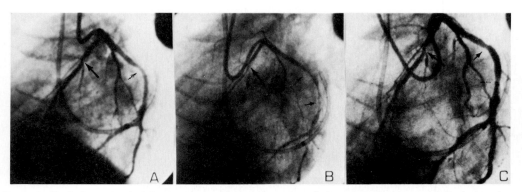

Figure 3. Single frame LAO, left coronary angiogram of a patient during a pain-free interval (*A*), during chest pain associated with ST segment elevation (*B*), and after the administration of sublingual nitroglycerin (*C*). Note the marked change in caliber of the LAD, diagonal, and circumflex coronary arteries (*arrows in B*) during spontaneous chest pain. The coronary stenoses in the LAD and circumflex arteries (*arrows in A and C*) persist after nitroglycerin is given (*arrows in C*).

emia occurs in the distribution of the anterior and precordial leads, as shown in Figure 4. Observations such as this add support to the hypothesis that rest angina and ST segment elevation are due to a regional decrease in myocardial oxygen delivery. Ricci and coworkers[6] reported similar observations in a patient during spontaneous chest pain and transient ST segment elevation. Coronary sinus blood flow fell from 96 to 46 ml per minute, whereas coronary sinus-arterial oxygen difference increased from 9.8 to 11.3 volumes percent. Parodi and

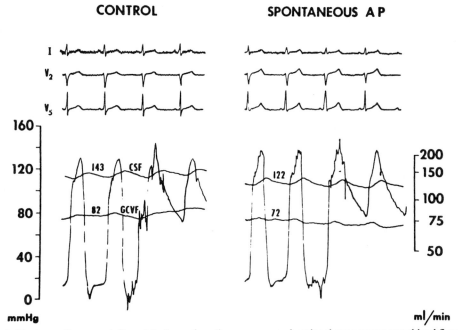

Figure 4. Electrocardiograms, left ventricular and aortic pressures, and regional coronary venous blood flow (continuous thermodilution) during a symptom-free interval (*left panel*) and at onset of spontaneous angina pectoris (AP) associated with anterior descending coronary artery spasm (*right panel*). Note increase of left ventricular end-diastolic pressure during angina with minimal ST segment elevation in leads I and V_2 and slight T wave peaking in V_5 as both coronary sinus flow (CSF) and great cardiac vein flow (GCVF) decline despite a slight increase in systolic pressure. (From Harvey, WP (ed): *Current problems in cardiology, vol. 4.* Yearbook Medical Publishers, Chicago, 1979, with permission.)

colleagues[7] have reported massive transmural perfusion defects occurring during pain and ST segment elevation. They noted a close correlation with location of the area of reduced thallium-201 uptake in the area predicted from ST segment elevation. Myocardial metabolic studies confirmed that hypoxia occurred with a reduction in coronary artery diameter observed before angiographic study. Myocardial lactate extraction was reduced, and in some instances myocardial lactate production occurred.

At the University of Florida, bolus injection of 0.2 mg or less of ergonovine maleate has been shown to produce chest pain and ST segment elevation in all patients with the clinical syndrome of variant angina. Heupler[8] reported a positive response to ergonovine in 34 of 35 variant angina patients; and in a review of the literature, he noted 110 positive tests occurring in 112 patients with the clinical syndrome of variant angina. In addition, Chahine[9] reported a "positive test" in 25 of 27 patients (95 percent) with variant angina. Bertrand and associates[10] noted a high incidence (93 percent) of positive responses to 0.4 mg ergonovine in 57 patients with variant angina.

Using ergonovine as a provocative agent in patients with chest pain, we evaluated coronary hemodynamics in 13 patients with variant angina and compared them with 19 patients with chest pain of uncertain etiology.[11] Both coronary sinus and great cardiac vein flow (continuous thermodilution), aortic and left ventricular pressure, and coronary artery diameters were measured before and after ergonovine administration. In patients with ergonovine-induced ST segment elevation of the "anterior" leads, we observed a greater than 50 percent diameter reduction of branches of the left coronary artery in all 10, associated with a 31 percent decrease in blood flow in the coronary sinus and 30 percent decrease in the great cardiac vein. In those patients with ergonovine-induced "inferior" ST segment elevation, there was 50 percent or greater diameter reduction of the right coronary artery; coronary sinus flow decreased in one whereas great cardiac vein flow was unchanged in all three patients.

In the 19 patients with chest pain of uncertain etiology, ergonovine induced chest pain in four patients, but none developed ST segment shifts. Only minor reduction in coronary artery diameter was noted, whereas coronary sinus and great cardiac vein flow increased 14 percent. These results are summarized in Table 1. Only one patient had a slight decrease in either great cardiac vein flow or coronary sinus flow. One can conclude from these studies that left coronary artery vasospasm induced by ergonovine significantly reduced total and anterior regional left ventricular blood flow. In contrast, right coronary artery vasospasm reduced total left ventricular blood flow but did not alter anterior regional blood flow. These results support the concept that ergonovine provokes a significant reduction in regional left ventricular myocardial oxygen delivery in variant angina patients coincident with angina pectoris in the distribution of the ST segment elevation on the electrocardiogram.

All the aforementioned physiologic studies fail to answer the question: What triggers variant angina? The most attractive hypothesis is related to localized hypersensitivity within the

Table 1. Effects of ergonovine on regional coronary blood flow

Variant Angina (13 Patients)
  LAD Vasospasm (10)
    CSF ↓ (31%)
    GCVF ↓ (30%)
  RCA Vasospasm (3)
    CSF ↓ in 1
    GCVF: No Change
Nonvariant Angina (19 Patients)
  Vasospasm (0)
    CSF ↑ (14%)
    GCVF ↑ (14%)

coronary artery wall to vasoconstrictor effects of various physiologic and pharmacologic stimuli. Perhaps this is somehow related to intracellular calcium and its effect on smooth muscle contraction. Strong support for the role of calcium in this process comes from data indicating that slow channel calcium blocking agents effectively prevent coronary artery spasm.

It must be remembered—and it may well be important pathophysiologically and clinically to consider—that the majority of patients with the syndrome of variant angina also have evidence of atherosclerotic coronary artery disease. In fact, when spasm occurs in these patients with obvious atherosclerotic obstruction, it often does so at the site of the atherosclerotic plaque.

CURRENT THERAPY OF VARIANT ANGINA

The goal of therapy for patients with variant angina should be prevention of myocardial ischemia rather than prevention of recurrent attacks of pain, because myocardial ischemia can occur in the absence of chest discomfort. Ideally it is desirable to have an objective endpoint of therapy, for example, reduction of the number of ST segment shifts with or without pain. Theoretically, prevention of myocardial ischemic episodes should result in a decrease of malignant ventricular arrhythmias and, possibly, a decrease in the incidence of myocardial infarction and sudden death.

Coronary vasodilators such as nitrates and slow calcium channel blocking agents are the drugs of choice. Examples of calcium channel blockers are diltiazem, nifedipine, and verapamil.

A reasonable approach to the patient with variant agina is to begin therapy with sublingual and long-acting nitrates. In patients who continue to experience recurrent myocardial ischemia despite therapy with nitrates, calcium channel antagonists should be tried.

Two studies performed at the University of Florida illustrate the effectiveness of these drugs.

DILTIAZEM. Initial short-term effects of diltiazem on angina frequency were examined in 12 patients with variant angina to determine if long-term responses could be predicted.[12] Initial responses were assessed using double-blind, placebo-controlled, cross-over protocols with 2-week exposure periods to diltiazem at 120 and 240 mg per day. Patients then took known diltiazem, and long-term responses were assessed and compared with initial responses. Ten of the twelve patients had significant (greater than 50 percent) decrease in angina frequency during short-term treatment. After 16 months mean followup (average 8 to 23 months), nine of the ten short-term responders continued to have a beneficial response. Six of these nine were asymptomatic during short-term therapy; and with long-term use, five remained asymptomatic and one had only rare angina episodes. One other patient continued to have a significant decrease in angina frequency, and the two others had a partial response. Only one short-term responder failed long-term treatment. To evaluate possible spontaneous remission, diltiazem was withdrawn in seven long-term responders, and angina recurred or increased in five of the seven patients evaluated. The two patients who were nonresponders during short-term therapy did not respond during long-term therapy. We concluded from this study that symptomatic responses during short-term diltiazem therapy accurately predict long-term responses in patients with variant angina.

NIFEDIPINE. Many investigators have shown effectiveness of nifedipine compared with placebo therapy in patients with variant angina. We undertook a study to compare the effectiveness of nifedipine with isosorbide dinitrate on angina frequency and nitroglycerin consumption in patients with variant angina.[13] Nineteen patients with proven coronary artery spasm were studied. A randomized, double-blind, cross-over design with dose titration (40 to 120 mg per day) and maintenance periods was used. Results indicated that one patient died suddenly during nifedipine therapy, one dropped out after an initial double-blind nifedipine trial, and one could not tolerate isosorbide dinitrate. In the other 16 patients, angina frequency decreased (p less than 0.05) during both nifedipine therapy (0.70 episode per day, mean) and isosorbide dinitrate therapy (0.77 episode per day) compared with control phase (1.70 episodes per day). Nitroglycerin consumption decreased similarly. Group angina frequency was similar with both nifedipine and isosorbide dinitrate. A greater than 50 percent decrease in angina frequency compared with control phase occurred in 72 percent of patients during nifedipine treatment and in 63 percent of patients during isosorbide dinitrate therapy (p not significant). During nifedipine therapy seven patients were better (greater than 50 percent decrease in angina frequency), comparing nifedipine with isosorbide dinitrate. However, six were better with isosorbide dinitrate, and three others were similar during nifedipine and isosorbide dinitrate therapies. No differences in effectiveness of either drug therapy occurred when comparing patients with or without severe coronary artery disease. We conclude from this study that though both nifedipine and isosorbide dinitrate were effective in certain patients with coronary artery spasm, neither drug appeared clearly superior.

Recently, Kimura and Kishida[14] reviewed data from 11 Cardiology Institutes in Japan to determine the effectiveness of drug therapy, especially slow calcium channel blocking agents, on variant angina patients. The subjects were 243 men and 43 women. Coronary artery disease was found in 92 of 162 patients (56.7 percent) in whom coronary angiography was performed. Table 2 is adapted from their report to indicate the effectiveness of calcium channel blockers. Regardless of the presence or absence of organic coronary artery lesions, these drugs were effective in 92.3 percent of the patients with normal or near normal coronary arteries and in 82.6 percent of those with stenosis of more than 50 percent of lumen diameter. The authors interpret these findings to suggest that the drugs are effective due to their antispasmodic action.

Our approach to the overall management of patients with variant angina is as follows:

Once the patient's condition is stabilized, cardiac catheterization and angiographic studies are performed to determine whether hemodynamically important atherosclerotic coronary artery disease is present. When possible, it is useful to determine the location and extent (local or diffuse) of the coronary artery spasm at the time of catheterization. If spasm does not occur spontaneously, it is provoked by administering ergonovine maleate intravenously. After this essential step in evaluation, nitrate therapy should be continued in a patient who has no significant atherosclerosis. If ischemia recurs, calcium blockers should be tried. If pain or asymptomatic myocardial ischemia persists despite medical therapy, the patient should be considered for coronary artery bypass surgery. However, despite this recommendation it must be recognized that current results of surgery for this condition may not be as good as those in patients whose recurrent myocardial ischemia is not obviously due to coronary artery spasm. In a survey of 89 patients who underwent surgery between 1971 and 1977 because of chest pain associated with ST segment elevation, the surgical myocardial infarction rate was 15 percent, and the surgical mortality was 13 percent.[15] There were 2 percent additional deaths over long-term followup, no reported myocardial infarctions, and a 27 percent incidence of recurrent angina pectoris during a mean followup period of 12.2 months. If surgery

Table 2. Calcium channel blockers in variant angina*

Therapy	Patients	Effective	Not effective
Nifedipine	149	140 (94%)	9 (6%)
Diltiazem	87	79 (90.8%)	8 (9.2%)
Nifedipine + Diltiazem	15	15 (100%)	0 (0%)
Verapamil	28	24 (85.7%)	4 (14.3%)
Total	279	258 (92.1%)	21 (7.9%)

*Adapted from Kimura and Kishida[14]

65

is performed, one must be aware that coronary artery spasm can occur distal to a fixed obstruction. Thus, coronary vasodilator therapy should be continued postoperatively in order to reduce the possibility of recurring coronary artery spasm distal to the bypass graft.

PROGNOSIS OF PATIENTS WITH VARIANT ANGINA

The two major endpoints of ischemic heart disease are death and myocardial infarction. When one notes the type and prevalence of severe arrhythmias associated with chest pain in patients with variant angina, it is not difficult to understand that ventricular arrhythmias can deteriorate into ventricular fibrillation and eventually can cause death of a patient (see Figure 2). In addition, there have been numerous anecdotal reports of patients with variant angina developing a myocardial infarction in the exact location corresponding to the site of their electrocardiographic changes. Unfortunately, there are no systematic studies that clearly establish the prognosis of patients with variant angina. Of the studies published, patient followup is usually one to three years, and in no study is average followup five or more years. In Prinzmetal's original description of variant angina, he reported that patients had many cardiovascular complications, including a high incidence of myocardial infarction and death.[1] Pathologic examination in a few patients demonstrated severe coronary atherosclerosis in each. Because there are no large studies available, it is appropriate to consider risk factors that are known to be important in patients with ischemic heart disease, for example, the degree of ventricular dysfunction and the extent of coronary artery disease. Unfortunately, no prognostic data are available in patients with previous myocardial infarction and continuing coronary artery spasm. However, if one extrapolates data from patients with other types of symptomatic ischemic heart disease to patients with variant angina, then the degree of ventricular dysfunction would be expected to greatly influence prognosis.

In a recent publication,[16] we reviewed eight studies describing the prognosis of patients with coronary artery spasm (Table 3). Sixty-six patients had normal coronary angiograms or coronary artery disease with narrowings of less than 50 percent. A total of 258 patients had coronary artery disease, that is, narrowing of 50 percent or greater. This simplistic angiographic separation of patients refers to both right and left coronary arteries. When stenosis of 50 percent or more was observed in one or more vessels, spasm usually occurred in one of the diseased vessels.

Approximately 8 percent of the patients with normal or mild coronary artery disease experienced a myocardial infarction during the followup period in these studies. By contrast, 23 percent of the patients with severe coronary artery disease had an acute myocardial infarction over a similar period of followup. The myocardial infarction occurred in the region of the ST segment elevation noted during attacks of rest angina. In the group of patients reported by Severi and associates,[17] many of the myocardial infarctions occurred in patients with severe coronary artery disease during their initial presentation. They treated these patients with nitrates and verapamil. In their experience, patient prognosis over the next year is relatively good if no major event occurs during the initial hospitalization. These studies suggest that the frequency of myocardial infarction in patients with rest angina and severe coronary artery disease is greater than in patients with lesser degrees of coronary artery disease or normal coronary angiograms.

Patients who die presumably do so because of ventricular fibrillation. Some of these patients have been defibrillated and successfully resuscitated. Selzer[18] reported a good prognosis in patients with normal coronary angiograms or only mild coronary artery disease, whereas the risk of sudden death was significantly higher in patients with severe coronary artery disease.

Based on selected reports, we believe that patients with coronary artery disease have a poorer overall prognosis with medical therapy than those with minimal or no coronary artery disease. However, prognosis of patients with variant angina and normal coronary arteries is not completely benign.

Table 3. Prognosis of patients with coronary artery spasm

Investigator	Normal coronary angiography[a]				Abnormal coronary angiography[a]			
	# of patients	Complications		Avg. dur. followup (yrs)	# of patients	Complications		Avg. dur. followup (yrs)
		Infarction	Deaths[c]			Infarction	Deaths	
Curry[19]	21	3	2	3.5	35 (16)	11	7	3.5
Selzer[18]	9	0	0	N.R.	20 (13)	9	3	N.R.
Heupler[20]	22	2	0	N.R.	0	—	—	—
Severi[17]	9	0	1	~3.5	129[d](13)	32	11	~3.5
Shubrooks[21]	3	0	1	1.5	17 (15)	1	2	1.5
Bertrand[22]	0	—	—	—	35 (35)	1	4	~3.0
McAlpin[23]	2	0	1	N.R.	17 (9)	2	0	N.R.
Silverman[24]	0	—	—	—	5 (2)	2	2	0.5
Total	66	5	5		258 (103)	58	29	

[a]Normal = <50% CAD.

[b]Abnormal = ≥50% CAD.

[c]Death = presumably due to ventricular fibrillation. A few patients were resuscitated.

[d]Only 98 of these 129 patients had coronary angiograms; therefore some may have had normal angiograms or narrowings <50%.

N.R. = Not reported.

Numbers in parentheses represent the subgroup of those with CAD who had surgical therapy.

SUMMARY

The diagnosis of variant angina is suspected from the history and confirmed by demonstrating transient ST segment elevation on the electrocardiogram during chest pain. Chest pain usually is unrelated to exertion, occurs primarily at rest, and may be cyclical in nature.

Pathophysiologic studies in patients with variant angina reveal that the majority of chest pain episodes are not preceded by any evidence of increased oxygen demand. From these observations, the assumption is made that clinical, electrocardiographic, and hemodynamic events are probably preceded by a transient decrease in diameter of an epicardial coronary artery.

Studies in man have documented changes in regional coronary blood flow during episodes of spontaneous variant angina. Most investigators report that the intravenous injection of ergonovine maleate will produce chest pain, ST segment elevation, and dynamic coronary stenosis in the majority of patients during the active phase of variant angina.

When patients with spontaneous variant angina and ergonovine-induced angina are compared, the clinical, electrocardiographic, hemodynamic, and regional blood flow findings are similar.

Despite a wealth of clinical and physiologic information on patients with variant angina, the triggering mechanism for myocardial ischemia in these patients remains unknown. The most attractive hypothesis relates to localized hypersensitivity within the coronary artery wall to vasoconstrictor effects of various physiologic and pharmacologic stimuli, that is, calcium, thromboxane, and so forth.

Current therapy of patients with variant angina involves the use of nitrates and calcium channel blocking agents. Coronary artery bypass surgery has been shown to be effective in many patients with obvious fixed obstructive coronary stenoses in addition to localized coronary artery spasm related to the underlying coronary artery lesion(s). However, results are not as good in these patients as in patients with fixed coronary artery stenosis and no evidence of coronary artery spasm.

Prognosis of patients on medical therapy seems to be related to the presence or absence of fixed coronary artery stenoses, that is, those with coronary stenoses have a poorer prognosis than those with normal coronary arteries. However, prognosis of patients with variant angina and normal coronary arteries is not entirely benign.

REFERENCES

1. PRINZMETAL, M, KEMNAMER, R, MERLISS, R, ET AL: *I. The variant form of angina pectoris.* Am J Med 27:375, 1959.

2. HERBERDEN, W: *Commentaries on the History in Care of Diseases.* Printed in London for T. Payne, Mews-Gate, by S. Hamilton, Falcon-Court, Fleet Street, 1802.

3. WILSON, F, AND JOHNSTON, F: *The occurrence in angina pectoris of electrocardiographic changes similar in magnitude and in kind to those produced by myocardial infarction.* Am Heart J 22:64, 1941.

4. CHIERCHIA, S, BRINELLI, C, SIMONETTA, I, ET AL: *Sequence of events in angina at rest: Primary reduction in coronary flow.* Circulation 61:759, 1980.

5. FELDMAN, RL, PEPINE, CJ, WHITTLE, JL, ET AL: *Coronary hemodynamic findings during spontaneous angina in patients with variant angina.* Circulation 64, 1981.

6. RICCI, D, ORLICK, A, DOHERTY, P, ET AL: *Reduction of coronary blood flow during coronary artery spasm occurring spontaneously and after provocation by ergonovine maleate.* Circulation 57:392, 1978.

7. PARODI, O, MASERI, A, AND SIMONETTI, I: *Management of unstable angina at rest by verapamil. A double blind cross-over study in coronary care unit.* Br Heart J 41:167, 1979.

8. HEUPLER, RA: *Provocative testing for coronary arterial spasm: Risk, method, and rationale.* Am J Cardiol 46:335, 1980.

9. CHAHINE, RA: *The provocation of coronary artery spasm.* Cath Cardiovasc Diag 6:1, 1980.

10. BERTRAND, ME, LABLANCHE, JM, AND TILMANT, PY: *Frequency of provoked coronary artery spasm in patients with chest pain.* Am J Cardiol 45:390, 1980.

11. FELDMAN, R, CURRY, R, PEPINE, C, ET AL: *Coronary hemodynamic effects of ergonovine in patients with and without variant angina.* Circulation 62:149, 1980.

12. FELDMAN, RL, PEPINE, CJ, WHITTLE, JL, ET AL: *Short and long-term responses to diltiazem in patients with variant angina.* Am J Cardiol 49:554, 1982.

13. HILL, JA, FELDMAN, RL, PEPINE, CJ, ET AL: *Randomized double-blind comparison of nifedipine and isosorbide dinitrate in patients with coronary artery spasm.* Am J Cardiol 49:431, 1982.

14. KIMURA, E, AND KISHIDA, H: *Treatment of variant angina with drugs: A survey of 11 Cardiology Institutes in Japan.* Circulation 63:844, 1981.

15. CONTI, CR, AND CURRY, RC: *Therapy of unstable angina.* In COHN, PF (ED): *Diagnosis and Therapy of Coronary Artery Disease.* Little, Brown & Co, Boston, 1979, p 333.

16. CONTI, CR, PEPINE, CJ, AND FELDMAN, RL: *Coronary artery spasm.* In MCINTOSH, HD (ED): *Baylor College of Medicine Cardiology Series, Vol. 4, # 2.* Cardiology Series, Princeton, 1981.

17. SEVERI, S, DAVIES, G, MASERI, A, ET AL: *Long term prognosis of variant angina with medical treatment.* Am J Cardiol 46:226, 1980.

18. SELZER, A, LANGSTON, M, RUGGEROLI, C, ET AL: *Clinical syndrome of variant angina with normal coronary arteriogram.* N Engl J Med 295:1343, 1976.

19. CURRY, RC, PEPINE, CJ, FELDMAN, RL, ET AL: *Frequency of myocardial infarction and sudden death in 44 variant angina patients: A high-risk ischemic heart disease subset.* Am J Cardiol 45:454, 1980.

20. HEUPLER, FA: *Syndrome of symptomatic coronary arterial spasm with nearly normal coronary arteriograms.* Am J Cardiol 45:873, 1980.

21. SHUBROOKS, S, BETE, J, HUTTER, A, ET AL: *Variant angina pectoris: Clinical and anatomic spectrum and results of coronary bypass surgery.* Am J Cardiol 36:142, 1975.

22. BERTRAND, M, LABLANCHE, JM, ROUSSEAU, MF, ET AL: *Surgical treatment of variant angina. Use of plexectomy with aortocoronary bypass.* Circulation 61:877, 1980.

23. MACALPIN, R, KATTUS, A, AND ALVARO, A: *Angina pectoris at rest with preservation of exercise capacity: Prinzmetal's variant angina.* Circulation 47:946, 1973.

24. SILVERMAN, ME, AND FLAMM, MD, JR: *Angina pectoris. Anatomic findings and prognostic implications.* Ann Intern Med 75:339, 1971.

The Role of Coronary Artery Spasm
in Unstable Angina Pectoris

John S. Schroeder, M.D.

Previous concepts that rest or unstable angina pectoris was the culmination of progressive occlusive coronary artery disease in patients who previously had only angina on exertion seemed a reasonable hypothesis, based on pathologic studies of patients dying from unstable angina and acute myocardial infarction. This concept included the proposal that there was progressive reduction in luminal diameter of the epicardial coronary arteries, finally reaching a point where minimal increases in myocardial oxygen demand outstripped coronary flow, even during periods of rest or inactivity. The explanations given for the minimal increases in myocardial oxygen demand at rest or during sleep included increases in central venous return and preload, REM sleep, and unexplained rises in sympathetic tone, which would cause changes in blood pressure or heart rate, precipitating the typical imbalance between fixed coronary flow and increased myocardial oxygen demand.

Latham and Osler, however, had suggested many years previously that spasm of a large coronary artery may play a role in typical angina pectoris.[1,2] Their early suggestions lay dormant until 1959 when Prinzmetal and coworkers reported on a small group of patients with "variant angina" who were observed to have repeated episodes of transient ST segment elevation on ECG, accompanied by typical angina pectoris, which always occurred spontaneously or at rest and was relieved by nitroglycerin.[3] Based on pathologic studies on one patient who died and subsequent studies in the animal laboratory, Prinzmetal proposed that spasm could occur spontaneously in areas of severe occlusive atherosclerotic disease, resulting in transmural ischemia and a current of injury pattern on the electrocardiogram—all which could be reversed by nitroglycerin. However, patients who had only unprovoked or spontaneous pain appeared rare, and Prinzmetal's syndrome was thought to be an unusual manifestation of angina pectoris until the 1970s, when coronary arteriography became commonplace in the evaluation of patients with rest or crescendo angina.

In many patients, there appeared to be a disparity between the severity of the patient's angina and the severity of the occlusive coronary artery disease at the time of coronary arteriography. Several other advances of the 1970s allowed further investigation into the relationships between rest or spontaneous angina and fixed versus dynamic coronary artery occlusion. Continuous electrocardiographic monitoring provided evidence that ST segment shifts may occur at times without chest pain.[4] Bedside hemodynamic monitoring utilizing a Swan-Ganz catheter and arterial line provided further insight into the sequence of events precipitating rest angina in patients with unstable angina.[5,6] Finally, in the mid-1970s the ability to reliably and safely provoke coronary artery spasm in the cardiac catheterization laboratory provided another diagnostic tool.[7-9] These studies over the past 10 years have provided dramatic and convincing evidence that coronary artery spasm plays an important role in unstable angina pectoris.

It is the purpose of this review to discuss the hemodynamic, radionuclide, and arteriographic findings that provide the basis for the current concept of the relationship between coronary artery spasm and unstable angina pectoris.

DEFINITIONS

Unstable angina pectoris is characterized by a progressive or crescendo pattern of pain frequency and intensity due to myocardial ischemia. There is often a nocturnal or rest component that appears to be unprovoked, and the patient may awaken from sleep with angina. The patient may report decreased responsiveness to antianginal medication or increased requirements of medications to maintain a pain-free state. The crescendo pattern may occur *de novo* or, more typically, on a background of previously stable, primarily exertional, angina. Because of the belief that many of these patients progressed to an acute myocardial infarction, a wide variety of syndromes and subcategories have been identified in the medical literature. Their names include crescendo angina, preinfarction angina, intermediate coronary syndrome, coronary insufficiency, and nocturnal angina, all which might preferably be called unstable angina pectoris.

Coronary artery spasm is a transient episode of focal spasm of an epicardial coronary artery of a sufficient degree to produce either subendocardial or transmural ischemia. This ischemia is generally, but not always, associated with angina pectoris and ST segment shifts that reverse after administration of sublingual nitroglycerin.

HEMODYNAMIC STUDIES

Early reports of hemodynamic changes during acute spontaneous episodes of angina usually reflected observations made either during a routine cardiac catheterization or while monitoring arterial pressure or the electrocardiogram alone. In 1967, Robinson reported on the relation of heart rate and systolic blood pressure to the onset of angina pectoris in 17 patients who were observed to have one or more spontaneous episodes of angina.[10] He reported that all patients had changes in their heart rate, blood pressure, or both of these variables, leading to an increase in myocardial work and oxygen demand that either accompanied or preceded angina pectoris. O'Brien and coworkers reported on circulatory changes associated with spontaneous angina pectoris and noted that hemodynamic changes, consisting of an increase in brachial artery pressure, usually preceded the onset of pain.[11] However, in these earlier studies, pulmonary artery pressures were not usually monitored, and it was difficult to ascertain whether measurements were made at the onset of clinically evident angina pectoris at a time when there may be sympathetic responses to the pain itself. These early observations, however, led to renewed interest in the pathophysiology of rest or spontaneous angina pectoris in patients with an unstable angina pectoris syndrome.

In 1974, Cannom and associates reported on 26 patients who were studied at Stanford University Hospital after admission to the Coronary Care Unit with unstable angina pectoris.[5] Within a few hours of admission, a Swan-Ganz catheter was positioned in the pulmonary artery, and a brachial artery line was placed for continuous hemodynamic monitoring. Both brachial and pulmonary artery pressures were recorded at least hourly, and during any episode of pain, on a Honeywell recorder. Patients were continuously monitored for 24 to 48 hours and then proceeded to coronary arteriography. The authors reported on the results of hemodynamic study during 56 episodes of spontaneous pain in 26 consecutive patients hospitalized with unstable angina. At the onset of clinical angina pectoris, marked rises in pulmonary wedge pressure were noted, as well as variable rises in heart rate and systolic pressure. In an effort to determine the hemodynamic changes at the onset of pain, it was found that one group of patients had rises either in heart rate or in systolic blood pressure that appeared to precede the clinical evidence of angina pectoris, whereas other patients had no hemodynamic abnormalities at a time when there was evidence of a pulmonary arterial end-diastolic pressure rise or clinical chest pain. Because cardiac output or index was not measured, the authors were unable to draw conclusions regarding the sequence of physiologic events that preceded the onset of pain but noted that there appeared to be several causes of spontaneous or rest pain.

In 1977 these observations at Stanford were clarified by Berndt and colleagues, who reported on hemodynamic changes at the onset of spontaneous versus pacing-induced angina.[6] Twenty-five patients with a clinical syndrome of unstable angina pectoris were studied after being hospitalized for progressive or crescendo chest pain. After myocardial infarction was excluded, all patients underwent hemodynamic monitoring for 24 to 72 hours in the Coronary Care Unit at Stanford University Hospital. Swan-Ganz catheter monitoring of pulmonary artery pressures, as well as cardiac output and arterial pressures, was maintained throughout the study. After controlled hemodynamic measurements were made during the pain-free resting state, right atrial pacing was started, usually at 90 beats per minute, and the pacing rate was increased in increments of 10 beats per minute after 3 minutes at each level. Measurements were made after 2½ minutes of pacing, at each heart rate level, or at the onset of definite ischemic pain that resembled the patient's spontaneous angina. Pain developed spontaneously in 7 of the 25 patients during the subsequent hemodynamic monitoring period. Table 1 compares the hemodynamic changes in the 7 patients at rest, at the onset of spontaneous angina pectoris, and at the onset of pacing-induced angina. At rest, all but one patient had normal cardiac outputs and normal right heart pressures. Angina pectoris developed in all patients at pacing rates between 100 and 120 beats per minute and was associated with a rise in pulmonary artery diastolic pressure and a slight decrease in cardiac output. These pulmonary artery pressures were similar at the onset of spontaneous episodes of chest pain, consistent with similar degrees of ischemia-induced left ventricular dysfunction.

It was of interest to us to note the calculated double and triple product at the onset of the spontaneous versus pacing-induced agina. Comparison of the double product to the pain-free resting state revealed an 87 percent increase at the onset of pacing-induced angina, compared with only a 12 percent increase at the onset of spontaneous angina. These observations were confirmed by calculation of triple product, with a 43.9 percent increase during pacing-induced angina from control, compared with a 16.9 percent increase during spontaneous angina. In fact, three of the seven patients had minimal if any increase in double or triple product at the earliest onset of pain. Other authors have shown that the level of tension time index at which recurrent episodes of either spontaneous, exercise-induced, or pacing-induced angina occurred is usually a consistent value.[11-14] This significantly lower index of myocardial oxygen demand consumption at the onset of spontaneous angina provided early circumstantial evidence that transient reductions in coronary artery flow, rather than increases in myocardial demand, were the etiology of rest angina in these patients with severe occlusive coronary disease and unstable angina pectoris.

Table 1. Hemodynamic values at rest and at the onset of pacing-induced and spontaneous angina pectoris

Case No.	Control double product (HR × SBP) at rest	% Change from control	
		During pacing	Spontaneous
1	6960	+64%	+41%
2	7020	+116%	+2%
3	6960	+109%	+46%
4	11,424	+108%	−3%
5	11,400	+108%	−11%
6	8192	+96%	+26%
7	13,920	+37%	+13%
Mean	9411	+87%	+12%

Guazzi and coworkers reported on 38 episodes of spontaneous angina in four patients with Prinzmetal's variant angina pectoris and noted that there were neither heart rate nor blood pressure changes that preceded angina pectoris or electrocardiographic abnormalities.[15]

More extensive studies have subsequently confirmed these early hemodynamic observations. Chierchia and associates reported on 137 transient ischemic episodes characterized by ST segment elevation in 28 episodes, ST segment depression in 3 episodes, and pseudonormalization of previously inverted or flat T waves in 106 patients with frequent angina at rest.[16] The authors noted that the onset of electrocardiographic and hemodynamic changes was preceded by a fall in coronary sinus oxygen saturation in all 132 episodes when ST-T wave changes occurred in the anterior leads. They also noted that the sequence of events indicated that there was no detectable increase in hemodynamic determinants of myocardial oxygen consumption prior to the fall in coronary sinus oxygen saturation, which was followed by signs of left ventricular function impairment. These important hemodynamic studies provided further evidence that a primary reduction in coronary perfusion, rather than a rising myocardial oxygen demand, plays a major role in rest angina.

Figueras and colleagues recently reported the results of hemodynamic monitoring in 23 patients with coronary artery disease and rest angina who were monitored from 11 to 43 hours.[17] Measurements were made every 2 hours and at the onset of relief of chest pain. They noted a consistent decline in arterial pressure during sleep, with general reductions in heart rate and slight decreases in cardiac indexing. Eleven patients developed acute ST-T wave abnormalities during pain. These patients showed changes in hemodynamic function that preceded the onset of pain by an average of 8 minutes, and the authors noted that the coronary sinus oxygen saturation was the first hemodynamic variable to change, with subsequent rises in arterial pressure after onset of clinical evidence of angina. The authors noted that myocardial oxygen demand, as judged by the product of heart rate times systolic blood pressure, increased in four patients at the onset of pain. However, at the onset of ischemic electrocardiographic changes the double product was unchanged in eight patients and increased minimally in four patients. These slight increases in double product are quite consistent with our previous observations.[5,6]

Smitherman and coworkers compared myocardial oxygen demands in 12 patients at the onset of spontaneous chest pain during unstable angina to myocardial oxygen demand during exercise-induced angina after resumption of a stable angina pattern 6 to 12 months later.[18] The authors noted that the rate pressure product of 95.8 ± 20 mm Hg per min per 10^2 just before spontaneous angina was significantly lower (p less than 0.001) than at the termination of bicycle ergometry in both the supine (RPP 141.8 ± 25.0 mm Hg per min per 10^2) and upright (RPP 143.0 ± 32.2 mm Hg per min per 10^2) positions.

Sharma and coworkers reported on left ventricular function during spontaneous angina pectoris occurring during cardiac catheterization.[19] They noted a significant increase in left ventricular end-diastolic pressure, left ventricular end-diastolic volume, and left ventricular and systolic volume consistent with marked systolic and diastolic dysfunction during spontaneous angina.

In summary, repeated observations by a number of investigators have now confirmed that there is no change or minimal rise in myocardial oxygen demand at the onset of spontaneous angina pectoris owing to occlusive coronary artery disease. These data provide circumstantial evidence that transient reductions in coronary flow and myocardial perfusion, rather than increases in oxygen demand, play an important pathophysiologic role in the unstable angina state.

MYOCARDIAL PERFUSION STUDIES

Maseri and associates reported on six patients who were admitted to coronary care units with coronary artery disease and frequent attacks of angina at rest, characterized by ST segment elevation.[20] The authors were able to obtain thallium-201 myocardial scintigrams during a spontaneous pain episode for comparison with pain-free scans. Tracer uptake was reduced by 15 to 40 percent in regional ischemic areas during angina corresponding to electrocardiographic location of the ST segment elevation. These studies were consistent with the hypothesis of transient transmural ischemia occurring during rest angina, presumably owing to focal spasm superimposed on an occlusive atherosclerotic lesion in the epicardial coronary arteries.

The relationship between transient electrocardiographic changes in patients with angina at rest and the proposed reduction in myocardial perfusion was investigated by Parodi and colleagues in patients with frequent angina attacks at rest.[21] Thallium-201 myocardial scintigrams were obtained during either spontaneous or ergonovine-induced angina attacks in 21 patients. During spontaneous and/or ergonovine-induced angina, 14 of these patients demonstrated ST segment depression, and in 7 patients there was normalization of previously negative T waves. Twelve of the fourteen patients showed a reduction in thallium-201 activity during pain. Scintigrams in the seven patients with T wave normalization during pain demonstrated large reductions in thallium-201 activity, corresponding to the area of the abnormal T waves. Furthermore, heart rate and systolic blood pressure were not significantly different from control pain-free states. These findings indicate that angina at rest is related to a reduction of myocardial perfusion rather than to an inadequate increase in coronary blood flow during a period of increased myocardial oxygen demand.

CORONARY ARTERIOGRAPHIC STUDIES

Maseri and coworkers reported on right and left ventricular pressure monitoring during 26 episodes of ST segment elevation in five patients with variant angina and recurrent episodes of spontaneous pain.[22] The authors noted no hemodynamic changes indicative of increased myocardial oxygen demand prior to the onset of electrocardiographic evidence of ischemia. The authors were able to perform coronary arteriography during a spontaneous episode of chest pain in four of these patients. They demonstrated complete occlusion of the proximal coronary artery corresponding to the area of ST segment elevation on the electrocardiogram. This occlusion was relieved by nitroglycerin administration and occurred superimposed on severe occlusive coronary disease in two of the four patients. These angiographic findings extended previous isolated reports of documented coronary artery spasm in patients who developed spontaneous angina during cardiac catheterization and coronary angiography.[23–25] These data provided evidence that coronary artery spasm could occur both in patients with severe occlusive coronary disease and in patients with more normal coronary arteries, and could cause unstable or rest angina. These studies were followed by Maseri's report in 1977 of coronary arteriography during 34 angina attacks in 30 patients who were hospitalized because of recurrent angina.[26] These 30 patients were admitted to the coronary care unit with frequent angina attacks at rest, consistent with an unstable angina pattern. The patients were noted to have a wide range of severity of occlusive coronary artery disease, even in areas where the vessel appeared to be subject to focal spasm. Nineteen spontaneous attacks of angina were documented during angiography, whereas 11 were documented during intravenous administration of ergonovine maleate. The authors noted focal spasm occurring both in areas that appeared to be entirely normal and in other areas of severe 90 percent fixed occlusion. These arteriographic studies confirmed that transmural reduction of myocardial perfusion during angina at rest associated with ST segment elevation was caused by severe focal coronary artery spasm. The broad range of severity of underlying coronary artery disease with superimposed spasm in patients admitted with unstable angina pectoris confirmed previous proposals that coronary artery spasm was an important factor in the unstable angina state. This arteriographic and anatomic evidence has substantiated the previous hemodynamic radionuclide studies by Maseri and Parodi.[20,21] Furthermore, it appears that coronary artery spasm

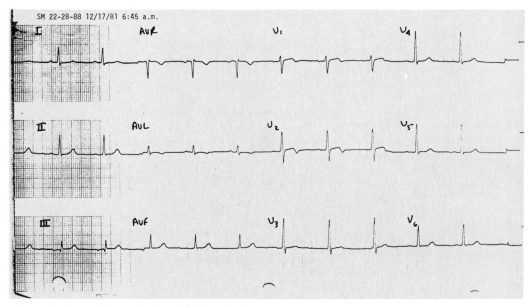

Figure 4. Same patient as in Figure 1. Normal serial ECGs obtained one day after those in Figure 3.

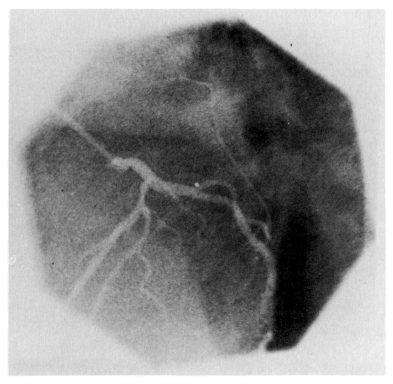

Figure 5. Same patient as in Figure 1. Coronary arteriogram performed while the patient was free of pain revealed a proximal 50 to 60 percent occlusion of the left anterior descending coronary artery.

further episodes of pain. Subsequent treadmill testing showed fair exercise tolerance to a heart rate of 140 beats per minute without ST-T wave abnormalities or occurrence of angina.

DISCUSSION

Technologic advances in the study of cardiovascular diseases have been essential to our understanding of the pathophysiology of rest or unstable angina pectoris. The ability to continuously monitor electrocardiographic and hemodynamic parameters during pain-free states and at the onset of unprovoked angina has now clarified the subsequent sequence of events. Unstable angina pectoris usually occurs in the setting of moderate or severe fixed occlusive coronary artery disease. For unclear reasons, focal areas of the diseased vessel are believed to become hypersensitive to either circulating or local vasoconstrictive influences which precipitate transient, further coronary occlusion. This primary reduction in coronary flow and myocardial perfusion is manifested by a rise in left ventricular end-diastolic pressure and pulmonary end-diastolic pressure as left ventricular ischemia occurs, with a reduction in left ventricular compliance. At this point there is minimal if any rise in myocardial oxygen demand (as manifested by the product of heart rate, systolic blood pressure, and ejection time). As myocardial ischemia continues, ST segment depression is encountered if nonocclusive, and ST segment elevation if occlusive, spasm occurs. These electrocardiographic manifestations may then be followed by complaints of angina by the patient, with subsequent rises in heart rate and blood pressure as a sympathetic response to pain. However, in many instances the sequence of transient coronary artery spasm, left ventricular dysfunction, and electrocardiographic ST segment shifts may occur so transiently (minutes) that the patient is not aware of the episode which resolved spontaneously. These cyclic events may recur, with some coming to clinical attention by causing angina or arrhythmias. Once pain is recognized by the patient, sublingual nitroglycerin usually rapidly corrects the problem by reversing the focal coronary artery spasm and allowing improved myocardial perfusion. Recently, the calcium channel antagonists have been demonstrated to have similar action at the time of coronary arteriography and ergonovine-induced spasm.

These observations are important, not only to understand the pathophysiology of the clinical syndrome of unstable angina pectoris but to guide therapeutic decisions. Because coronary artery spasm appears to play an important etiologic role in precipitating the "unstable" state, nitrates and calcium channel antagonists can be used to prevent these transient episodes and to restabilize the patient. Once stabilized, further therapeutic decisions can be made on the basis of functional limitations and arteriographic coronary anatomy.

REFERENCES

1. LATHAM, P: *Collected Works, vol 1*. New Sydenham Society, London, 1876.
2. OSLER, W: *The Lumleian lectures on angina pectoris*. Lancet 1:697, 1910.
3. PRINZMETAL, M, KENNAMER, R, MERLISS, R, ET AL: *Angina pectoris. I. The variant form of angina pectoris.* Am J Med 27:375, 1959.
4. ROBERTSON, D, ROBERTSON, RM, NIES, AS, ET AL: *Variant angina pectoris: Investigation of indexes of sympathetic nervous system function.* Am J Cardiol 43:1080, 1979.
5. CANNOM, DS, HARRISON, DC, AND SCHROEDER, JS: *Hemodynamic observations in patients with unstable angina pectoris.* Am J Cardiol 33:17, 1974.
6. BERNDT, TB, FITZGERALD, J, HARRISON, DC, ET AL: *Hemodynamic changes at the onset of spontaneous versus pacing-induced angina.* Am J Cardiol 39:784, 1977.
7. SCHROEDER, JS, BOLEN, JL, QUINT, RA, ET AL: *Provocation of coronary spasm with ergonovine maleate. New test with results in 57 patients undergoing coronary arteriography.* Am J Cardiol 40:487, 1977.
8. HEUPLER, FA: *Provocative testing for coronary arterial spasm: Risk, method and rationale.* Am J Cardiol 46:335, 1980.

9. CONTI, CR, CURRY, RC, CHRISTIE, LG, ET AL: *Clinical use of provocative pharmacoangiography in patients with chest pain.* Adv Cardiol 26:44, 1979.

10. ROBINSON, BF: *Relation of heart rate and systolic blood pressure to the onset of pain in angina pectoris.* Circulation 35:1073, 1967.

11. O'BRIEN, KP, HIGGS, LM, GLANCY, DL, ET AL: *Hemodynamic accompaniments of angina. A comparison during angina induced by exercise and atrial pacing.* Circulation 39:735, 1969.

12. PARKER, JO, LEDWICH, JR, WEST, RO, ET AL: *Reversible cardiac failure during angina pectoris. Hemodynamic effects of atrial pacing in coronary artery disease.* Circulation 39:745, 1969.

13. PARKER, JO, CHIONG, MA, WEST, RO, ET AL: *Sequential alterations in myocardial lactate metabolism, ST segments, and left ventricular function during angina induced by atrial pacing.* Circulation 40:113, 1969.

14. SOWTON, GE, BALCON, R, CROSS, D, ET AL: *Measurements of the angina threshhold using atrial pacing. A new technique for the study of angina pectoris.* Cardiovasc Res 1:301, 1967.

15. GUAZZI, M, POLESE, A, FLORENTINI, C, ET AL: *Left ventricular performance and related hemodynamic changes in Prinzmetal's variant angina pectoris.* Br Heart J 33:84, 1971.

16. CHIERCHIA, S, BRUNELLI, C, SIMONETTI, I, ET AL: *Sequence of events in angina at rest: Primary reduction in coronary flow.* Circulation 61:759, 1980.

17. FIGUERAS, J, SINGH, BN, GANZ, W, ET AL: *Mechanism of rest and nocturnal angina: Observations during continuous hemodynamic and electrocardiographic monitoring.* Circulation 59:995, 1979.

18. SMITHERMAN, TC, HILLERT, MC, NARAHARA, KA, ET AL: *Evidence of transient limitations in coronary blood flow during unstable angina pectoris: Hemodynamic changes with spontaneous pain at rest versus exercise-induced ischemia following stabilization of angina.* Clin Cardiol 3:309, 1980.

19. SHARMA, B, HODGES, M, ASINGER, RW, ET AL: *Left ventricular function during spontaneous angina pectoris: Effect of sublingual nitroglycerin.* Am J Cardiol 46:34, 1980.

20. MASERI, A, PARODI, O, SEVERI, S, ET AL: *Transient transmural reduction of myocardial blood flow diminished by thallium-201 scintigraphy, as a cause of variant angina.* Circulation 54:280, 1976.

21. PARODI, O, UTHURRALT, N, SEVERI, S, ET AL: *Transient reduction of regional myocardial perfusion during angina at rest with ST-segment depression or normalization of negative T waves.* Circulation 63:1238, 1981.

22. MASERI, A, MIMMO, R, AND CHIERCHIA, S: *Coronary artery spasm as a cause of acute myocardial ischemia in man.* Chest 68:625, 1975.

23. OLIVA, RB, POTTS, DE, AND PLUSS, RG: *Coronary arterial spasm in Prinzmetal angina: Documentation by coronary arteriography.* N Engl J Med 288:745, 1973.

24. ROSE, RJ, JOHNSON, AD, AND CARLETON, RA: *Spasm of the left anterior descending coronary artery.* Chest 66:719, 1974.

25. SCHROEDER, JS, SILVERMAN, JF, AND HARRISON, DC: *Right coronary arterial spasm causing Prinzmetal's variant angina.* Chest 65:573, 1974.

26. MASERI, A, PESOLA, A, MARZILLI, M, ET AL: *Coronary vasospasm in angina pectoris.* Lancet 713 (April), 1977.

The Role of Coronary Artery Spasm in Exercise-Induced Angina

Carl J. Pepine, M.D.

Traditionally, angina evoked by exercise stress has been thought to be caused by increasing oxygen demands that cannot be met owing to limitations of oxygen delivery imposed by the presence of atherosclerotic coronary artery narrowings. The physiologically important atherosclerotic narrowings encountered in patients with effort angina frequently involve multiple large coronary arteries. These anatomic findings are often associated with ST segment depression during exercise-induced angina. In contrast, coronary artery spasm, with or without physiologically important atherosclerotic narrowings, has been implicated in a variety of other syndromes seen in patients with ischemic heart disease.[1]

Coronary artery spasm has been confirmed in many patients as the basis for angina at rest associated with ST segment elevation.[2] More recently, however, coronary artery spasm has also been described in certain patients with exercise-induced angina.[3,4] These cases have prompted a reconsideration of traditional concepts relative to the pathophysiologic basis for exercise-evoked angina.[5] The purpose of this chapter is to examine critically the possible role of coronary artery spasm in the genesis of exercise-induced angina.

BACKGROUND INFORMATION

A review of selected materials suggests that there is a rational basis for the consideration of coronary artery spasm in exercise angina. Data from patients with variant angina (i.e., ST segment elevation and rest angina) are considered first.

Patients with Variant Angina Who Also Have Effort Angina

Prinzmetal and associates noted that "it is not uncommon for both the variant and classic forms of angina pectoris to occur together in the same patient."[6] These workers correctly predicted coronary artery spasm as the basis for ischemic findings occurring at rest. The effort component of ischemia they thought was due to a different mechanism related to increasing oxygen demands of exercise in the presence of atherosclerotic obstructions. Electrocardiograms during exercise-induced angina in the patients that they described had either ST depression or no ST shift. They concluded that "exercise tests were of little value" in the evaluation of variant angina patients. Similarly, in subsequent studies of patients with variant angina, attention focused upon the rest angina syndrome, although some patients also were described to have exercise angina. Details about exercise testing were, in general, brief or absent in this subset of patients with variant angina. In one of our series, exercise angina occurred in five of eight patients subsequently found to have variant angina.[7] Exercise testing evoked pain and ST segment depression in three of these five patients. We did not study their coronary arteries during exercise-evoked angina, which we assumed was due to associated atherosclerotic obstruction.

Patients with Coronary Artery Disease Who Have ST Segment Elevation during Exercise

Approximately a decade after Prinzmetal's report, Fortuin and Friesinger summarized findings relative to ST segment elevation during exercise testing.[8] These findings, and reports by others on larger groups of patients,[9] indicated that ventricular akinesis or dyskinesis was present in many of these cases studied by angiography. More recently, exercise-induced ST segment elevation was recognized to occur in approximately one out of every hundred patients undergoing exercise testing.[10] Electrophysiologically, it is believed that currents of injury, created by an electrical gradient between the normal and dyskinetic cardiac tissue, give rise to ST segment elevation. It has been suggested that during exercise the relative differences between ischemic and nonischemic regions probably become magnified.[10] Another probably related variation is ST segment depression during exercise, replaced by ST segment elevation following exercise. Lahiri and coworkers[11] found five patients in a review of 1500 exercise tests who had ST segment depression during exercise with ST segment elevation during the recovery period. Each had severe coronary artery disease, but no mention about ventricular wall motion was made. Although no direct evidence for coronary artery spasm, either at rest or during exercise, was given, these workers suggested that these cases represent part of the spectrum of variant angina.

Patients without Coronary Artery Disease Who Have Exercise-Induced ST Segment Elevation

Could a mechanism other than left ventricular dyskinesis, in the presence of severe coronary artery disease, explain exercise-induced ST segment elevation? One of Fortuin and Friesinger's patients had 4 to 9 mm of ST segment elevation induced by exercise.[8] This patient did not have coronary artery disease or left ventricular dyskinesis, and chest pain was described as atypical for angina pectoris. The authors suggested that this was a "false-positive" ECG response. Waters and coworkers described seven patients with variant angina, without physiologically important narrowing and with normal left ventricular wall motion, who developed ST segment elevation during treadmill exercise testing.[12] In all cases, the ST segment elevation occurred in the same leads during exercise testing as during spontaneous attacks of rest angina. Five of these patients also had coronary artery spasm during angiography. In each of these cases, the artery developing spasm supplied the left ventricular region reflected in the ECG leads showing ST segment elevation. In addition, thallium perfusion scans during exercise testing associated with ST segment elevation showed a large perfusion defect in the myocardial region corresponding to the site localized from the leads showing ST segment elevation. Inasmuch as coronary artery disease was not present, these perfusion defects strongly suggest that a reduction in coronary artery flow occurred during exercise, most likely due to coronary artery spasm. These studies indicated that coronary artery spasm was probably responsible for effort-induced angina. Cheng and associates described one patient with normal coronary angiography and variant angina who developed ST segment elevation with exercise.[13] Similarly, a few cases of patients with variant angina and normal coronary arteriograms who developed ST segment elevation, either during or immediately after exercise, were described by others.[14-17]

Patients with Documented Coronary Artery Spasm during Exercise

Yasue and colleagues described 13 patients with variant angina who also had exercise-induced ST segment elevation and angina.[18] Attacks of angina could be induced repeatedly in the morning, but not in the afternoon, in 11 of these patients. Coronary arteriograms done during rest pain and ST segment elevation showed spasm involving arteries that supplied the left ventricular region, reflecting ST segment elevation during effort angina. Seven of these patients performed arm exercise in the catheterization laboratory, and three of them developed angiographic evidence of spasm. In one of these three cases, an angiographically normal right coronary artery became completely occluded during exercise. In the other two cases, physiologically important atherosclerotic stenosis was present in the left anterior descending artery; this vessel became completely or nearly completely occluded during exercise. Two of the remaining four patients, in whom angina could not be induced during exercise, had spasm after exercise, involving a large coronary artery with a physiologically important atherosclerotic stenosis. In each of these five cases, angiographic evidence for spasm disappeared after nitroglycerin administration. Furthermore, the authors could induce attacks during arm exercise in only one patient in the afternoon. The measured coronary artery diameters of the patients in whom the angiograms were done in the morning were compared with diameters of those patients exercised in the afternoon. All coronary diameters increased after nitroglycerin administration, but the change in diameter was significantly greater in the patients studied in the morning compared with those studied in the afternoon (74 vs 12 percent). This was taken to indicate that the tone of the large coronary arteries was increased in the early morning compared with the afternoon. These workers suggested that there was a circadian variation in the tone of the large coronary arteries in patients with variant angina. The variation in tone may explain the variation in exercise capacity and may relate to effort-induced angina occurring in the morning.

Simultaneously with the former report, Specchia and coworkers described four patients with variant angina who exhibited reproducible exercise-induced angina with ST segment elevation.[4] Coronary angiograms documented spasm in a normal-appearing right coronary artery after termination of exercise in two patients. In another patient, spasm involving a right coronary artery that already had a 50 percent stenosis occurred after ergonovine stimulation, which evoked ST segment elevation in the inferior leads. During exercise-induced angina, ST segment elevation was localized to the leads showing ST segment elevation with ergonovine. In a fourth case, a 75 percent left anterior descending artery narrowing progressed to 99 percent during exercise-induced angina associated with anterior lead ST segment elevation. In some of these cases, coronary angiographic evidence for spasm was identified after exercise was terminated. Freedman and coworkers[19] reported six patients with variant angina who had ST segment elevation with exercise. They observed exercise-induced spasm involving the left anterior descending artery of a man with a 50 percent stenosis at rest. These investigators inferred the presence of spasm on the basis of ST segment elevation or thallium perfusion defects during exercise-induced angina. These cases had no evidence for important atherosclerotic obstructions.

All these findings indicate that coronary artery spasm may occur infrequently during or after exercise in selected patients with variant angina. Exercise-induced spasm may be localized to vessels with or without important atherosclerotic stenosis.

Coronary Spasm as the Basis for Classic Effort-Induced Angina in Patients without Variant Angina

Isolated episodes of coronary artery spasm documented at rest have been reported in patients with classic effort angina syndrome. Nevertheless, a cause and effect relationship between spasm and effort angina is unclear in patients without variant angina. Recently, however, Yasue and coworkers presented four cases with exercise-induced angina associated with ST segment depression.[3] Each patient had coronary artery spasm documented during or shortly after exercise-induced angina. Two of these cases had spasm involving the left anterior descending artery superimposed on normal or nearly normal coronary arteries. Two others had physiologically important atherosclerotic-type narrowings in two of the three major coronary arteries. In each of the latter two cases, spasm occurred with exercise about the site of an important atherosclerotic narrowing. No mention was made about the possible coexistence of ST segment elevation or rest pain. More recently, Fuller and associates described exercise-related spasm in two patients with exercise-induced ST segment elevation.[20] In these patients, coronary angiography demonstrated spasm involving the left anterior descending artery, which showed only mild irregularities before exercise. Both patients, however, had rest pain, and one had spontaneous spasm with total occlusion of the left anterior descending artery during such an episode. Neither the electrocardiographic findings nor coronary angiographic findings during spontaneous pain were described in the second patient. Thus, it is not totally clear whether or not some or all the aforementioned patients would be considered by others to have variant angina.

These findings prompted a series of studies in our laboratory to further define the possible role of coronary artery spasm in stress-induced angina.[5] These studies were divided into three phases. In the initial phase we examined coronary artery responses during angina evoked by pacing-induced tachycardia in patients with classic effort angina. Thirteen men with classic angina were studied. Each had ischemic-type ST segment depression associated with angina during exercise testing on a treadmill. No patient had rest angina or ST segment elevation. Twelve of the thirteen patients had atherosclerotic coronary artery disease defined as one or more areas showing 50 percent or more diameter narrowing. In five patients, coronary artery disease involved three vessels; in three patients, two vessels; and in four others only one vessel was involved. The remaining patient had only lumen outline irregularities, with 20 to 30 percent diameter narrowing involving the left anterior descending and right coronary arteries. All studies were conducted in the morning while these patients took their beta-blocking drugs to enhance the possibility of detecting coronary artery spasm, as suggested by recent reports.[18] Furthermore, no sedation, atropine, or nitrates were used prior to study. A control coronary angiogram was performed and followed by institution of an atrial pacing stress test in which heart rate was increased by increments of 10 beats per minute. At the onset of angina associated with ST segment depression, angiograms of both coronary arteries were repeated. Thirty-nine coronary artery segments and eight narrowed segments were measured, using techniques summarized elsewhere.[21] We found a mean increase in coronary diameter of 7 percent—a change of borderline statistical significance (p equals 0.05). More importantly, no patient had a decrease in coronary artery diameter or stenosis diameter during tachycardia-induced angina. From these initial studies we concluded that there was no evidence to suggest coronary artery spasm in the genesis of angina evoked by tachycardia stress in patients with effort angina. Furthermore, the increased oxygen demands accompanying increasing tachycardia may be associated with a small increase in size of the large epicardial coronary arteries. Moreover, this increase in size was detectable in individuals who were all taking beta-adrenergic blocking drugs at the time of the study. These findings are consistent with animal studies relative to the regulation of large coronary artery size by increases in myocardial metabolic demands.[22]

In the next phase of investigation, we examined coronary size before and during exercise-induced angina in seven patients with classic effort angina. Each of these patients was studied in the previously outlined manner, except that supine bicycle exercise replaced pacing as the form of stress. Twenty-five coronary arteries and six coronary narrowings were measured. During exercise-induced angina we observed a 21 percent mean increase in coronary artery diameter (p less than 0.05). Furthermore, in no patient did coronary artery diameter or stenosis diameter decrease during exercise-induced angina. In contrast to findings during pacing-induced tachycardia stress, exercise also increased both left ventricular systolic and end-diastolic pressures. These findings are consistent with the conclusion that the coronary arteries increase in diameter during exercise-induced angina.

In a final investigation, this work was extended to evaluate the possibility that stress (either exercise or tachycardia) evokes increases in coronary resistance that would not necessarily be detectable by coronary angiography. In these studies, nine patients with classic exercise-induced angina were studied during both pacing- and exercise-induced angina. Coronary resistance was calculated from the ratio of aortic pressure to regional coronary venous blood flow measured by thermodilution.[23] In these individuals, both the total and regional coronary flow increased during each form of stress-induced angina. Coronary resistance in regions supplied by stenosed coronary arteries and in regions supplied by nonstenosed coronary arteries declined during stress-induced angina. Small doses (100 μg) of intracoronary nitroglycerin were administered first into the left coronary artery and then into the right coronary artery of each of these individuals as exercise stress continued. This dose of nitroglycerin administered directly into a coronary artery relieves coronary artery spasm and dilates coronary arteries, with only a minimal systemic effect.[24] No patient had relief of stress-induced angina with intracoronary nitroglycerin. When nitroglycerin was infused systemically as exercise continued, angina was relieved only after left ventricular systolic and end-diastolic pressures declined. These observations support the concept that coronary artery spasm does not play an important role in the genesis of stress-induced angina in patients without variant angina.

CONCLUSIONS

From the foregoing reports, it appears that coronary artery spasm plays an infrequent role in the genesis of exercise-induced angina in selected patients. In this regard, the patient almost always has other evidence suggesting spasm (that is, rest angina with ST segment elevation) and is likely to have a widely variable exercise threshold. Although exercise-induced spasm occurs in these patients with variant angina, in our experience the rest angina component of the symptom complex predominates over the effort component. Furthermore, it seems likely that coronary artery spasm does not play an important role in the genesis of exercise-induced angina in most patients with only a classic angina syndrome. Exercise in these individuals appears to increase coronary artery size and to dilate many coronary artery stenoses. It is possible that other vascular factors (e.g., platelet aggregation, prostanoids, microvascular constriction) operate to transiently reduce myocardial oxygen supply in patients with exercise-induced angina.[25]

REFERENCES

1. PEPINE, CJ, and CONTI, CR: *Acute and chronic heart disease—coronary artery spasm: An important pathophysiologic consideration.* In ROSEN, KM (ED): *Current Cardiology,* 2. Houghton Mifflin, Boston, 1980, p 295.
2. CURRY, RC, PEPINE, CJ, SABOM, MB, ET AL: *Effects of ergonovine in patients with and without coronary artery disease.* Circulation 56:803, 1977.
3. YASUE, H, OMOTE, S, TAKIZAWA, A, ET AL: *Exertional angina pectoris caused by coronary arterial spasm: Effects of various drugs.* Am J Cardiol 43:647, 1979.
4. SPECCHIA, G, DE SERVI, S, FALCONE, C, ET AL: *Coronary arterial spasm as a cause of exercise-induced ST-segment elevation in patients with variant angina.* Circulation 59:948, 1979.
5. PEPINE, CJ, FELDMAN, RL, and CONTI, CR: *Observations on the role of coronary artery spasm in stress-induced angina.* Circulation 62(Suppl 2):99, 1980.
6. PRINZMETAL, M, KENNAMER, R, MERLISS, R, ET AL: *Angina pectoris. I. A variant form of angina pectoris.* Am J Med 27:375, 1959.
7. CURRY, RC, PEPINE, CJ, SABOM, MB, ET AL: *Similarities between ergonovine-induced and spontaneous attacks of variant angina.* Circulation 59:307, 1979.
8. FORTUIN, JJ, and FRIESINGER, GC: *Exercise-induced ST-segment elevation.* Am J Med 49:459, 1970.
9. MANVI, KN, and ELLESTAD, MH: *Elevated ST segments with exercise in ventricular aneurysm.* J Electrocardiol 5:317, 1972.

10. ELLESTAD, MH: *Stress Testing.* FA Davis, Philadelphia, 1976, p 120.

11. LAHIRI, A, SUBRAMANIAN, B, MILLAR-CRAIG, M, ET AL: *Exercise-induced S-T segment elevation in variant angina.* Am J Cardiol 45:887, 1980.

12. WATERS, DD, CHAITMAN, BR, DUPRAS, G, ET AL: *Coronary artery spasm during exercise in patients with variant angina.* Circulation 59:580, 1979.

13. CHENG, TO, BASHOUR, T, KELSER, GA, JR, ET AL: *Variant angina of Prinzmetal with normal coronary arteriograms. A variant of the variant.* Circulation 47:476, 1973.

14. WHITING, RB, KLEIN, MD, VANDER VEER, J, ET AL: *Variant angina pectoris.* N Engl J Med 282:709, 1970.

15. MACALPIN, RN, KATTUS, AA, and ALVARO, AB: *Angina pectoris at rest with preservation of exercise capacity: Prinzmetal's variant angina.* Circulation 47:946, 1973.

16. CHAHINE, RA, RAIZNER, AE, and LUCHI, RJ: *Coronary arterial spasm in classic angina pectoris.* Cath Cardiovasc Diag 1:337, 1975.

17. BETRIU, A, SOLIGNAC, A, and BOURASSA, MG: *The variant forms of angina: Diagnostic and therapeutic implications.* Am Heart J 87:272, 1974.

18. YASUE, H, OMOTE, S, TAKIZAWA, A, ET AL: *Circadian variation of exercise capacity in patients with Prinzmetal's variant angina: Role of exercise-induced coronary arterial spasm.* Circulation 59:938, 1979.

19. FREEDMAN, B, DUNN, RF, RICHMOND, D, ET AL: *Coronary artery spasm during exercise treatment with verapamil.* Circulation 64:68, 1981.

20. FULLER, GM, RAIZNER, AE, CHAHINE, RA, ET AL: *Exercise-induced coronary arterial spasm: Angiographic demonstration, documentation of ischemia by myocardial scintigraphy and results of pharmacologic intervention.* Am J Cardiol 46:500, 1980.

21. FELDMAN, RL, PEPINE, CJ, CURRY, RC, ET AL: *Quantification of coronary arteriography using 105 mm photospot angiography and an optical magnifying device.* Cath Cardiovasc Diag 5:195, 1979.

22. MACHO, P, HINTZE, TH, and VATNER, SF: *Regulation of large coronary arteries by increases in myocardial metabolic demands in conscious dogs.* Circ Res 49:594, 1981.

23. PEPINE, CJ, MEHTA, J, WEBSTER, WW, ET AL: *In vivo validation of a thermodilution method to determine regional left ventricular blood flow in patients with coronary disease.* Circulation 58:795, 1978.

24. PEPINE, CJ, FELDMAN, RL, and CONTI, CR: *Action of intracoronary nitroglycerin in refractory coronary artery spasm.* Circulation 66:411, 1982.

25. PEPINE, CJ, AND FELDMAN, RL: *The concept of dynamic coronary blood flow reduction: Spasm, arteriolar constriction, platelet aggregation, prostanoids and other supply side considerations.* Int J Cardiol, March, 1983 (in press).

Value and Limitations of Provocative Testing to Assess the Efficacy of Treatment in Variant Angina

David D. Waters, M.D.

PROBLEMS IN THE ASSESSMENT OF TREATMENT FOR VARIANT ANGINA

In patients with stable effort angina, the efficacy of antianginal drugs can be evaluated and compared with an acceptable degree of precision. Usual features of such studies include randomization, crossover, and double-blinding; a placebo control period is mandatory because placebo improves many cases of stable effort angina. Angina frequency and nitroglycerin consumption may be used as endpoints, but exercise testing provides more objective and discriminative measurements that may also provide an insight into the mechanism of drug action. Because effort angina occurs when coronary blood flow is limited by relatively fixed[1] organic stenoses, exercise tests in the same patient yield reproducible results if other factors are not changed.[2] In most patients, the severity of organic lesions remains stable over the weeks or months of a study. Even in individual patients with effort angina, repeat exercise testing during treatment can be helpful clinically to optimize medical therapy.

In variant angina, many problems complicate the evaluation of antianginal drugs, both in clinical trials and in the treatment of individual patients. The clinical course of variant angina is characterized by frequent spontaneous remissions[3] and exacerbations; because clinical manifestations are episodic, symptoms decrease greatly or disappear within weeks or months in many patients.[4] This feature of the syndrome may explain why an uncontrolled study[5] concluded that propranolol was beneficial in variant angina and two controlled studies[6,7] later demonstrated that propranolol aggravated variant angina.

Myocardial infarction is a frequent complication in the active phase of variant angina,[8,9] and patients with arrhythmias during attacks are at high risk for sudden death.[10] Since uncontrolled studies suggest that calcium channel blockers are highly effective in preventing attacks,[11] placebo administration to patients with active symptoms has been avoided by some investigators for ethical reasons.[11] Others have compared placebo administration with active drug therapy over weeks or months in outpatients with infrequent symptoms; the results of such studies are useful and important but may not be directly applicable to the patient with many attacks per day.

Myocardial ischemia caused by coronary artery spasm may occur silently;[9] therefore, nitroglycerin usage and patient diaries may not accurately reflect the effect of treatment. Holter monitoring partially overcomes this problem by detecting asymptomatic ST segment shifts;[12] but in patients with infrequent attacks, repeated Holter recordings usually do not coincide with symptoms and thus do not provide objective corroboration. Patients with variant angina and organic stenoses may also experience effort angina not due to coronary spasm; studies of drug efficacy in these patients measure total angina episodes and do not distinguish between these two mechanisms.

In spite of these limitations, several carefully designed, placebo-controlled, crossover studies have clearly demonstrated that calcium channel blockers[12-16] and long-acting nitrates[17,18] effectively prevent spontaneous attacks of variant angina. Studies comparing one drug to another have not shown important differences.[19-21]

Because of the aforementioned limitations, the efficacy of treatment in variant angina has been assessed by other methods. Although the cause of spontaneous episodes of coronary artery spasm is not known, attacks can be induced by ergonovine,[22] exercise,[23] cold,[24] and hyperventilation.[25] Spontaneous and induced attacks share similar clinical, electrocardiographic, hemodynamic, and angiographic characteristics.[26] For this reason, a drug that blocks provoked attacks might also effectively block spontaneous attacks. Provocative testing has been used to assess treatment for variant angina in several studies, and these investigations will be reviewed in the remainder of this chapter.

COMPARISON OF PROVOCATIVE TESTS

The ideal provocative test to assess treatment should be safe, reproducible, easy to perform, easily repeated, have an endpoint that can be quantitated, and be sensitive and specific for coronary artery spasm or variant angina. No single test fulfills all these criteria or is as good as exercise testing is for stable effort angina. The provocation of coronary artery spasm with severe transmural ischemia is unlikely to ever be completely free of complications, no matter what provocative maneuver is employed. Deaths have been reported with ergonovine testing,[27] and myocardial infarction has been encountered after a cold pressor test.[28] The risk of complications can be greatly reduced with appropriate precautions.[22,27,29]

The sensitivity of provocative tests in variant angina depends upon the degree of disease activity.[3,23] In a group of 34 patients with active variant angina, all of whom had the three tests, the sensitivity was 94 percent for ergonovine, 29 percent for exercise, and 9 percent for the cold pressor test, using ST segment elevation as the criterion for positivity.[30] Sensitivity decreases with less frequent symptoms. In our experience, the cold pressor test is not useful in the evaluation of treatment because the control test before therapy is almost always negative. An exception is illustrated in Figure 1. In this patient, the cold pressor test induced angina with ST segment elevation in leads AVL and V_1 through V_4, but this response was blocked with diltiazem. The number of spontaneous attacks also decreased during treatment with diltiazem.

Provocative tests in variant angina may not be reproducible owing to cyclic changes in disease activity. Spontaneous episodes of variant angina exhibit circadian variation. Similarly, Yasue and coworkers demonstrated that exercise provoked ST segment elevation in 13 of 13 cases in the early morning but in only 2 of the 13 in the afternoon.[31] In addition, De Servi and associates described a widely variable threshold for effort angina in some patients with variant angina.[32] Many patients with a positive ergonovine test during the active phase of variant angina will become asymptomatic later off treatment, and their ergonovine test reverts to negative.[3] When ergonovine testing is performed in the coronary care unit using incremental doses,[29] the results correlate roughly with the degree of clinical activity, as illustrated in Figure 2.[33,34] The test is positive at low ergonovine doses in patients with frequent spontaneous attacks, whereas negative tests or tests positive at high dose levels occur in angina-free patients. As illustrated in Figure 3, the results of the ergonovine test are fairly reproducible if the tests are done within a short time interval and the degree of disease activity does not change. When a positive test becomes negative with treatment, a corresponding improvement in symptoms can be expected. The change in both the test and the symptoms may have been caused either by treatment or by a coincidental spontaneous decrease in disease activity.

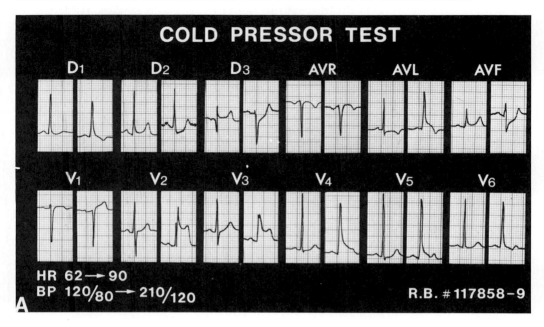

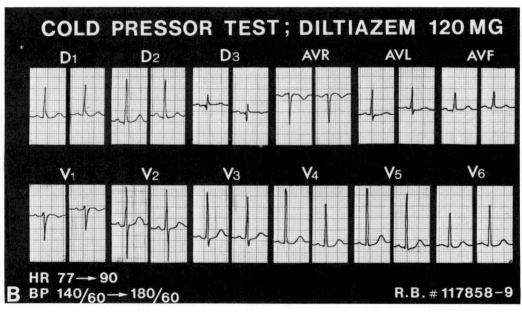

Figure 1. *A,* Results of the cold pressor test from a 56-year-old man with active variant angina and a 70 percent stenosis of the left anterior descending artery. ST segment elevation occurred in leads AVL and V₁ through V₄ both during spontaneous episodes and during the cold pressor test. Angina and ST segment elevation disappeared within 2 minutes of nitroglycerin administration. *B,* When repeated during treatment with diltiazem 120 mg three times daily, the cold pressor test induced neither angina nor electrocardiographic changes. Diltiazem only partially prevented the increase in heart rate and blood pressure caused by the test.

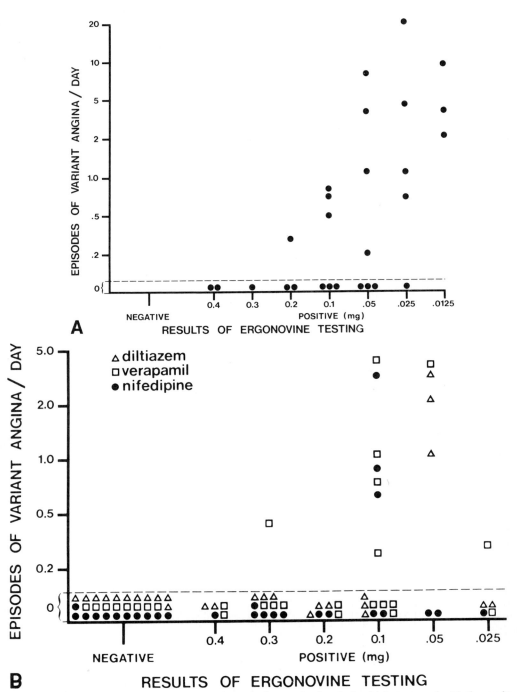

Figure 2. *A,* The average number of variant angina episodes per day (vertical axis) is compared with the results of the ergonovine test (horizontal axis) for 27 hospitalized patients with active variant angina during a control period before treatment. *B,* A similar comparison for each of three treatment periods in the same 27 variant angina patients. The ergonovine test is positive at low doses in periods containing frequent spontaneous attacks. Negative tests occur only in asymptomatic periods. Tests positive at high doses, 0.2 to 0.4 mg, occur most often in periods with no spontaneous attacks. Thus, the results of the ergonovine test before and during treatment correlate roughly with the degree of spontaneous clinical activity. (From Waters et al,[34] with permission.)

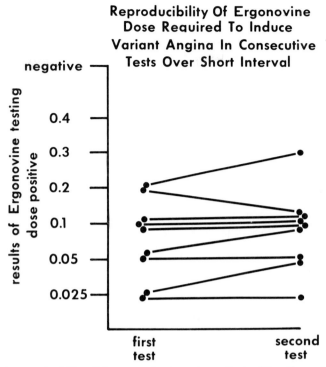

Figure 3. To assess the reproducibility of the ergonovine test, nine patients with active variant angina underwent two tests within a 1-week period. All patients were untreated, and the tests were performed at the same time of day. No important change in symptoms occurred between the tests. In five patients, the two tests were positive with angina and ST segment elevation at the same ergonovine dose level; in the other four, the second test was positive at the adjacent dose. (From Waters et al,[34] with permission.)

Ergonovine Testing

Ergonovine testing has been used extensively to assess the effect of treatment in patients with variant angina and coronary artery spasm.[33-40] Théroux and coworkers[33] studied 10 hospitalized patients with variant angina during a control period and during successive periods of treatment with nifedipine and perhexiline maleate. All 10 patients had a positive ergonovine test during the control period, but in 9 of the 10 the test was negative during nifedipine treatment. During the perhexiline treatment period, two tests were negative, six tests remained positive, and two were not repeated. The clinical response was similar: 3.9 ± 4.7 episodes of variant angina per patient per day occurred during the control period, 0.09 ± 0.15 during nifedipine treatment (p less than 0.02 vs control), and 2.3 ± 3.2 during the perhexiline period (p less than 0.05 vs nifedipine but not significantly different from control). Among the 12 ergonovine tests that were positive at 0.1 mg or less, 11 occurred during periods with more than one episode per day, whereas all 16 negative tests or tests positive only at 0.2 mg or more occurred during periods with less than one episode per day of variant angina. This study concluded not only that nifedipine was highly effective for variant angina but also that the results of ergonovine testing during treatment correlated with the short-term clinical response to therapy.

The same investigators compared the efficacy of nifedipine, diltiazem, and verapamil in 27 hospitalized patients with variant angina using a similar study design.[34] The ergonovine test during the control period before treatment provoked ST segment elevation in all 27 cases. All patients completed three short treatment periods, with nifedipine, diltiazem, and verapamil administered in a variable order. The ergonovine test was negative for 11 patients treated with nifedipine, for 11 with diltiazem, and for 8 with verapamil. The test result improved by two or more ergonovine dose levels for 11 patients, each treated with nifedipine and diltiazem, and for 10 with verapamil. The test was unimproved during nifedipine treatment in five patients, during diltiazem treatment in five, and during verapamil treatment in nine. As in the previous study, the ergonovine test results correlated with the clinical response during control and treatment periods, as illustrated in Figure 2. The electrocardiograms from the ergonovine tests of a typical patient in this study are shown in Figure 4. In 12 of the 27 patients, the three drugs produced dissimilar effects upon the ergonovine test. One patient had an unimproved test with all three drugs; five patients had two drugs and 12 patients had at least one drug that did not improve their ergonovine test result by two or more dose levels compared with the control test. Diltiazem and nifedipine were the best drugs in five patients each, and verapamil was superior in two cases. These findings suggest that it may be reasonable to try another calcium antagonist drug in the patient whose symptoms persist during treatment with the drug chosen initially. During the 7-month followup period of this study, 14 of 15 patients treated with a drug that had converted the ergonovine test response to negative remained angina-free, compared with only 4 of 12 treated with a drug associated with a persistently positive test (p less than 0.01). The initial clinical response to treatment was

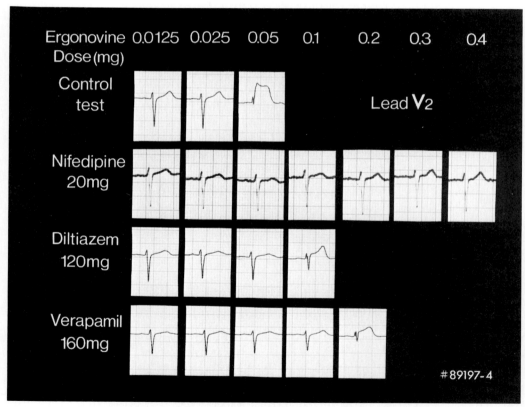

Figure 4. Results of ergonovine tests during control and treatment periods for a typical patient with variant angina. All tracings are from lead V_2. Angina and ST segment elevation developed during the control ergonovine test at a dose of 0.05 mg. No angina or ST segment abnormalities occurred when the test was repeated during the nifedipine treatment period. Angina and ST segment elevation appeared at the 0.1 mg dose when the test was repeated during treatment with diltiazem and at the 0.2 mg dose during treatment with verapamil. (From Waters et al,[34] with permission.)

not as good as the ergonovine test in predicting the result of treatment during the followup period.

Using a similar study design, Bory and colleagues[35] studied 20 patients with coronary artery spasm during coronary angiography but without organic lesions greater than 50 percent; 12 had ST segment elevation, 5 had ST segment depression, and 3 had T wave changes during spasm. Spasm was spontaneous in 1 case and provoked by ergonovine in the other 19. When the ergonovine test was repeated in the coronary unit using electrocardiographic endpoints, 3 of 14 patients had negative tests during placebo treatment, 4 of 15 had negative tests during propranolol treatment, 12 of 18 had negative tests during verapamil treatment, and 12 of 19 had negative tests during diltiazem treatment. Propranolol was not significantly better than placebo. Both calcium channel blockers were superior to placebo and propranolol, with little difference between them.

Bertrand and coworkers[36] used ergonovine testing as part of the assessment of 13 patients with variant angina treated with nifedipine. All 13 had angiographically normal coronary arteries or minimal lesions, and all exhibited coronary artery spasm after ergonovine administration. Complete suppression of anginal attacks was achieved in 11 of the 13 cases, and 12 of the 13 had no ischemic attacks during 24-hour Holter monitoring. One patient had persistent angina, ST segment elevation during the Holter recording, and a persistently positive ergonovine test. The ergonovine test was negative in the other 12 patients. These results confirm that nifedipine can block ergonovine-induced episodes of variant angina and that the results of the ergonovine test during treatment correlate with the clinical response.

Rutitzky and associates[37] treated three patients with vasospastic angina with the coronary vasodilator amiodarone and performed ergonovine tests before and during treatment. Clinical improvement was noted in each case, and the dose of ergonovine required to induce an attack increased concomitantly.

Tiefenbrunn and colleagues[39] performed coronary arteriography during ergonovine testing before and after the sublingual administration of 20 mg of nifedipine in four patients with vasospastic angina. Before nifedipine, ergonovine provoked coronary artery spasm in all four cases with angina and electrocardiographic changes in three. After nifedipine, no chest pain, electrocardiographic changes, or coronary artery spasm occurred following ergonovine administration.

No complications caused by ergonovine testing were reported in any of these studies. In spite of differences in methodology, the results of these studies are generally in agreement.

The Hyperventilation Test

Girotti and coworkers[41] have used the hyperventilation test extensively to assess therapy in patients with variant angina. Unlike Yasue and coworkers,[25] who administered Tris buffer intravenously during hyperventilation to augment systemic alkalosis, the former group used hyperventilation alone and demonstrated that a positive response often follows peak alkalosis by several minutes. In their experience the test had a sensitivity of 70 percent in patients with active variant angina but was less likely to be positive if performed during coronary arteriography.

The hyperventilation test was repeated during treatment with a variety of drugs. In only one of seven cases did the test become negative during treatment with phentolamine, but isosorbide dinitrate effectively blocked attacks induced by hyperventilation in each of the six cases where it was assessed. In six of eight patients treated with propranolol, the test remained positive; in four of these six, propranolol increased the frequency of spontaneous attacks or increased the positive response to hyperventilation or both. Amiodarone converted the test to negative in four of eight patients. Calcium channel blockers were more effective: Four of five patients treated with verapamil and eight of ten treated with nifedipine had negative hyperventilation tests during treatment. Seventeen of eighteen negative tests performed under the influence of a long-acting drug coincided with a total remission of angina episodes when the drug was continued on a short- or long-term basis. In contrast, angina persisted in 13 of the 17 treatment periods associated with a positive test. This correlation with the clinical response to treatment is similar to that discussed previously for ergonovine testing. The 10 study patients were treated with a drug that had blocked attacks provoked by hyperventilation, and none died or developed myocardial infarction during a followup of nearly one year.

Weber and associates[42] have used alkalosis produced by Tris buffer infusion and hyperventilation as a diagnostic test for coronary artery spasm. The test induced ST segment elevation in 10 patients and ST segment depression in 14. At coronary arteriography, 21 of these 24 patients had organic stenoses of 70 percent or more; the other three developed coronary artery spasm after ergonovine administration. Coronary artery spasm was not proven to be the cause of myocardial ischemia for all patients in this study. The alkalosis test was repeated during treatment with nifedipine in 16 of these patients, and in each instance the second test was negative. Thus, nifedipine appears capable of blocking attacks provoked by alkalosis or hyperventilation as well as those provoked by ergonovine.

Exercise Testing

ST segment elevation during an exercise test is most often associated with a previous myocardial infarction.[43] As shown by Specchia and coworkers,[44] coronary artery spasm is the likely cause of exercise-induced ST segment elevation in patients without previous infarction. Overall, ST segment elevation occurs during exercise in 30 percent of variant angina patients, but this incidence varies depending upon the degree of disease activity in the patients studied.[23] Coronary artery spasm has been directly observed during exercise in a few patients;[45,46] spasm not severe enough to cause ST segment elevation can cause ST segment depression during exercise.[47]

The variability of exercise-induced coronary artery spasm or ST segment elevation should be considered in studies examining the influence of drugs upon this phenomenon. Exercise-induced ST segment elevation exhibits circadian variation,[31] a variable threshold,[32] and disappears entirely during spontaneous remissions of variant angina.[23]

Yasue and coworkers have reported the largest series of patients with variant angina and exercise-induced ST segment elevation retested after administration of various drugs.[48] Their results are summarized in Table 1. In 30 patients retested during propranolol therapy, exercise-induced ST segment elevation was worsened compared with the control test in 13, was unchanged in 11, and was improved in 6. In no instance did propranolol completely suppress exercise-induced ST segment elevation. The results with phentolamine were somewhat better. This drug eliminated exercise-induced attacks in 10 cases, improved the test in 9, produced no change in 3, and worsened in 2. The best results were obtained with calcium channel blockers. Nifedipine completely suppressed attacks in 16 cases and improved the result in the other 3. Diltiazem eliminated the attacks in 22 patients, and the other 8 had an improved result.

Table 1. Effect of drugs upon variant angina attacks provoked by exercise

	Propranolol N = 30	Phentolamine N = 24	Diltiazem N = 30	Nifedipine N = 19
Attack eliminated	0	10	22	16
Improvement	6	9	8	3
No change	11	3	0	0
Worsening	13	2	0	0

Adapted from Yasue et al.[48]

Other studies of smaller numbers of patients generally support these findings. Waters and associates[23] retested 12 patients with variant angina during treatment with nifedipine, diltiazem, or a combination of both drugs. Eight of the twelve had no ST segment abnormality during the second test, despite equivalent or longer treadmill times in all eight and higher pressure-rate products in five. Two of the patients with ST segment elevation during their first test developed ST segment depression during the repeat test on treatment; in both, the ST segment depression could be attributed to organic stenoses greater than 70 percent. The remaining two patients had ST segment elevation during the second test in spite of treatment; neither had a critical organic lesion or left ventricular contraction abnormality to explain this finding. Eleven of the twelve patients had no spontaneous variant angina attacks during treatment; the one exception was one of the two patients whose ST segment elevation recurred during the repeat test.

Freedman and colleagues[49] retested six patients with variant angina and exercise-induced ST segment elevation during treatment with verapamil. Each patient reached a higher workload and had no ischemia during the verapamil test. In two patients who underwent multiple tests, plasma verapamil concentration correlated roughly with the presence and severity of ST segment elevation during exercise. In contrast to these findings, Fuller and coworkers[50] described two patients with exercise-induced coronary artery spasm that could be prevented by nitrates but not by verapamil.

Miwa and associates[51] have demonstrated that large doses of aspirin may increase the frequency of variant angina attacks. As part of their patient assessment, exercise tests were done in the morning and afternoon before and after aspirin administration. In some patients, exercise provoked attacks after aspirin, but not before, corresponding to the observed increase in spontaneous attacks.

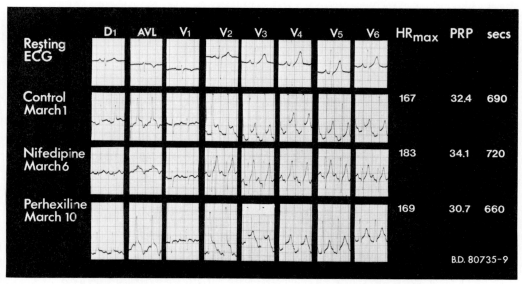

Figure 5. Exercise tests from a 32-year-old man with active variant angina. During spontaneous attacks ST segment elevation appeared in leads D_1, AVL, and V_2 through V_6. Spontaneous spasm developed during arteriography at the site of a 40 percent left anterior descending artery stenosis. No other coronary lesions were present; left ventriculography was normal. The ST segments are normal in the resting tracing *(top line)*. Angina and ST segment elevation developed at a heart rate of 167 during the control exercise test off medication. During treatment with nifedipine, ST segment elevation recurs with exercise but to a lesser degree and at higher heart rate, pressure-rate product, and treadmill time. Perhexiline maleate, a weak and ineffective calcium channel blocker, does not affect exercise-induced angina and ST segment elevation *(bottom line)*.

Figure 5 illustrates the exercise tests from a 32-year-old diabetic with active variant angina. Spontaneous spasm had developed at the site of a 40 percent stenosis in the proximal left anterior descending coronary artery during arteriography. No other coronary lesions were present, and left ventriculography was normal. During spontaneous and exercise-induced attacks, ST segment elevation was recorded in leads D_1, AVL, and V_2 through V_6. Nifedipine decreased the frequency of spontaneous attacks and improved the exercise test result, but did not completely block exercise-induced ST segment elevation. Perhexiline maleate was ineffective.

CLINICAL IMPLICATIONS

Should all patients with variant angina undergo a provocative test at the start of treatment to assess its effect? None of the studies cited in this chapter recommends such a plan of management. Provocative testing is unnecessary for diagnostic purposes in patients with documented attacks of spontaneous ST segment elevation that is rapidly relieved by nitroglycerin without evidence of myocardial necrosis. Such patients require coronary arteriography because some will have multiple, critical organic stenoses for which bypass surgery is probably indicated. A good response to treatment with a calcium channel blocker can be expected in most of the remainder of these patients.[11] If rest angina persists, a long-acting nitrate or another calcium channel blocker should be added, or the original calcium channel blocker should be changed. In our experience, provocative testing is clinically useful to assess the effect of treatment in patients who are refractory to more than one drug or in patients with atypical symptoms where the response to treatment cannot otherwise be accurately evaluated. Provocative testing may also be useful to decide when treatment can be safely discontinued.[3] Further studies are required to define the role of provocative testing in these circumstances. When the pathophysiology of this syndrome is better understood, a less cumbersome procedure, perhaps a simple blood test, might replace provocative testing as a method of assessing disease activity.

CONCLUSIONS

Provocative testing is a useful research tool to assess the effect of treatment in variant angina. Usually, provoked and spontaneous attacks are affected similarly by a drug, both in general and in a specific patient. Thus, if spontaneous attacks persist during treatment, a provocative test is likely to remain positive; and if treatment eliminates all spontaneous attacks, provoked attacks are likely to be suppressed as well. Exceptions occur when the provocative stimulus is either very weak or very strong; for example, the cold pressor test is a weak stimulus and may revert to negative with a level of treatment that does not eliminate spontaneous attacks. On the other hand, large doses of ergonovine may sometimes provoke attacks in treated, asymptomatic patients.

The results of studies using ergonovine, hyperventilation-alkalosis, and exercise are generally consistent. Propranolol either has no effect or aggravates provoked attacks, and calcium channel blockers either partially or completely block attacks in nearly all cases. Prognosis during treatment is probably better for patients in whom treatment suppresses provoked attacks.

REFERENCES

1. BROWN, BG, BOLSON, E, PETERSEN, RB, ET AL: *The mechanism of nitroglycerin action: Stenosis vasodilatation as a major component of the drug response.* Circulation 64:1089, 1981.
2. REDWOOD, DR, ROSING, DR, GOLDSTEIN, RE, ET AL: *Importance of the design of an exercise protocol in the evaluation of patients with angina pectoris.* Circulation 43:618, 1971.

3. WATERS, DD, SZLACHCIC, J, THÉROUX, P, ET AL: *Ergonovine testing to detect spontaneous remissions of variant angina during long-term treatment with calcium antagonist drugs.* Am J Cardiol 47:179, 1981.

4. PRINZMETAL, M, KENNAMER, R, MERLISS, R, ET AL: *Angina pectoris. I. A variant form of angina pectoris. Preliminary report.* Am J Med 27:375, 1959.

5. GUAZZI, M, MAGRINI, F, FIORENTINI, C, ET AL: *Clinical, electrocardiographic, and haemodynamic effects of long-term use of propranolol in Prinzmetal's variant angina pectoris.* Br Heart J 33:889, 1971.

6. ROBERTSON, RM, WOOD, AJJ, VAUGHN, WK, ET AL: *Exacerbation of vasotonic angina pectoris by propranolol.* Circulation 65:281, 1982.

7. TILMANT, PY, LABLANCHE, JM, THIEULEUX, FP, ET AL: *Comparison of beta blockers and calcium antagonists in the treatment of patients with coronary artery spasm.* Am J Cardiol 49:976, 1982.

8. WATERS, DD, SZLACHCIC, J, MILLER, D, ET AL: *Clinical characteristics of patients with variant angina complicated by myocardial infarction or death within 1 month.* Am J Cardiol 49:658, 1982.

9. MASERI, A, SEVERI, S, DeNES, M, ET AL: *"Variant" angina: One aspect of a continuous spectrum of vasospastic myocardial ischemia. Pathogenetic mechanisms, estimated incidence and clinical and coronary arteriographic findings in 138 patients.* Am J Cardiol 42:1019, 1978.

10. MILLER, DD, WATERS, DD, SZLACHCIC, J, ET AL: *Clinical characteristics associated with sudden death in patients with variant angina.* Circulation 66:588, 1982.

11. KIMURA, E, and KISHIDA, H: *Treatment of variant angina with drugs: A survey of 11 cardiology institutes in Japan.* Circulation 63:844, 1981.

12. JOHNSON, SM, MAURITSON, DR, WILLERSON, JT, ET AL: *A controlled trial of verapamil for Prinzmetal's variant angina.* N Engl J Med 304:862, 1981.

13. PARODI, O, MASERI, A, and SIMONETTI, I: *Management of unstable angina at rest by verapamil. A double-blind cross-over study in coronary care unit.* Br Heart J 41:167, 1979.

14. PREVITALI, M, SALERNO, JA, TAVAZZI, L, ET AL: *Treatment of angina at rest with nifedipine: A short-term controlled study.* Am J Cardiol 45:825, 1980.

15. ROSENTHAL, SJ, GINSBURG, R, LAMB, IH, ET AL: *Efficacy of diltiazem for control of symptoms of coronary arterial spasm.* Am J Cardiol 46:1027, 1980.

16. PEPINE, CJ, FELDMAN, RL, WHITTLE, J, ET AL: *Effect of diltiazem in patients with variant angina: A randomized double-blind trial.* Am Heart J 101:719, 1981.

17. DISTANTE, A, MASERI, A, SEVERI, S, ET AL: *Management of vasospastic angina at rest with continuous infusion of isosorbide dinitrate. A double cross over study in a coronary care unit.* Am J Cardiol 44:533, 1979.

18. SALERNO, JA, PREVITALI, M, MEDICI, A, ET AL: *Treatment of vasospastic angina pectoris at rest with nitroglycerin ointment: A short-term controlled study in the coronary care unit.* Am J Cardiol 47:1128, 1981.

19. JOHNSON, SM, MAURITSON, DR, WILLERSON, JT, ET AL: *Comparison of verapamil and nifedipine in the treatment of variant angina pectoris: Preliminary observations in 10 patients.* Am J Cardiol 47:1295, 1981.

20. HILL, JA, FELDMAN, RL, PEPINE, CJ, ET AL: *Randomized double-blind comparison of nifedipine and isosorbide dinitrate in patients with coronary arterial spasm.* Am J Cardiol 49:431, 1982.

21. GINSBURG, R, LAMB, IH, SCHROEDER, JS, ET AL: *Randomized double-blind comparison of nifedipine and isosorbide dinitrate therapy in variant angina pectoris due to coronary artery spasm.* Am Heart J 103:44, 1982.

22. HEUPLER, FA, JR: *Provocative testing for coronary arterial spasm: Risk, method and rationale.* Am J Cardiol 46:335, 1980.

23. WATERS, DD, SZLACHCIC, J, BOURASSA, MG, ET AL: *Exercise testing in patients with variant angina: Results, correlation with clinical and angiographic features and prognostic significance.* Circulation 65:265, 1982.

24. RAIZNER, RE, CHAHINE, RA, ISHIMORI, T, ET AL: *Provocation of coronary artery spasm by the cold pressor test. Hemodynamic, arteriographic and quantitative angiographic observations.* Circulation 62:925, 1980.

25. YASUE, H, NAGAO, M, OMOTE, S, ET AL: *Coronary arterial spasm and Prinzmetal's variant form of angina induced by hyperventilation and Tris buffer infusion.* Circulation 58:56, 1978.

26. CURRY, RC, JR, PEPINE, CJ, SABOM. MB, ET AL: *Similarities of ergonovine-induced and spontaneous attacks of variant angina.* Circulation 59:307, 1979.

27. BUXTON, A, GOLDBERG, S, HIRSHFELD, JW, ET AL: *Refractory ergonovine-induced coronary vasospasm: Importance of intracoronary nitroglycerin.* Am J Cardiol 46:329, 1980.

28. SHEA, DJ, OCKENE, IS, and GREENE, HL: *Acute myocardial infarction provoked by a cold pressor test.* Chest 80:649, 1981.

29. WATERS, DD, THÉROUX, P, SZLACHCIC, J, ET AL: *Ergonovine testing in a coronary care unit.* Am J Cardiol 46:922, 1980.

30. WATERS, DD, SZLACHCIC, J, BONAN, R, ET AL: *Comparative sensitivity of exercise, cold pressor and ergonovine testing in provoking attacks of variant angina in patients with active disease.* Circulation (in press).

31. YASUE, H, OMOTE, S, TAKIZAWA, A, ET AL: *Circadian variation of exercise capacity in patients with Prinzmetal's variant angina: Role of exercise-induced coronary arterial spasm.* Circulation 59:938, 1979.

32. DE SERVI, S, SPECCHIA, G, CURTI, MT, ET AL: *Variable threshold of angina during exercise: A clinical manifestation of some patients with vasospastic angina.* Am J Cardiol 48:188, 1981.

33. THÉROUX, P, WATERS, DD, AFFAKI, GS, ET AL: *Provocative testing with ergonovine to evaluate the efficacy of treatment with calcium antagonists in variant angina.* Circulation 60:504, 1979.

34. WATERS, DD, THÉROUX, P, SZLACHCIC, J, ET AL: *Provocative testing with ergonovine to assess the efficacy of treatment with nifedipine, diltiazem and verapamil in variant angina.* Am J Cardiol 48:123, 1981.

35. BORY, M, FRANCK, R, BÉNICHOU, M, ET AL: *Le test à l'ergométrine dans l'évaluation des thérapeutiques de l'angor spastique.* Arch Mal Coeur 74:901, 1981.

36. BERTRAND, ME, LABLANCHE, JM, and TILMANT, PY: *Treatment of Prinzmetal's variant angina. Role of medical treatment with nifedipine and surgical coronary revascularization combined with plexectomy.* Am J Cardiol 47:174, 1981.

37. RUTITZKY, B, GIROTTI, AL, and ROSENBAUM, MB: *Efficacy of chronic amiodarone therapy in patients with variant angina pectoris and inhibition of ergonovine coronary constriction.* Am Heart J 103:38, 1982.

38. RICH, S, FORD, LE, and AL-SADIR, J: *The angiographic effect of ergonovine and nifedipine in coronary artery spasm.* Circulation 62:1127, 1980.

39. TIEFENBRUNN, AJ, SOBEL, BE, GOWDA, S, ET AL: *Nifedipine blockade of ergonovine-induced coronary arterial spasm: Angiographic documentation.* Am J Cardiol 48:184, 1981.

40. PHANEUF, DC, WATERS, DD, DAUWE, F, ET AL: *Refractory variant angina controlled with combined drug therapy in a patient with a single coronary artery.* Cath Cardiovasc Diag 6:413, 1980.

41. GIROTTI, LA, CROSATTO, JR, MESSUTI, H, ET AL: *The hyperventilation test as a method for developing successful therapy in Prinzmetal's angina.* Am J Cardiol 49:832, 1982.

42. WEBER, S, PASQUIER, G, GUIOMARD, A, ET AL: *Application clinique du test de provocation par l'alcalose du spasme artériel coronaire.* Arch Mal Coeur 74:1389, 1981.

43. WATERS, DD, CHAITMAN, BR, BOURASSA, MG, ET AL: *Clinical and angiographic correlates of exercise-induced ST-segment elevation. Increased detection with multiple ECG leads.* Circulation 61:286, 1980.

44. SPECCHIA, G, DE SERVI, S, FALCONE, C, ET AL: *Significance of exercise-induced ST-segment elevation in patients without myocardial infarction.* Circulation 63:46, 1981.

45. SPECCHIA, G, DE SERVI, S, FALCONE, C, ET AL: *Coronary arterial spasm as a cause of exercise-induced ST-segment elevation in patients with variant angina.* Circulation 59:948, 1979.

46. YASUE, H, OMOTE, S, TAKIZAWA, A, ET AL: *Exertional angina pectoris caused by coronary arterial spasm: Effect of various drugs.* Am J Cardiol 43:647, 1979.

47. YASUE, H, OMOTE, S, TAKIZAWA, A, ET AL: *Comparison of coronary arteriographic findings during angina pectoris associated with S-T elevation or depression.* Am J Cardiol 47:539, 1981.

48. YASUE, H: *Pathophysiology and treatment of coronary arterial spasm.* Chest 78:216, 1980.

49. FREEDMAN, B, DUNN, RF, RICHMOND, DR, ET AL: *Coronary artery spasm during exercise: Treatment with verapamil.* Circulation 64:68, 1981.

50. FULLER, CM, RAIZNER, AE, CHAHINE, RA, ET AL: *Exercise-induced coronary arterial spasm: Angiographic demonstration, documentation of ischemia by myocardial scintigraphy and results of pharmacologic intervention.* Am J Cardiol 46:500, 1980.

51. MIWA, K, KAMBARA, H, and KAWAI, C: *Exercise-induced angina provoked by aspirin administration in patients with variant angina.* Am J Cardiol 47:1210, 1981.

Provocative Testing for Coronary Artery Spasm: Specific Methodology

Sheldon Goldberg, M.D.

Coronary artery spasm is the predominant physiologic mechanism in variant angina[1-3] and may play a role in other acute ischemic syndromes ranging from exertional angina to acute myocardial infarction.[4,5] The current availability of specific, potent therapy for vasospastic angina[6,7] makes the precise diagnosis of coronary vasospasm critical. The diagnostic steps involved in attributing specific ischemic episodes to coronary artery spasm include noninvasive modalities such as ECG monitoring and thallium scintigraphy during episodes of pain.[8,9] However, noninvasive diagnostic techniques may be frustrating in patients with infrequent episodes of pain. Definitive diagnosis of coronary artery spasm may be difficult with electrocardiographic techniques for several reasons. First, the clinical events may be episodic and therefore easily missed by ambulatory or coronary care unit monitoring. Furthermore, pain episodes may be associated with nonspecific ECG changes[10] such as subtle alterations in T waves and ST segment depression rather than the usual finding of ST segment elevation. Though the demonstration of a normal or nearly normal coronary arteriogram in a patient with ischemic pain and recurrent, transient ST segment elevation obviates the clinical need for provocative testing, a substantial number of patients remain with a less clearcut clinical situation in which proper diagnosis is crucial for correct management. Moreover, provocative testing has been shown to be useful in selection of drug therapy in the management of variant angina.[11-13] For these reasons, knowledge of the types of provocative tests available and their relative usefulness is important.

TYPES OF PROVOCATIVE TESTS

Induction of coronary vasospasm has been achieved with many methods. Alpha-adrenergic stimulation by use of the cold pressor test,[6,14] hyperventilation,[15] exercise,[16-20] and ergonovine maleate[21-28] have been employed as methods for stimulating coronary artery spasm in patients with variant angina.

Using the cold pressor test, Raizner and coworkers provoked coronary artery spasm in four of six patients with variant angina.[14] Yasue and associates used hyperventilation plus Tris buffer infusion in nine patients with variant angina and succeeded in provoking coronary spasm in eight.[15] Pco_2 decreased from a mean of 38 torr in the control state to 20 torr during hyperventilation, with a concomitant rise in pH from 7.42 to 7.65. In the eight patients, chest pain was accompanied by ischemic ECG changes (ST segment elevation in seven and ST segment depression in one). In all four patients who underwent selective coronary arteriography during this study, coronary vasospasm appeared with hyperventilation and resolved following the administration of sublingual nitroglycerin. These investigators hypothesized the cause of hyperventilation-induced coronary artery spasm as follows: With a reduction in hydrogen ion content, more calcium ion is left to act unopposed on myofibrillar ATPase; as a result, vascular smooth muscle contraction ensues. These investigators further postulated that production of hydrogen ions decreases at rest, thus providing the clinical explanation for nocturnal attacks in Prinzmetal's angina. The use of the exercise test in the detection of coronary artery spasm is of particular interest. Yasue and associates performed treadmill testing in 13 patients with variant angina.[16] The tests were carried out early in the morning and in the afternoon of the same day. In that small series, attacks with ST segment elevation were induced in all 13 patients in the morning, but in only 2 patients undergoing afternoon exercise. In all four patients who underwent coronary angiography and arm exercise, coronary artery spasm occurred in association with the ST segment elevation. The authors concluded that there was a circadian variation of exercise capacity in variant angina. They suggested that a daily variation in hydrogen ion concentration might be responsible for their findings.

The use of the ergonovine maleate test for provoking coronary artery spasm has received particular attention. As a provocative test, it is sensitive and specific for coronary spasm,[10,21-28] producing pain, ST segment changes, and angiographically demonstrable spasm in more than 90 percent of patients with variant angina. Recently, Waters and colleagues compared the sensitivity of exercise, cold pressor, and ergonovine testing in provoking attacks of variant angina in patients with active disease.[10] The sensitivity of these three tests was compared in the same population of 34 hospitalized patients with documented variant angina who had recently undergone coronary arteriography. The three tests were performed on three consecutive days. Angina was provoked by ergonovine in all 34 cases, by exercise in 17, and by the cold pressor test in only 5. ST segment elevation developed during the ergonovine test in 32 (94 percent), during exercise in 10 (29 percent), and during the cold pressor test in only 3 (9 percent). Therefore, the sensitivity of the ergonovine test is very high in comparison with the other tests.

For clinical purposes, it would seem that the ergonovine maleate test is the most useful diagnostic test for coronary artery spasm. The vasospasm induced by ergonovine has usually been readily reversible by sublingual or intravenous nitroglycerin, and the test has been performed successfully outside the cardiac catheterization laboratory with only clinical and electrocardiographic monitoring available. If vasospasm were predictably reversible in every instance, the ergonovine maleate test could be safely performed in the noninvasive laboratory or coronary care unit setting. In early reports describing experience with ergonovine provocation, there were no serious complications. These studies all noted relief of myocardial ischemia due to coronary artery spasm within 5 to 10 minutes of administration of nitroglycerin, and one review of coronary artery spasm stated that "ergonovine induced coronary vasospasm is quickly relieved by nitroglycerin."[29] On the basis of such studies, it was proposed that provocative testing with ergonovine be done in the coronary care unit rather than in the cardiac catheterization laboratory because of the added risk of catheterization, the possible difficulties of interpreting coronary angiograms due to catheter-induced spasm, and the masking of coronary spasm due to the vasodilating effect of angiographic dye.[30,31] However, recent reports have indicated that the ergonovine test is not benign and may cause severe coronary vasospasm that is unresponsive to sublingual and intravenous nitroglycerin, though it may be reversed by *intracoronary* nitroglycerin.[32] The following illustrative examples underscore the importance of performing provocative testing in the cardiac catheterization laboratory. Cases A through C are taken from our original report.[32]

Patient A

A 58-year-old man was admitted to the hospital for evaluation of exertional and resting angina pectoris of 1½ years' duration. Therapy with nitroglycerin and propranolol was unsuccessful, and frequent episodes of chest pain continued. The physical examination and electrocardiogram at rest were normal. At cardiac catheterization, the left ventricular end-diastolic pressure was 20 mm Hg. The left ventriculogram was normal, with an ejection fraction of 71 percent. Coronary arteriography revealed a mixed dominant system with luminal irregularities of both coronary arteries but no obstructing lesions (Fig. 1A).

Ergonovine maleate was then infused intravenously in three sequential doses of 0.05, 0.10, and 0.15 mg at 3-minute intervals for a total dose of 0.3 mg. After the third dose the patient noted chest pain, and ST segment elevation in leads V_1 to V_6 occurred. Left coronary arteriography after administration of ergonovine revealed spasm with obliteration of the entire left coronary system (Fig. 1B). Three doses of 0.3 mg nitroglycerin were administered sublingually, but progressive hypotension and electromechanical dissociation occurred. Attempts at resuscitation were unsuccessful, and the patient died.

COMMENT. This case demonstrates the progressive hemodynamic deterioration caused by refractory coronary vasospasm, in this instance causing death. When hemodynamic collapse occurs, administration of sublingual nitroglycerin has no significant effect, because inadequate circulation precludes delivery of enough nitroglycerin to the target site, that is, the coronary smooth musculature.

The next illustrative example demonstrates that even severe refractory spasm of both coronary arteries can be effectively reversed by intracoronary nitroglycerin.

Patient B

A 36-year-old woman was well until two months before hospital admission, when severe anginal pain awakened her from sleep. Serial electrocardiograms and serum enzyme determinations were compatible with a nontransmural myocardial infarction. Treatment with nitroglycerin ointment was instituted, and because nocturnal angina continued she was readmitted two months later for cardiac catheterization. Physical examination was normal, as was a resting electrocardiogram, with the exception of a prolonged Q-T interval. Cardiac catheterization revealed a left ventricular end-diastolic pressure of 15 mm Hg, but otherwise normal hemodynamic status. A left ventriculogram was normal, with an ejection fraction of 59 percent. Coronary arteriography performed using the Judkins technique showed minor irregularities of the left anterior descending artery and the mid right coronary artery. The patient was then given two doses of ergonovine maleate, 0.05 mg each, intravenously, 3 minutes apart. Three minutes after the second dose the patient experienced severe chest pain accompanied by 4 mm ST segment elevation in lead V_1. A repeat left coronary arteriogram demonstrated a 99 percent occlusion of the left anterior descending coronary artery that subsided within 4 minutes after administration of three sublingual nitroglycerin tablets, 0.4 mg each.

Two days later the patient returned to the cardiac catheterization laboratory for evaluation of nifedipine therapy. After baseline measurements, the patient was given 20 mg of nifedipine buccally. Twenty-five minutes later, two 0.05 mg doses of ergonovine maleate were given intravenously in the same manner as two days earlier. Within two minutes the patient complained of substernal discomfort, and minor ST segment elevation was noted in lead V_1. Coronary arteriography now demonstrated diffuse spasm of the left coronary artery. Nitroglycerin (0.4 mg) was given sublingually and the dose repeated twice, but the chest pain persisted, ST segment elevation in lead V_1 increased, ST segment elevation in lead II was noted, and systemic hypotension developed. An intravenous nitroglycerin infusion (300 μg per minute) was immediately begun, but the systemic blood pressure rapidly decreased to 60 mm Hg. Complete atrioventricular block and electromechanical dissociation developed (Fig. 2A), and the patient had a cardiopulmonary arrest. Cardiopulmonary resuscitation was initiated, and a mixture of Renografin-76 and nitroglycerin, 300 μg, was injected twice directly into the left coronary artery. Repeat left coronary arteriography revealed resolution of coronary vasospasm, but asystole persisted. Right coronary arteriography revealed severe, diffuse vasospasm. A mixture of Renografin-76 and nitroglycerin, 300 μg, was then injected into the right

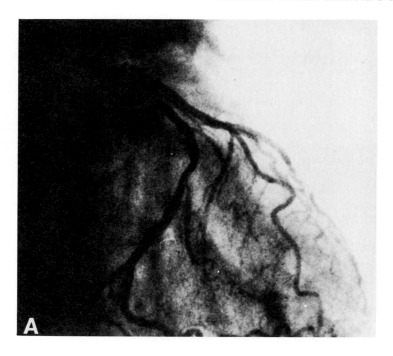

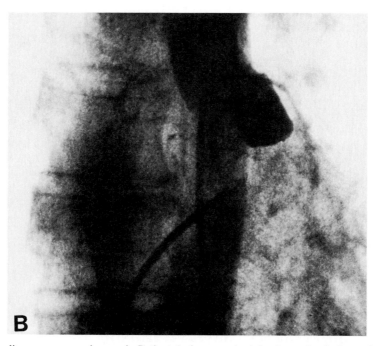

Figure 1. *A*, Baseline coronary angiogram in Patient A shows a mixed dominant circulation and no obstructing lesions. *B*, Following ergonovine administration, there is obliteration of the entire left coronary system. (From Am J Cardiol 46:329, 1980, with permission.)

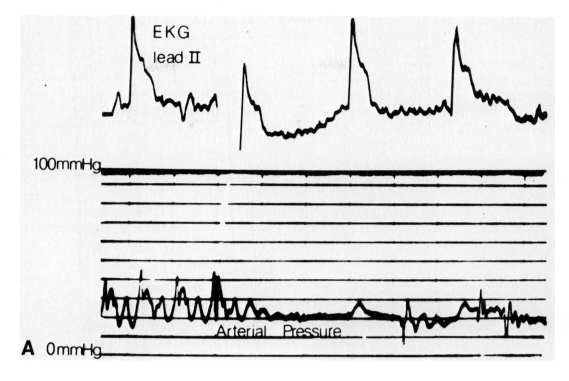

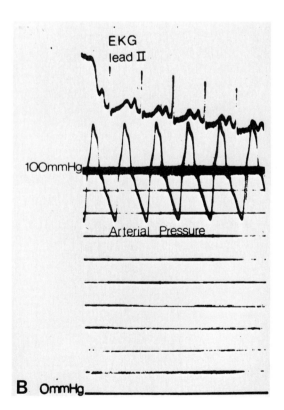

Figure 2. *A*, Electrocardiogram and pressure tracing taken during cardiovascular collapse following ergonovine administration in Patient B. *B*, Electrocardiogram and arterial pressure tracing taken following reversal of spasm with intracoronary nitroglycerin. (From Am J Cardiol 46:329, 1980, with permission.)

coronary artery, and subsequent injections revealed relief of the vasospasm. The ST segment elevation gradually resolved, and systemic arterial pressure increased. During resolution of vasospasm, the patient had three episodes of ventricular tachycardia that responded to electric cardioversion. Approximately 1½ hours after the initial cardiac arrest the patient regained sinus rhythm and normal blood pressure (120/80 mm Hg) (Fig. 2B). A postarrest electrocardiogram showed T wave inversions in leads V_1–V_6. Subsequent recovery was uneventful. The patient remained asymptomatic and well on nitrate therapy 12 months after this event.

Patient C

A 48-year-old woman was admitted for evaluation of variant angina. The baseline right coronary angiogram was normal (Fig. 3A). The patient was given three 0.05 mg intravenous bolus injections of ergonovine at 5-minute intervals. Severe angina developed after the last dose, and a second angiogram revealed progressive, severe spasm of the right coronary artery accompanied by ST segment elevation in the inferior leads and hypotension (systolic blood

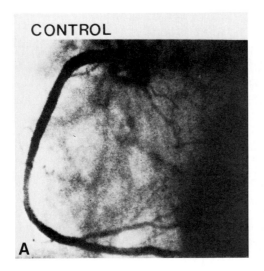

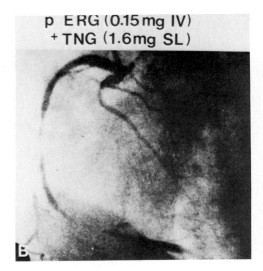

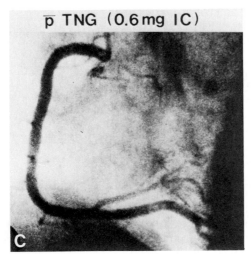

Figure 3. *A,* Baseline right coronary angiogram in Patient C is normal. *B,* After ergonovine, severe spasm of the right coronary artery persists despite 1.6 mg of nitroglycerin administered sublingually. *C,* Right coronary artery spasm is reversed by 0.6 mg of nitroglycerin infused directly into the artery. (From Am J Cardiol 46:329, 1980, with permission.)

pressure 50 mm Hg) followed by complete AV block. Spasm persisted after administration of four 0.4 mg sublingual nitroglycerin tablets (Fig. 3*B*). Therefore, 0.6 mg of nitroglycerin was slowly infused directly into the right coronary artery, resulting in complete resolution of angiographic evidence of spasm and reversal of electrocardiographic changes and hypotension (Fig. 3*C*).

Patient D

A 34-year-old man sustained an acute anteroseptal myocardial infarction. Several days later, he developed recurrent angina associated with ST segment elevation in the inferior leads. He was treated with intravenous nitroglycerin, nitroglycerin ointment, and isosorbide dinitrate, but he continued to have recurrent, severe ischemia. Cardiac catheterization was performed. Ventriculography revealed anterior dyskinesis. Figure 4*A* shows the control ECG, arterial and right ventricular pressure tracings, and the left coronary angiogram (left dominant circulation); the QS pattern in V_1 reflects the recent anteroseptal infarction. The left coronary arteriogram showed total occlusion of the left anterior descending coronary artery and a critical narrowing of the dominant circumflex vessel. With a right ventricular Zucker pacing catheter in place, and intracoronary nitroglycerin prepared, ergonovine maleate was given in four divided doses of 50 μg each, for a total dose of 200 μg. Following the last 50 μg dose (Fig. 4*B*), chest pain occurred and ST segment elevation developed in lead II, accompanied by a fall in arterial pressure and a rise in right ventricular systolic pressure (reflecting left ventricular dysfunction). The angiogram now revealed spastic obliteration at the site of the stenosis in the dominant circumflex artery. Nitroglycerin, 600 μg, was immediately given directly into the left coronary artery. This resulted in complete relief of pain; return of ST segments, arterial pressure, and right ventricular pressure toward the baseline; and the circumflex coronary artery spasm was relieved (Fig. 4*C*).

DIFFERING EFFECTS OF ERGONOVINE IN PATIENTS WITH AND WITHOUT CORONARY SPASM

Patients with atypical chest pain syndrome have a very different pattern of response to provocative testing with ergonovine than do patients with variant angina pectoris.[25-27] In the former group, administration of ergonovine maleate may or may not cause chest discomfort. When it does occur, it can be on the basis of esophageal spasm. The electrocardiogram does *not* exhibit signs of myocardial ischemia. There is a mild rise in arterial pressure, and this rise is usually accompanied by a proportionate increase in coronary blood flow. Coronary angiography in this group displays mild, diffuse narrowing of the epicardial coronary arteries; however, there is no evidence of focal spasm. By contrast, in patients with variant angina, their typical discomfort is usually reproduced. The pain is usually accompanied by ischemic ST-T wave changes. Classically, ST segment elevation occurs, but more subtle alterations can appear; these include T wave peaking, ST segment depression, T wave inversion, and "pseudonormalization" of the ST-T wave segment. Less often, ST segment changes may be difficult to detect. There is a variable arterial pressure response, with some patients developing hypotension secondary to spasm-induced ventricular dysfunction, whereas in others there is a hypertensive response or no important change in blood pressure. Regional myocardial blood flow is reduced during coronary artery spasm. Coronary angiography in this group shows severe focal spasm or total spastic obliteration of one or more epicardial coronary arteries.

Whereas ergonovine maleate does not generally cause clinically deleterious effects in patients without variant angina, it can cause severe myocardial ischemia, myocardial infarction, and even death in patients with the syndrome of variant angina.

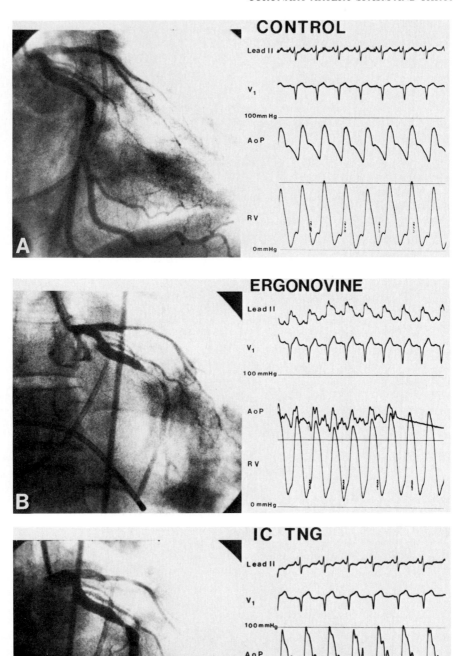

SUBLINGUAL OR INTRAVENOUS NITROGLYCERIN VERSUS INTRACORONARY NITROGLYCERIN

Some patients may develop spasm refractory to sublingual or intravenous nitroglycerin that responds to intracoronary nitroglycerin. Intracoronary nitroglycerin appears to be the method of choice for reversing coronary artery spasm. The reason for the enhanced efficacy of intracoronary nitroglycerin as compared with other routes of administration is twofold: First, if coronary artery spasm results in such severe myocardial ischemia as to cause systemic hypotension, sublingual or intravenous nitroglycerin may cause venodilatation and further reduction of cardiac output, which may in turn worsen spasm-induced ischemia. Second, under these conditions, the nitroglycerin may not reach its critical site of action, that is, the coronary arteries. Nitroglycerin injected directly into the coronary artery has much less systemic effect, and a much greater concentration of drug reaches the critical site of action.

RECOMMENDED GUIDELINES FOR THE PERFORMANCE OF THE ERGONOVINE TEST

In light of the aforementioned considerations, the following recommendations are offered for the conduct of provocative testing for coronary artery spasm with ergonovine:

1. Testing should be performed in those individuals in whom there is genuine doubt concerning the role of spasm in the patient's symptoms. In cases of clear-cut variant angina, provocative testing is usually unnecessary.
2. Testing should be performed only with full hemodynamic and electrocardiographic monitoring in a fully equipped cardiac catheterization laboratory by physicians who are experienced in provocative testing.
3. A right ventricular pacing catheter should be in place in case atrioventricular block develops, as often occurs during spasm of a dominant right or circumflex coronary artery.
4. After demonstration of baseline coronary anatomy, ergonovine is given in serial intravenous doses of 50 μg each, separated by an adequate period to observe response (5 minutes), and with test arteriograms performed before administration of the next dose. Ergonovine is given until clinical, ECG, or angiographic evidence of spasm develops, with no further doses given after signs or symptoms of ischemia develop. The ECG is continuously observed for ST segment depression, T wave changes, and "pseudonormalization of T waves,"[10] as well as for ST segment elevation. All these changes have been observed with severe coronary artery spasm. The maximal total dose should be 200 μg.
5. If signs or symptoms of myocardial ischemia develop, no further ergonovine is given and immediate angiography is performed. The vessel supplying the affected myocardial zone is visualized first. If spasm is demonstrated, intracoronary nitroglycerin is given in doses of 100 to 300 μg and repeated until spasm and ECG changes resolve. The other coronary artery is then visualized. If no ECG changes occur, both coronary arteries should be visualized nonetheless. Arrhythmias in this setting are due to ischemia, and therapy should be directed primarily to reverse the spasm.

Figure 4. *A*, Baseline coronary angiogram, electrocardiogram (leads II and V$_1$), and pressure tracings in Patient D. AoP = aortic pressure, RV = right ventricular pressure. *B*, Administration of ergonovine maleate results in spastic obliteration of the circumflex coronary artery, ST segment elevation in lead II, and severe hypotension. In addition, right ventricular systolic pressure is elevated, reflecting left ventricular dysfunction. *C*, Following intracoronary nitroglycerin administration, spasm is relieved, the electrocardiogram shows resolution of ST segment elevation, and arterial pressure is restored. In addition, right ventricular systolic pressure declines toward the baseline.

Because the conditions necessary for the conduction of a useful and safe provocative test are available only in the cardiac catheterization laboratory, I recommend its use only after careful consideration of the risks/benefit ratio. Certainly, provocative testing should be performed under the safest conditions.

REFERENCES

1. PRINZMETAL, M, KENNANER, R, MERLISS, R, ET AL: *Angina pectoris I. A variant form of angina pectoris. A preliminary report.* Am J Med 27:375, 1959.

2. OLIVA, PB, POTTS, DE, and PLUSS, RG: *Coronary arterial spasm in Prinzmetal angina. Documentation by coronary arteriography.* N Engl J Med 288:745,1973.

3. MASERI, A, SEVERI, S, DENES, M, ET AL: *Variant angina: One aspect of a continuous spectrum of vasospastic myocardial ischemia. Pathogenetic mechanisms, estimated incidence and clinical and coronary arteriographic findings in 138 patients.* Am J Cardiol 42:1019, 1978.

4. OLIVIA, PB, and BRECKINRIDGE, JC: *Arteriographic evidence of coronary arterial spasm in acute myocardial infarction.* Circulation 56:366, 1977.

5. MASERI, A, L'ABBATE, A, BAROLDI, G. ET AL: *Coronary vasospasm as a possible cause of myocardial infarction: A conclusion derived from the study of "preinfarction" angina.* N Engl J Med 299:1271, 1978.

6. GOLDBERG, S, REICHEK, N, MULLER, J, ET AL: *Nifedipine therapy for Prinzmetal's (variant) angina.* Am J Cardiol 44:804, 1979.

7. ANTMAN, E, MULLER, J, GOLDBERG, S, ET AL: *Nifedipine therapy for coronary spasm: Experience in 127 patients.* N Engl J Med 302:1269, 1980.

8. MASERI, A, PARODI, O, SEVERI, S, ET AL: *Transient transmural reduction of myocardial blood flow, demonstrated by thallium-201 scintigraphy, as a cause of variant angina.* Circulation 54:280, 1976.

9. DOHERTY, PW, GORIS, ML, ORLICK, AE, ET AL: *Thallium-201 imaging for identifying patients with coronary artery spasm.* Circulation 58 (Suppl 2):135, 1978.

10. WATERS, DD, SZLACHCIC, J, BANON, R, ET AL: *Comparative sensitivity of exercise, cold pressor and ergonovine testing in provoking attacks of variant angina in patients with active disease.* Circulation (in press).

11. THEROUX, P, WATERS, DD, AFFAKI, GS, ET AL: *Provocative testing with ergonovine to evaluate the efficacy of treatment with calcium antagonists in variant angina.* Circulation 60:504, 1979.

12. WATERS, DD, THÉROUX, P, SZLACHCIC, J, ET AL: *Provocative testing with ergonovine to assess the efficacy of treatment with nifedipine, diltiazem and verapamil in variant angina.* Am J Cardiol 48:123, 1981.

13. WATERS, DD, SZLACHCIC, J, THÉROUX, P, ET AL: *Ergonovine testing to detect spontaneous remissions of variant angina during long-term treatment with calcium antagonist drugs.* Am J Cardiol 47:179, 1981.

14. RAIZNER, AE, CHAHINE, RA, ISHIMORI, T, ET AL: *Provocation of coronary artery spasm by the cold pressor test. Hemodynamic, arteriographic and quantitative angiographic observations.* Circulation 62:925, 1980.

15. YASUE, H, MASAO, N, OMOTE, S, ET AL: *Coronary arterial spasm and Prinzmetal's variant form of angina induced by hyperventilation and Tris buffer infusion.* Circulation 58:56, 1978.

16. YASUE, H, OMOTE, S, TAKIZAWA, A, ET AL: *Circadian variation of exercise capacity in patients with Prinzmetal's variant angina. Role of exercise-induced coronary arterial spasm.* Circulation 59:938, 1979.

17. DE SERVI, S, FALCONE, C, GAVAZZI, A, ET AL: *The exercise test in variant angina: Results in 114 patients.* Circulation 64:684, 1981.

18. WATERS, DD, SZLACHCIC, J, BOURASSA, MG, ET AL: *Exercise testing in patients with variant angina: Results, correlation with clinical and angiographic features, and prognostic significance.* Circulation 65:265, 1982.

19. WATERS, DD, CHAITMAN, BR, BOURASSA, MG, ET AL: *Clinical and angiographic correlates of exercise-induced ST segment elevation. Increased detection with multiple ECG leads.* Circulation 61:286, 1980.

20. SPECCHI, G, DE SERVI, S, FALCONE, C, ET AL: *Significance of exercise-induced ST-segment elevation in patients without myocardial infarction.* Circulation 63:46, 1981.

21. SCHROEDER, JS, BOLEN, JL, QUINT, RA, ET AL: *Provocation of coronary spasm with ergonovine maleate. New test with results in 57 patients undergoing coronary arteriography.* Am J Cardiol 40:487, 1977.

22. HEUPLER, FA, JR, PROUDFIT, WL, RAZAVI, M, ET AL: *Ergonovine maleate—provocative test for coronary arterial spasm.* Am J Cardiol 41:631, 1978.

23. CURRY, RC, JR, PEPINE, CJ, SABOM, MB, ET AL: *Hemodynamic and myocardial metabolic effects of ergonovine in patients with chest pain.* Circulation 58:648, 1978.

24. WATERS, DD, THÉROUX, P, SZLACHCIC, J, ET AL: *Ergonovine testing in a coronary care unit.* Am J Cardiol 46:922, 1980.

25. GOLDBERG, S, LAM, W, MUDGE, GH, ET AL: *Coronary hemodynamics with myocardial metabolic alterations accompanying coronary spasm.* Am J Cardiol 43:481, 1979.

26. CURRY, RC, JR, PEPINE, CJ, SABOM, MB, ET AL: *Effects of ergonovine in patients with and without coronary disease.* Circulation 56:803, 1977.

27. RICCI, DR, ORLICK, AE, DOHERTY, PW, ET AL: *Reduction of coronary blood flow during coronary artery spasm occurring spontaneously and after provocation by ergonovine maleate.* Circulation 57:392, 1978.

28. CIPRIANO, PR, GUTHANER, DF, ORLICK, AE, ET AL: *The effects of ergonovine maleate on coronary arterial size.* Circulation 59:82, 1979.

29. HILLIS, LD, and BRAUNWALD, E: *Coronary arterial spasm.* N Engl J Med 299:695, 1978.

30. NELSON, C, NOWAK, B, CHILDS, H, ET AL: *Provocative testing for coronary arterial spasm: Rationale, risk and clinical illustrations.* Am J Cardiol 40:624, 1977.

31. HELFANT, RH: *Coronary arterial spasm: Provocative testing in ischemic heart disease.* Am J Cardiol 41:787, 1978.

32. BUXTON, A, GOLDBERG, S, HIRSHFELD, JW, ET AL: *Refractory ergonovine induced coronary vasospasm: Importance of intracoronary nitroglycerin.* Am J Cardiol 46:329, 1980.

Postoperative Coronary Vasospasm

V. Paul Addonizio, M.D., Alden H. Harken, M.D., and Sheldon Goldberg, M.D.

CORONARY SPASM FOLLOWING MYOCARDIAL REVASCULARIZATION

As has been pointed out in other chapters in this book, the consequences of coronary artery spasm range from asymptomatic ST segment changes and angina easily relieved by nitroglycerin to arrhythmias, hypotension, myocardial infarction, and cardiovascular collapse.[1-8] We have recently reported a group of patients who developed cardiovascular collapse due to coronary artery spasm following successful myocardial revascularization for fixed obstructive coronary artery disease.[9] The recognition, pathophysiologic mechanisms, and therapy of this clinical syndrome are the subject of this chapter.

Illustrative Cases

CASE A. A 39-year-old woman underwent cardiac catheterization for the evaluation of angina during exercise and at rest. Episodes of angina were accompanied by ST segment depression in the anterior leads. Coronary arteriography revealed a 90 percent fixed obstructive lesion of the left main coronary artery, with noncritical luminal irregularities of the left anterior descending and circumflex arteries. The right coronary artery was dominant and normal (Fig. 1).

The patient underwent uneventful saphenous vein bypass grafting to the left anterior descending and circumflex coronary arteries, and cardiopulmonary bypass was terminated without difficulty. Two hours after surgery, inferior ST segment elevation (Fig. 2 *top*) and then atrioventricular block developed, with a fall in systolic arterial pressure to 30 mm Hg from baseline levels of 140/100 mm Hg. Intravenous nitroglycerin infusion (dose range, 0.3 mg per minute initially to a 1.0 mg bolus) transiently reversed the ST segment elevation, but the hypotension persisted, and external cardiac massage was initiated. ST segment elevation, accompanied by high-grade atrioventricular block, ventricular tachycardia, and hypotension, recurred nine times but was partly reversed by intravenous boluses of nitroglycerin. In spite of these measures, severe hypotension persisted, and while external cardiac massage was continued the patient was taken to the cardiac catheterization laboratory. Angiography of the right coronary artery revealed spastic obliteration of the right coronary artery (Fig. 2 *bottom*). Nitroglycerin (0.5 mg as a bolus) was then infused directly into the right coronary artery. Repeat angiography showed partial relief of right coronary artery spasm. After 7.0 mg of intracoronary nitroglycerin was given over 15 minutes, the right coronary artery spasm was relieved, sinus rhythm was restored, and the systolic blood pressure returned to 170 mm Hg. An electrocardiogram showed resolution of the ST segment elevation in the inferior leads.

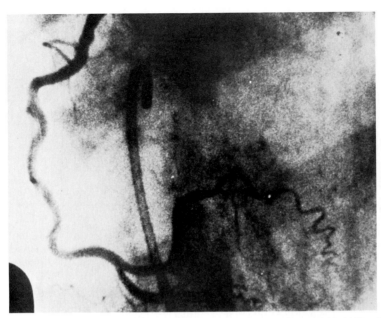

Figure 1. Normal right coronary artery in Patient A. (From New Engl J Med 304:1249, 1981, with permission.)

Right coronary artery spasm then recurred, and intracoronary nitroglycerin infusion was resumed. After an additional 30 mg of nitroglycerin was infused into the right coronary artery, vasospasm was completely relieved (Fig. 3). Nifedipine (30 mg every 6 hours by naso-gastric tube) was begun, and the dose of intravenous nitroglycerin (0.1 mg per minute) was tapered over 24 hours.

A postoperative electrocardiogram showed T wave inversions in the inferior leads but no Q waves, and further recovery was uneventful. After 15 months, the patient is now free of angina and has returned to her usual occupation.

CASE B. A 49-year-old man presented to Thomas Jefferson University Hospital with rest angina and transient ST segment elevation in the precordial leads. These ischemic episodes were accompanied by ventricular tachycardia. Cardiac catheterization revealed a normal resting left ventricular end-diastolic pressure. Left ventricular wall motion was normal, and the ejection fraction was 64 percent. The resting ECG, arterial pressure, and left coronary arteriogram are depicted in Figure 4. In the control state, the patient was pain-free, and the ECG was normal. There was a long, eccentric fixed 90 percent stenosis in the proximal left anterior descending coronary artery.

The patient underwent provocative testing with ergonovine maleate as follows: With a Zucker pacing catheter in the right ventricle and constant ECG and arterial pressure moni-toring, two 0.05 mg doses of ergonovine maleate were given 5 minutes apart. Shortly after the second dose, the patient experienced his typical angina. The ECG, arterial pressure, and left coronary angiogram at this point are shown in Figure 5. Despite no important change in blood pressure or heart rate, there was now ST segment elevation in the precordial lead. The left coronary angiogram revealed total occlusion of the left anterior descending coronary artery at the site of the 90 percent fixed lesion. Intracoronary nitroglycerin, 300 μg, was immediately injected into the left coronary ostium, with rapid resolution of the patient's angina, return of the ST segment elevation to baseline, and restoration of antegrade coronary flow in the left anterior descending artery (Fig. 6). The right coronary artery was normal and did not develop spasm.

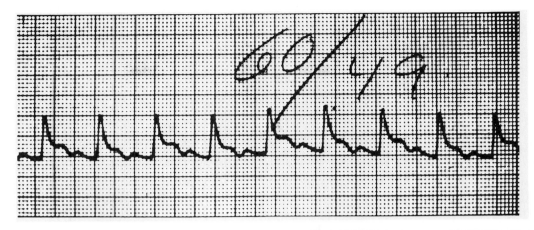

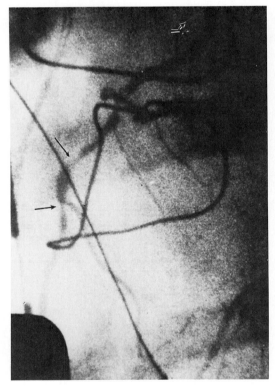

Figure 2. *Top,* Electrocardiographic lead II tracing from Patient A, during an episode of spasm immediately after operation. The blood pressure was 60/49 at the time. *Bottom,* Right coronary artery spasm after saphenous vein bypass to the left coronary artery. The right coronary angiogram was performed during cardiovascular collapse in Patient A. The upper arrow points to the right coronary artery catheter. The lower arrows indicate areas of severe focal spasm. (From New Engl J Med 304:1249, 1981, with permission.)

Despite medical therapy, the patient's symptoms continued, and he underwent saphenous vein bypass graft surgery to the left anterior descending artery. After the vein graft was successfully placed and the patient came off bypass, ST segment elevation was noted and the left ventricle became flaccid. Nitroglycerin was injected into the vein graft to the left anterior descending coronary artery. Several doses of 500 to 1000 μg of nitroglycerin were given. The ST segment elevation returned to baseline, and left ventricular function improved markedly. Several minutes later, ST segment elevation in lead II developed, accompanied by directly visualized spasm of the *right* coronary artery and poor contraction of both the left and right ventricles. Again nitroglycerin was given, at first into the aortic root (500 μg) and then

113

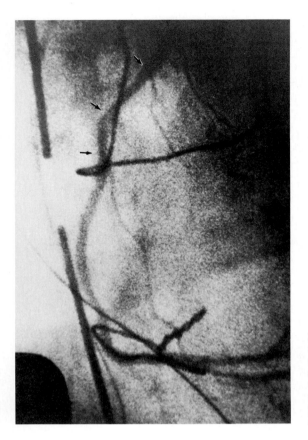

Figure 3. Resolution of coronary artery spasm after administration of intracoronary nitroglycerin. The angiogram shows the left anterior oblique view after intracoronary nitroglycerin, with spasm resolved *(arrows)*. The electrocardiographic changes reverted to normal, and the patient recovered completely. (From New Engl J Med 304:1249, 1981, with permission.)

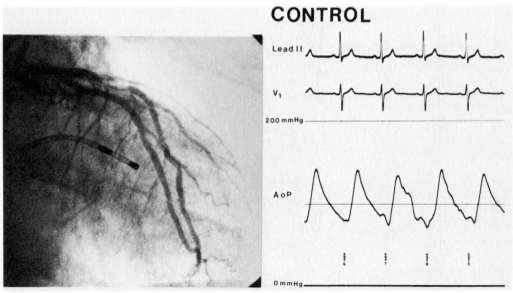

Figure 4. Control ECG, arterial pressure, and left coronary angiogram in Patient B. There is a 90 percent eccentric fixed lesion in the left anterior descending coronary artery. The patient was pain-free at this time.

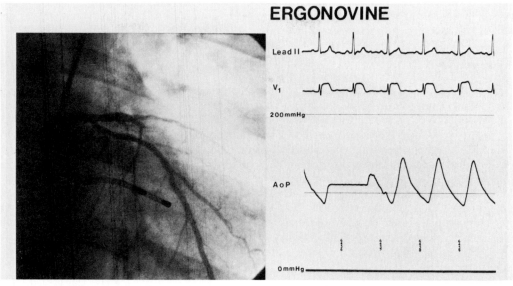

Figure 5. The ECG, arterial pressure, and left coronary angiogram during ergonovine-induced spasm. The patient developed angina. There was ST segment elevation in V_1 and no significant change in heart rate or arterial pressure. The left coronary angiogram now shows spastic obliteration of the left anterior descending artery at the site of the fixed lesion.

directly into the right coronary artery. After approximately 2,000 μg of intracoronary nitroglycerin, spasm resolved, the ST segment elevation returned to baseline, and function of both ventricles improved. An intravenous nitroglycerin drip was begun, and the patient was returned to the intensive care unit without incident. The intravenous nitroglycerin was continued for two days. The patient made a full recovery, without any ECG evidence of myo-

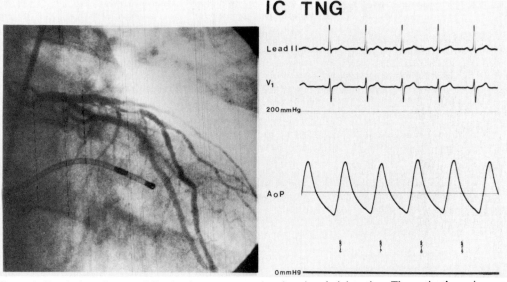

Figure 6. Resolution of spasm following intracoronary nitroglycerin administration. The patient's angina was relieved. The ECG shows resolution of ST segment elevation, and the angiogram shows re-establishment of flow in the left anterior descending coronary artery. The fixed lesion remains unchanged.

115

cardial infarction. He was discharged on nitrates and nifedipine; both medications were discontinued without any recurrence of symptoms 17 months later.

Comment

We recently described six patients who experienced sudden cardiovascular collapse within two hours of myocardial revascularization.[9] Case A is taken from this series. The clinical characteristics of these six cases are summarized in Table 1.

In these six cases, the electrocardiographic pattern of acute transmural myocardial ischemia (ST segment elevation) developed in a myocardial zone perfused by a coronary artery that was not critically diseased. In Case B presented above, ST segment elevation occurred in two zones: the anterior wall supplied by the grafted vessel and subsequently in the inferior wall, supplied by a noncritically diseased right coronary artery. The myocardial ischemia was severe, acute in onset, and recurrent. The marked hemodynamic compromise resulting from coronary artery spasm noted in these subjects is similar to that observed in other patients during spontaneous and provoked attacks of vasospastic angina.[10]

Etiology of Postoperative Coronary Vasospasm

As with variant angina, the stimulus provoking an episode of coronary vasospasm in the postoperative period remains unknown. In both clinical settings, the spastic segment may be diffuse or discrete and may occur in an angiographically normal or noncritically diseased vessel. Multiple factors might alter the threshold for coronary vasospasm in the perioperative

Table 1. Clinical characteristics of right coronary artery spasm occurring after coronary bypass grafting*

Case	Anginal pattern and coronary pathology†	ECG findings and blood pressure	Treatment	Outcome
1	Exertional angina; 90% obstruction of left main coronary artery	Inferior ST segment elevation; hypotension	Intravenous nitroglycerin; intra-aortic balloon pulsation; nifedipine	Death
2	Exertional and variant angina; 80% obstruction of left anterior descending artery	Inferior ST segment elevation; hypotension; sinus bradycardia	Intravenous nitroglycerin, intra-aortic balloon pulsation	Death
3	Variant angina with anterior ST segment elevation; 95% obstruction of left anterior descending artery	Inferior ST segment elevation; hypotension	Intravenous nitroglycerin; nifedipine	Death
4	Rest and exertional angina; 90% obstruction of left main coronary artery	Inferior ST segment elevation; hypotension; atrioventricular block; ventricular tachycardia	Intracoronary and intravenous nitroglycerin; nifedipine	Recovery
5	Exertional angina; 99% obstruction of left anterior descending artery; 90% obstruction of left circumflex artery	Inferior ST segment elevation; hypotension; atrioventricular block	Intracoronary and intravenous nitroglycerin; nifedipine; intra-aortic balloon pulsation	Recovery
6	Rest and exertional angina; 90% obstruction of left anterior descending artery; 70% obstruction of diagonal artery	Inferior ST segment elevation; hypotension; atrioventricular block; ventricular tachycardia	Intravenous nitroglycerin; nifedipine; phentolamine	Recovery

*From New Engl J Med 304:1249, 1981, with permission.
†Obstruction of arteries refers to narrowing by atherosclerotic obstructions.

period. These stimuli include physical manipulation of the vessel at the time of surgery with or without unsuspected internal injury, chronic changes in the vasa vasorum leading to local hypoxia,[11] the presence of endothelial cell damage, or a local defect in prostacyclin production (see below).[12] Furthermore, a fall in the hydrogen ion concentration in the microenvironment of the vascular smooth muscle cell and increased alpha-adrenergic activity[13,14] are associated with coronary vasospasm, and both conditions frequently exist following open cardiac surgery.

The recent discovery that activated platelets release both serotonin and an extremely potent vasoconstrictor, thromboxane A_2, has stimulated increased interest in the role of platelets in the genesis of vasotonic ischemic heart disease.[15] Indeed, this potential relationship appears to be the logical extension of work implicating platelets and thrombosis in myocardial infarction,[16] lethal arrhythmias,[17] and sudden cardiac death.[18]

Even minor erosions, tears, or fissures in arterial intima caused by hemodynamic stress, catheters, or immunologic insult are followed quickly by platelet adhesion to the exposed subendothelium.[13,14] Adherent platelets may then undergo the release reaction with extrusion of the contents of at least three types of granules: dense, alpha, and lysosomal.[19] Released adenine nucleotides from dense granules serve to recruit additional platelets to the growing aggregate (Fig. 7). Released proteins from alpha granules may antagonize the anticoagulant properties of heparin[20] or contribute to the coagulation cascade via fibrinogen and factors V and VIII. Acutely, arachidonate metabolism is initiated with release of thromboxane A_2, which causes vasoconstriction and further platelet recruitment.[21]

Thromboxane A_2 is a vascular smooth muscle constrictor in all species so far examined.[22,23] As little as 30 picomoles of thromboxane A_2 cause profound constriction of rabbit aorta, making thromboxane A_2 the most potent vasoconstrictor known.[24] Furthermore, thromboxane A_2 is essential for one pathway leading to platelet activation.[25] Thus, in view of the potent proaggregating and vasoactive properties of thromboxane A_2, it has been suggested that thromboxanes may be involved in the propagation of vasotonic angina, either locally or downstream after release from activated platelets. Consistently, enhanced thromboxane synthesis has been observed in patients with variant angina,[26] during acute myocardial infarction,[27] during coronary vasospasm,[28] and during pacing-induced myocardial ischemia.[29]

It is now clear, however, that thromboxane synthesis and release are only one component of complex platelet-vessel wall interactions. Prostacyclin and not thromboxane is the major product of arachidonate metabolism in blood vessels, thus differing from platelets.[30] Prostacyclin balances thromboxane by being as potent an antiaggregating and vasodilating agent as thromboxane is proaggregating and vasoconstrictive.[31] Indeed, the mechanism by which intact endothelium remains nonthrombogenic is in part due to the synthesis and release of prostacyclin. It is postulated that segmental vasoconstriction may result from platelet activation on an area of angiographically undetectable endothelial damage and reduced prostacylin synthesis. In fact, the inability to document in clinical studies the relative contribution of the thromboxane-prostacyclin axis to coronary vasospasm may be due to the inadvertent interference of prostacyclin synthesis, which often results from platelet inhibition.[32] An imbalance between prostacyclin and thromboxane synthesis may thus be fundamental to the genesis of vasospasm and thrombosis.

Platelet Activation During Open Cardiac Surgery

As noted previously, the metabolic alterations associated with variant angina may be sequelae of open cardiac surgery. Furthermore, the necessary introduction of blood to the synthetic surfaces of an extracorporeal circuit is followed by extensive alterations in platelet function, including release of thromboxanes.[33–35] Only a minority of circulating platelets are actually activated to the point of granule release.[35] The remainder circulate with reduced sensitivity to standard platelet agonists. The reduced sensitivity of circulating platelets, however, does not preclude platelet adhesion. In fact, within the extracorporeal circuit surface-mediated and

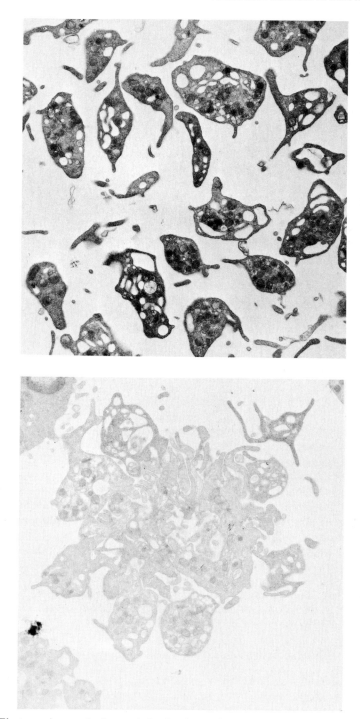

Figure 7. *Top,* Electron micrograph of normal platelets (×12,000, reduced 35 percent). *Bottom,* Electron micrograph of evolving platelet aggregation. Note that central platelets have released their granule contents (×12,000, reduced 35 percent).

thromboxane-mediated platelet activation can actually be distinguished,[34] making it conceivable that platelet adhesion to an area of minimally damaged endothelium could be followed at a later time by thromboxane synthesis and platelet activation.[28] Thus, open cardiac surgery would appear to provide an ideal milieu for platelet-induced coronary vasospasm. Perhaps it is only the polypharmacy required for open cardiac surgery that reduces the frequency of postoperative coronary vasospasm by providing effective inhibition of platelet function.[34]

Therapeutic Implications

Physicians involved in the intraoperative and postoperative care of patients undergoing myocardial revascularization procedures need to be aware that coronary artery spasm in this setting, although potentially lethal, is reversible. Coronary artery spasm should be suspected in the patient who has signs of acute transmural myocardial ischemia manifested by ST segment elevation, either in the operating room or in the intensive care area in the early hours following revascularization. In our recent report, we reviewed cases of sudden circulatory collapse following coronary bypass grafting.[9] There were 19 cases of cardiovascular collapse occurring in 784 bypass operations. In 6 of these 19 cases, coronary artery spasm was implicated as the mechanism of circulatory failure.

What should the physician do when confronted by a patient with new transmural injury current and resulting hemodynamic instability? If the situation occurs in the operating room, nitroglycerin can be instilled directly into either the vein graft or the coronary artery supplying the affected myocardial zone. As demonstrated in Case B (above), this approach may result in rapid reversal of spasm and concomitant improvement in ventricular performance. It is important to point out that attempts to stabilize such patients by the infusion of catecholamines may be ineffective. In fact, these agents may cause further deterioration in the clinical situation because of their potential to worsen coronary vasoconstriction. Though intra-aortic balloon counterpulsation may decrease myocardial dysfunction in patients with transmural ischemia, the use of the balloon pump alone does not deal with the primary derangement in this setting. If patients develop coronary artery spasm after they leave the surgical suite, effective therapy may be difficult. Intravenous nitroglycerin infusion may be attempted. However, if profound circulatory collapse is present, this form of therapy may be suboptimal. The reasons for the lack of efficacy of sublingual, transdermal, or intravenous nitroglycerin may be several. First, the venodilating properties of the drug, when administered in this fashion, may exacerbate arterial hypotension. Second, in a hemodynamically compromised patient, an ineffective concentration of drug may reach its target site, that is, the coronary smooth muscle. Therefore, if standard treatment with intravenous nitroglycerin fails, it may be necessary to return the patient to the catheterization suite and administer *intracoronary* nitroglycerin, with repeated doses given until there is angiographic relief of spasm, accompanied by resolution of ST segment elevation and stabilization of blood pressure. This sequence of events was dramatically demonstrated by the patient in Case A (above). By our experiences with ergonovine-induced coronary spasm,[10] we were led to the idea that intracoronary nitroglycerin might be more efficacious than intravenous nitroglycerin in the setting of refractory spasm. We have given intracoronary nitroglycerin in repeated boluses of 0.1 to 1.0 mg with striking beneficial effects.

Previous experience indicates that myocardial revascularization is less effective in relieving symptoms in patients with variant angina as opposed to classical angina pectoris.[36] Also, sudden death and perioperative myocardial infarction occur with greater frequency in patients with variant angina who undergo coronary bypass surgery.[3,6,37-39] In light of our current experience, we can postulate that severe perioperative spasm might be accountable for some of these events.

Although perioperative coronary artery spasm is not common, when it does occur, the consequences can be lethal. Therefore, preoperative identification of patients at risk for developing this complication would be valuable. Certainly, patients with a history of variant angina who undergo bypass surgery should be prophylactically treated with calcium blockers[40] and nitrates. Preoperative provocative testing in all patients does not seem practical or logical. The factors responsible for coronary artery spasm in the perioperative phase may be present only transiently, and therefore preoperative provocative testing may lack sensitivity. Also, such testing is not without risk. The use of prophylactic calcium channel blockers and nitrates might therefore be useful in the majority of patients undergoing myocardial revascularization procedures.

In summary, if ST segment elevation develops in the operating room, the surgeon should be prepared to administer intracoronary and/or intravein-graft nitroglycerin. If spasm and hemodynamic compromise develop in the intensive care unit soon after surgery, coronary angiography may be needed in certain instances. In the catheterization suite, the mechanism responsible for reduced coronary flow can be established with certainty. If coronary artery spasm and/or intraluminal thrombus[16,41,42] are contributing to interruption of coronary flow, then specific, effective therapy may be undertaken.

REFERENCES

1. MASERI, A, L'ABBATE, A, BAROLDI, G, ET AL: *Coronary vasospasm as a possible cause of myocardial infarction: A conclusion derived from the study of "preinfarction" angina.* N Engl J Med 299:1271, 1978.

2. MASERI, A, SEVERI, S, NES, MD, ET AL: *"Variant" angina: One aspect of a continuous spectrum of vasospastic myocardial ischemia: Pathogenetic mechanisms, estimated incidence and clinical and coronary arteriographic findings in 138 patients.* Am J Cardiol 42:1019, 1978.

3. OLIVA, PB, and BRECKINRIDGE, JC: *Arteriographic evidence of coronary arterial spasm in acute myocardial infarction.* Circulation 56:366, 1977.

4. OLIVA PB, POTTS, DE and PLUSS, RG: *Coronary arterial spasm in Prinzmetal angina: Documentation by coronary arteriography.* N Engl J Med 288:745, 1973.

5. MACALPIN, RN, KATTUS, AA and ALVARO, AB: *Angina pectoris at rest with preservation of exercise capacity: Prinzmetal's variant angina.* Circulation 47:946, 1973.

6. BETRIU, A, SOLIGNAC, A and BOURASSA, MG: *The variant form of angina: Diagnostic and therapeutic implications.* Am Heart J 87:272, 1974.

7. SILVERMAN, ME, and FLAMM, MD, JR: *Variant angina pectoris: Anatomic findings and prognostic implications.* Ann Intern Med 75:339, 1971.

8. PICHARD, AD, AMBROSE, J, MINDICH, B, ET AL: *Coronary artery spasm and perioperative cardiac arrest.* J Thorac Cardiovasc Surg 80:249, 1980.

9. BUXTON, AE, GOLDBERG, S, HARKEN, A, ET AL: *Coronary artery spasm immediately after myocardial revascularization: Recognition and management.* N Engl J Med 304:1249, 1981.

10. BUXTON, AE, GOLDBERG, S, HIRSHFELD, JW, ET AL: *Refractory ergonovine induced coronary vasospasm: Importance of intracoronary nitroglycerin.* Am J Cardiol 46:329, 1980.

11. YOKOAMA, M, and HENRY, PD: *Sensitization of isolated coronary arteries to calcium ions after exposure to cholesterol.* Circ Res 45:479, 1979.

12. DEMBINSKE-KIEC, A, GRYGLEWSKY, T, ZUNDE, A, ET AL: *The generation of prostacyclin by arteries and by the coronary vascular beds is reduced in experimental atherosclerosis in rabbit.* Prostaglandins 14:1025, 1977.

13. BARMGARTNER, HR, MUGGLE, R, TSCHOPP, TB, ET AL: *Platelet adhesion, release, and aggregation in flowing blood: Effects of surface properties and platelet function.* Thromb Haemost, 35:124, 1976.

14. GROVES, HM, KINLOUGH-RATHBONE, RL, RICHARDSON, M, ET AL: *Platelet interaction with damaged rabbit aorta.* Lab Invest 40:194, 1979.

15. HAMBERG, M, SVENSSON, J, and SAMUELSON, B: *A new group of biologically active compounds derived from prostaglandin endoperoxides.* Proc Nat Acad Sci 72:2994, 1975.

16. RENTROP, P, BLANKE, H, KARSCH, KR, ET AL: *Selective intracoronary thrombolysis in acute myocardial infarction and unstable angina pectoris.* Circulation 63:307, 1981.

17. JORGENSON, C, ROWSELL, HC, HONIG, T, ET AL: *Platelet aggregation and myocardial infarction in swine.* Lab Invest 17:616, 1967.

18. Haerem, JW: *Sudden unexpected coronary death*. Acta Path Micro Suppl 265, 1978.
19. Weiss, HJ: *Platelet physiology and abnormalities of platelet function*. N Engl Med 293:531, 1975.
20. Niewiarowski, S: *Proteins secreted by platelets*. Thromb Haemost 38:924, 1977.
21. Smith, JB, Ingerman, C, Kocsis, JJ, et al: *Formation of an intermediate in prostaglandin biosynthesis and its association with the platelet release reaction*. J Clin Invest 53:1468, 1974.
22. Ellis, EF, Oclz, O, Roberts, LJ, et al: *Coronary arterial smooth muscle contraction by a substance released from platelets: Evidence that it is thromboxane A₂* (In press).
23. Svensson, J, and Hamberg, M: *Thromboxane A₂ and prostaglandin H₂: Potent stimulators of the swine coronary artery*. Prostaglandins 12:943, 1976.
24. Needleman, P, Minkes, MS, and Raz, A: *Thromboxane selective biosynthesis and distinct biological properties*. Science 193:163, 1976.
25. Charo, IF, Feinman, RD, and Detwiler, TC: *Interrelations of platelet aggregation and secretion*. J Clin Invest 60:866, 1977.
26. Mehta, J, Mehta, P, and Conti, CK: *Platelet function studies in coronary heart disease. Increased platelet prostaglandin generation and abnormal platelet sensitivity to prostacyclin and endoperoxide analog in angina pectoris*. Am J Cardiol 46:943, 1980.
27. Szczezklik, A, Gryglewski, RJ, Muscal, J, et al: *Thromboxane generation and platelet aggregation in survivals of myocardial infarction*. Thromb Haemost 40:66, 1978.
28. Lewy, RI, Smith, JB, Silver, MJ, et al: *Detection of thromboxane B₂ in peripheral blood of patients with Prinzmetal's angina*. Prostaglandins Med 5:243, 1979.
29. Lewy, RI, Weiner, L, Walinsky, P, et al: *Thromboxane release during pacing-induced angina pectoris: Possible vasoconstrictor influence on the coronary vasculature*. Circulation 61:1165, 1980.
30. Needleman, P, and Kaley, G: *Cardiac and coronary prostaglandin synthesis and function*. N Engl J Med 300:1142, 1979.
31. Moncada, S, Herman, AG, Higgs, EA, et al: *Differential formation of prostacyclin by layers of the arterial wall*. Thromb Res 11:323, 1977.
32. Kelton, JG, Hirsch, J, Carter, CJ, et al: *Thrombogenic effect of high-dose aspirin in rabbits*. J Clin Invest 62:892, 1978.
33. Addonizio, VP, Macarak, EJ, Niewiarowski, S, et al: *Preservation of human platelets with prostaglandin E-1 during in vitro simulation of cardiopulmonary bypass*. Circ Res 44:350, 1979.
34. Addonizio, VP, Smith, JB, Guiod, LR, et al: *Thromboxane synthesis and platelet protein release during simulated extracorporeal circulation*. Blood 54:371, 1979.
35. Addonizio, VP, and Colman, RW: *Platelet alterations during extracorporeal circulation*. Biomaterials (In press).
36. Hillis, LD, and Braunwald, E: *Coronary-artery spasm*. N Engl J Med 299:695, 1978.
37. Gaasch, WH, Lufschanowski, R, Leachman, RD, et al: *Surgical managment of Prinzmetal's variant angina*. Chest 66:614, 1974.
38. Johnson, AD, Stroud, HA, Vieweg, WVR, et al: *Variant angina pectoris: Clinical presentations, coronary angiographic patterns, and the results of medical and surgical management in 42 consecutive patients*. Chest 73:786, 1978.
39. Wiener, L, Kasparian, H, Duca, PR, et al: *Spectrum of coronary arterial spasm: Clinical, angiographic and myocardial metabolic experience in 29 cases*. Am J Cardiol 38:945, 1976.
40. Goldberg, S, Reichek, N, Wilson, J, et al: *Nifedipine in the treatment of Prinzmetal's (variant) angina*. Am J Cardiol 44:804, 1979.
41. Mathey, DG, Kuck, K-H, Tilsner, V, et al: *Nonsurgical coronary artery recanalization in acute transmural myocardial infarction*. Circulation 63:489, 1981.
42. Leinbach, RC, and Gold, HK: *Regional streptokinase in myocardial infarction*. Circulation 63:489, 1981.

Clinical Pharmacology of Calcium Entry Blockers

C. Paul Bianchi, Ph.D.

Calcium entry blockers are a new class of drugs designed to restrict or to limit the entry of calcium into cells. Cells contain a low intracellular content of calcium and a high content of magnesium. Magnesium serves as the major intracellular divalent ion and forms soluble complexes with ATP and serves as a necessary metal cofactor for many enzymes. Calcium forms insoluble complexes with phosphates and must be maintained at intracellular concentrations below the solubility product for intracellular calcium phosphate complexes. The unique distribution of calcium (high extracellular and low intracellular concentration) allows calcium entry into the cell or release from intracellular-bound stores to play a key modulating role for changing the functional state of the cell. In muscle cells, intracellular calcium plays a key role in regulation of both anabolic and catabolic physiologic states and leads to cell death if the intracellular concentration exceeds a limit of 10^{-5} M. Figure 1 shows the changes in functional states of muscles (smooth, cardiac, and skeletal) as regulated by changes in intracellular calcium concentration expressed as pCa_i ($-\log Ca_i^{2+}$). As the intracellular calcium concentration rises from a pCa_i of 9 to 7, no contraction is observed; but a marked increase in aerobic metabolism occurs associated with an increase in glycogen synthesis, glucose uptake, amino acid transport, and enhanced uptake of potassium. Insulin may be considered as a prototype hormone that regulates the anabolic state in muscle via a calcium-dependent step. As the intracellular calcium concentration rises from a pCa_i of 7 to 5, contraction and catabolic processes take place, that is, breakdown of glycogen, creatine phosphate, and protein.[1] The catabolic state can be maintained only for relatively short periods of time before feedback mechanisms occur to restore the intracellular calcium level to a level associated with relaxation and anabolic processes. If intracellular calcium rises above 10^{-5} M (pCa_i 5), mitochondrial calcium overload occurs, ATP production is inhibited, and Ca-ATPases are activated leading to a wastage of ATP; moreover, phospholipases and proteases are activated, with loss of membrane structure and loss of intracellular soluble enzymes. A sustained increase in myoplasmic free calcium above 10^{-5} M leads to cell death. The mechanisms that protect against calcium overload of the cell are (1) restriction of calcium entry across the membrane and (2) calcium removal from the cell by transport systems in the cell membrane. The major protective mechanism is restriction of calcium entry because less energy is used by the cell to keep calcium out of the cell than to transport calcium from within.

The regulation of calcium entry into smooth muscle cells is shown in Figure 2. The intracellular calcium concentration in the sarcoplasm is below 10^{-7} M when the muscle is at rest. The intracellular calcium concentrations can be increased above 10^{-7} M by (1) calcium entry through slow calcium channels opened by membrane depolarization, that is, voltage-depen-

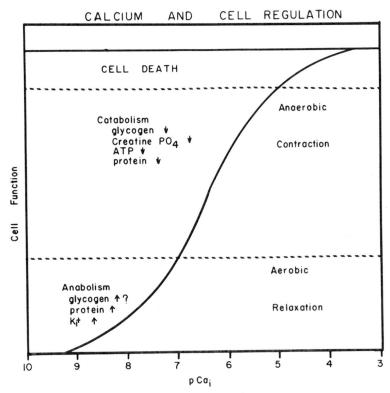

Figure 1. Regulation of cell function by increases in the cytoplasmic free calcium. Free calcium is plotted on the abscissa as pCa_i ($-$ log Ca_i). Anabolic processes and relaxation of smooth and skeletal muscles occur at pCa_i between 9 and 7. Catabolic processes and contraction occur between pCa_i 7 and 5. If catabolic processes are not reversed, slow cell death can occur. At pCa_i below 5, cell death and destruction are rapid.

dent channels (VDC), (2) calcium entry through receptor-dependent calcium channels (RDC), or (3) calcium release from receptor-dependent storage and release sites associated with the surface membrane. The free calcium level is decreased by uptake into storage and release sites and also into storage sites from which extrusion across the membrane occurs. The alpha 1 receptor in smooth muscle, when activated by norepinephrine, opens a receptor-dependent channel and causes smooth muscle contraction. The alpha 2 receptor activated by norepinephrine causes release of calcium from an internal storage site and also causes contraction of smooth muscle.[2] Removal of calcium from the smooth muscle cell is associated with activation of adenyl cyclase by the beta 2 receptor, stimulated by epinephrine. Restriction of calcium entry into cells may be expected to be of benefit in preventing smooth muscle spasm and in protecting cells from cell death due to calcium overload.

A new class of drugs clinically useful for the treatment of angina and cardiac arrhythmias has been developed in recent years. These drugs act as calcium entry blockers by restricting calcium entry through voltage and receptor-dependent calcium channels of smooth muscle and cardiac muscle cells. The net result of blocking calcium channels in vascular smooth muscle is vasodilation, and in cardiac muscle a slowing of conduction through the AV node and a negative inotropic effect.[3,4]

Calcium entry blockers were earlier called calcium antagonists, based on the finding by Fleckenstein[5,6] that verapamil mimicked the cardiac effects of lowered extracellular calcium. The negative inotropic effect of verapamil was antagonized by increasing extracellular calcium. The main features of the action of verapamil on cardiac muscle are: reduction in cal-

124

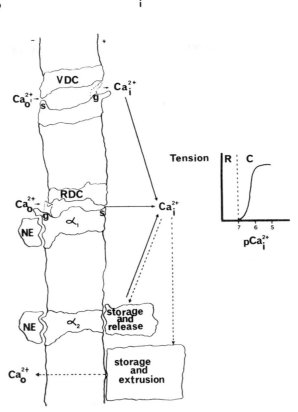

Figure 2. Schematic view of calcium entry and exit from a smooth muscle cell. Calcium can enter through voltage-dependent channels (VDC) which contain a selectivity filter site which is specific for calcium (s) and a voltage-dependent gate (g) which allows calcium entry. Entry of calcium through receptor-dependent channels is regulated by a receptor-dependent gate (g) and a selectivity filter (s). Calcium can also enter the cytoplasm from storage and release sites; release is triggered by an agonist interaction with an alpha 2 receptor. Storage and extrusion sites for calcium efflux are activated by beta 2 adrenergic receptor stimulation. Tension is pictured in the insert as a function of pCa_i^{2+}. Relaxation (R) occurs above pCa_i^{2+} 7 and contraction (C) occurs below pCa_i^{2+} 7.

cium-dependent contractile force without a major change in the cardiac action potential, reduction of Ca^{2+}-dependent high-energy phosphate utilization of the beating heart, and reduction of extra oxygen consumption during contraction.

The important therapeutic actions of calcium entry blockers on the heart are (1) protection of myocardium against intracellular calcium overload during ischemia—a major factor in myocardial cell death, (2) decrease of calcium-dependent automaticity caused by slow calcium channel ectopic cardiac pacemakers, (3) delay of conduction through the AV node with protection of the ventricles against supraventricular tachycardia, and (4) relaxation of coronary vasospasm.

All the aforementioned actions are dependent upon the ability of calcium entry blockers to decrease calcium influx into the cell through calcium channels. Fleckenstein[4] divides the calcium entry blockers into two groups. The calcium entry blockers in group A are capable of inhibiting calcium-dependent excitation-contraction coupling of the mammalian ventricular myocardium by 90 percent before inhibiting the fast sodium influx that occurs during the rise of the cardiac action potential. Group B drugs inhibit the fast sodium influx at concentrations that depress calcium-dependent contraction of papillary muscles by 50 to 70 percent. A tabulation of drugs in groups A and B is shown in Table 1.

Table 1. Calcium entry blockers

Drug	Molecular weight
Group A. Inhibitors of calcium entry	
Verapamil	454.59
Nifedipine	346.34
Niludipine	490.55
Nimodipine	418.45
Diltiazem	414.52
Group B. Inhibitors of both calcium and sodium channels	
Prenylamine	329.46
Fendiline	315.46
Terodiline	381.00
Perhexiline	277.50

At present, the three major drugs that exhibit therapeutic promise as coronary vasodilators are verapamil, nifedipine, and diltiazem. Nimodipine shows good promise as a cerebral vasodilator.[7]

Verapamil, as a prototype calcium channel blocker, causes bradycardia by its direct action on the SA node, and it exerts an antagonistic action to the tachycardia caused by beta 1 adrenergic receptor stimulation. The inward depolarizing current of the SA node is depressed by verapamil and enhanced by norepinephrine. Conduction through the AV node, which is regulated by slow inward currents (upstroke velocity 2 to 7 V per second), is also depressed by verapamil.[8,9] Conduction in the atrial and ventricular myocardium is not depressed by verapamil at concentrations that depress the firing rate of the SA node or the conduction through the AV node. The fast sodium channels (upstroke velocity 170 to 400 V per second) responsible for rapid conduction of the cardiac action potential are uninfluenced by verapamil at concentrations below 10^{-5} M.

Ectopic foci in atrial and ventricular myocardial cells are associated with low resting potentials because of accumulation of potassium at the cell surface. In ischemic regions of the myocardium, insufficient energy is present in the cells to maintain intracellular potassium at normal physiologic levels. As potassium accumulates at the surface, the cells depolarize, and the resting membrane potential falls. The fast sodium channels inactivate, but at sufficient levels of depolarization the slow calcium channels become activated. The membrane potential begins to oscillate between depolarization caused by slow calcium inward currents and repolarization induced by potassium outward currents. These conditions set the stage for automaticity with rapid firing rates.[3] Verapamil blockade of slow calcium channels is frequency dependent, that is, verapamil interacts with a receptor in the slow calcium channel primarily when the channel is in an open configuration[10] (see Fig. 2). As a consequence of blockade of the open calcium channel, ectopic cells firing at relatively high rates will be depressed in preference to the SA node, and sinus rhythm can be restored.

In a recent study[11] on the influence of the severity of ventricular dysfunction on hemodynamic responses to intravenously administered verapamil in ischemic heart diseases, it was found that patients with chronic angina (N = 15) exhibited reductions in systolic and diastolic pressures, mean arterial pressure, and systemic vascular resistance. In addition, the stroke work index was reduced by 13 percent. Patients with uncomplicated acute myocardial infarction (N = 7) behaved in a similar manner to the patients with chronic angina. However, in three patients with pulmonary capillary wedge pressures in the range of 20 to 29 mm Hg, verapamil increased the pulmonary wedge pressure by 7 to 10 mm Hg; in all three patients the mean arterial pressure was reduced. Overall, verapamil was found to exert only a minor myocardial depressant effect in patients with normal or moderately reduced ventricular function. However, when the left ventricular ejection fraction is severely reduced or pulmonary capillary pressure is substantially elevated, verapamil may lead to enhanced cardiac decompensation. In the latter instances, the reduction in ventricular afterload is not sufficient to overcome the depressant effect on cardiac contractility.

Verapamil is metabolized in the liver, thereby markedly reducing the amount of drug that reaches the heart following oral administration.[12] Patients with impaired liver function should be treated with lower doses of verapamil; otherwise, severe hypotension may ensue. Thirteen patients, aged 6 weeks to 16 years, with uncontrolled recurrent supraventricular tachycardia, were given intravenous verapamil (0.1 mg per kg over 30 seconds) to abolish the arrhythmia.[13] In seven patients, conversion to sinus rhythm occurred after parenteral administration of verapamil, and, subsequently, four of the seven were maintained on oral verapamil. Two of the patients, 6 weeks and 8 months old, with junctional ectopic foci, suffered severe hypotension following intravenous administration of verapamil. Each patient had to receive intravenous injections of calcium chloride to counteract the severe hypotension. Caution should be used in treating patients under one year old because we have no information on the rate of metabolism of verapamil by such young persons, nor do we know the volume of distribution. The intravenous injection of verapamil was administered to these young patients over a 30-second period, which may be too short an interval, allowing the bolus concentration reaching the heart to increase to a toxic range. Administration over a 2-minute interval, as used in the previously cited study in adults,[11] would appear to be a safer method.

The primary hemodynamic effects of diltiazem are related to systemic vasodilation, and the drug appears to be a more selective vasodilator for the coronary and cerebral circulations.[14] With large oral doses (180 to 270 mg) or intravenous administration, systemic vasodilation predominates. Lower doses administered orally decrease the heart rate and produce a slight negative inotropic effect in patients with no significant ventricular dysfunction. However, diltiazem exhibits less negative inotropic effect than verapamil.[15]

Diltiazem is almost completely absorbed (95 percent) after oral administration and undergoes extensive hepatic metabolism. The primary metabolite, desacetyl diltiazem, has 25 to 50 percent of the activity of diltiazem. Diltiazem is highly protein-bound, with 20 percent bound to albumin and 60 percent to alpha 2 glycoprotein. After oral administration, peak plasma levels are reached in 1 to 2 hours, and the plasma half-life is 4 to 5.5 hours.

Nifedipine is also almost completely absorbed (90 percent) after oral administration and is metabolized in the liver to a pyridine derivative that shows no pharmacologic activity. Nifedipine is strongly bound to albumin (92 percent) and is highly unstable when exposed to light. Peak levels are reached between 1 and 2 hours after oral administration. Disappearance from plasma occurs in two phases. The first phase of disappearance has a half-life of 50 minutes during the first 3 hours and a half-life of 2.5 hours over the next 8 hours.

Nifedipine exerts a more potent negative inotropic effect than either diltiazem or verapamil; however, this does not appear to be of major clinical significance. The primary effects encountered after oral administration are a fall in blood pressure, an increase in cardiac output, and a reduction in left ventricular filling pressure.[15]

In addition to the effects on smooth and cardiac muscles, calcium entry blockers may exhibit other potentially useful therapeutic actions on peripheral circulatory disturbances. The viscosity of blood is determined in part by the deformability of red blood cells, especially in the microcirculation. Hypoxia causes an increase in blood viscosity, and this effect can be reduced by calcium entry blockers. However, it is not known whether the decrease in viscosity is due to an effect on the red blood cells or on platelets. In some instances, changes in capillary permeability may be due to a change in shape of capillary endothelial cells, thereby increasing the leakage of albumin into tissue spaces. Such changes may be related to calcium action in endothelial cell actomyosin-like proteins. Calcium entry blockers have been shown to decrease peripheral edema formation in some cases, suggesting that increased calcium entry into endothelial cells may underlie certain types of peripheral edema.[16]

REFERENCES

1. NAYLOR, WG, AND GRINWALD, P: *Calcium entry blockers and myocardial function*. Fed Proc 40:2855, 1981.

2. VANHOUTTE, PM: *Differential effects of calcium entry blockers on vascular smooth muscle*. In WEISS, GB (ED): *New Perspectives on Calcium Antagonists*. Clinical Physiology Series, American Physiological Society, Bethesda, Maryland, 1981, p. 109.

3. FLECKENSTEIN-GRUN, G AND FLECKENSTEIN, A: *Calcium-Antagonisus, ein Grundprinzip der Vasodilation*. In FLECKENSTEIN, A, AND RASKAMM, H (EDS): *Calcium-Antagonismas*. Springer-Verlag, Berlin, Heidelberg, New York, 1980, p. 191.

4. FLECKENSTEIN, A: *Pharmacology and electrophysiology of calcium antagonists*. In *Calcium Antagonism in Cardiovascular Therapy: Experience with Verapamil. International Symposium, Florence, October 2–4*. Excerpta Medica, Amsterdam, Oxford, Princeton, 1980.

5. FLECKENSTEIN, A: *Die Bedeutung der energiereichen Phosphate fur Kontraktilitat und toluen des Myokards*. Verh Disch Ges inn Med 70th Congress, 1964, p 80.

6. FLECKENSTEIN, A: *Specific inhibitors and promoters of calcium action in excitation-contraction coupling of heart muscle and their role in the prevention or production of myocardial lesions*. In HARRIS, P AND OPIE, L (EDS): *Calcium and the Heart*. Academic Press, London, New York, 1971, p. 135.

7. KAYADA, S: *Pharmacology of dihydropyridines*. Symposium on Calcium Antagonists, New York, June 19–20. Sponsored by Miles Institute for Preclinical Pharmacology, New Haven, 1980, p 7.

8. CRANFIELD, P: *The Conduction of the Cardiac Impulse*. Futura Publishing, Mt Kisco, New York, 1975.

9. REUTER, H: *Properties of two inward membrane currents in the heart*. Ann Rev Physiol 44:413, 1979.

10. TRITTHART, N, FLECKENSTEIN, B, and FLECKENSTEIN, A: *Some fundamental actions of antiarrhythmic drugs on the excitability and the contractility of single myocardial fibers*. Naunyn-Schmiedebergs Arch Pharmacol 269:212, 1971.

11. CHRISTOPHER, YC, HECHT, HS, COLLETT, JT, ET AL: *Influence of severity of ventricular dysfunction on hemodynamic response to intravenously administered verapamil in ischemic heart disease*. Am J Cardiol 47:917, 1981.

12. WILLENS, H, and ARONSON, RS: *Cardiac antiarrhythmic agents, 1981*. Cardiovascular Reviews and Reports 2:826, 1981.

13. PORTER, JC, GILLETTE, PC, GARSON, A, ET AL: *Effects of verapamil on supraventricular tachycardia in children*. Am J Cardiol 48:487, 1981.

14. ZELIS, R, AND SCHROEDER, JS: *Calcium, calcium antagonists and cardiovascular disease*. Chest 78:121, 1980.

15. FLAIM, SF, and ZELIS, R: *Clinical use of calcium entry blockers*. Fed Proc 40:2877, 1981.

16. VAN HOUTTE, PM: *Calcium entry blockers and cardiovascular failure*. Fed Proc 40:2882, 1981.

Treatment of Vasospastic Angina*

Rex MacAlpin, M.D.

INTRODUCTION

Definition

In a broad sense, the term "vasospastic angina" as used in this chapter encompasses all transient reversible episodes of myocardial ischemia due to severe coronary artery obstruction resulting wholly or in part from short-lived, active contraction of the coronary artery vascular smooth muscle. These episodes include symptomatic attacks as well as those without symptoms, which in some patients may be more numerous than those with symptoms.[1] Because most vasospastic angina is associated with the superimposition of coronary artery constriction on organic atherosclerotic disease, the possibility exists that in sufficiently diseased vessels physiologic degrees of strategically located coronary arterial smooth muscle constriction can produce enough obstruction to cause ischemia.[2,3] Many prefer to reserve the term "spasm" for an unphysiologic contraction. Hence there are some who favor the term "vasotonic angina."[4] The use of vasospastic angina in the following discussion is a convenience, a concession to common contemporary usage. Though it is not currently possible in most cases to determine clinically whether one is dealing with physiologic or nonphysiologic vascular smooth muscle activity, and though this distinction at present has few therapeutic implications, the reader is cautioned that such a distinction may assume practical importance in the future when more is known about the pathophysiologic mechanisms responsible for coronary artery constriction that causes myocardial ischemia.

Clinical Syndromes Included

The term vasospastic angina no longer applies just to variant angina.[1] It is now realized that coronary artery constriction can contribute to the production of a variety of clinical anginal syndromes. Spontaneous angina (angina with no apparent provoking cause) with either elevation or depression of the ST segment on the ECG is frequently due to coronary spasm.[1,5] This will include a large percentage of patients with "unstable angina."[1] In occasional cases, pure effort angina can be due to coronary spasm.[6] The sharp separation of variant and classic angina is usually not possible because many patients present a mixed picture in which classic and variant angina coexist. It is not rare for patients with spontaneous angina

*Supported in part by Grant HL 17591 from the National Institutes of Health and by a grant from Marion Laboratories, Kansas City, Missouri.

to have ST segment elevation during some attacks but ST segment depression in the same leads in others. Careful questioning of patients with classic angina frequently elicits clues suggesting a variable degree of coronary obstruction, for example, marked variability in effort tolerance from day to day or angina primarily on first effort of the day. This is not surprising in view of angiographic evidence that 30 to 40 percent of organic coronary stenoses in patients with classic anginal syndromes are not "fixed" but can change their dimensions under the influence of vasoactive drugs.[7-9]

Spasm of small, resistance coronary arterioles may occur and be an as yet undocumented cause of myocardial ischemia in the presence of normal large, epicardial coronary arteries.

Importance of Making a Firm Diagnosis

In devising a treatment program for a patient who is suspected of having vasospastic angina, it is essential first to make sure the diagnosis rests on the best objective documentation obtainable. Coronary vasospasm is becoming a popular diagnosis to pin on patients with atypical chest pain and no or mild coronary disease. The enormous medical, psychologic, and economic consequences of labeling a patient as having coronary heart disease must be appreciated before the fact. As far as possible, *objective* electrocardiographic, scintographic, or angiographic confirmation should be sought that the patient's symptom is indeed associated with myocardial ischemia. Noncardiac causes of chest pain that can mimic vasospastic angina, such as esophageal spasm, are common and hence will frequently coexist in patients with organic coronary disease. Noncardiac chest pain is often difficult to abolish by *any* measures in patients who because of pending litigation or other reason have little motivation to be relieved of symptoms.

When sure that myocardial ischemia is the cause of symptoms, it is further helpful to get some idea of the relative contributions of organic coronary obstruction and dynamic coronary constriction in the genesis of a patient's symptoms. In patients with angina at rest and an unlimited, symptom-free exercise capacity documented at treadmill testing, coronary artery spasm is usually the most important factor. Even when significant effort-induced angina accompanies frequent spontaneous anginal attacks, demonstration of a good, angina-free exercise capacity with treadmill testing done after premedication with an effective dose of nitroglycerin or a calcium channel blocker suggests the possibility of a significant role for coronary artery spasm and a good chance of abolishing all symptoms with vasodilator medication, even if important organic coronary obstruction is present. In such patients there is little to be gained from the use of beta-adrenergic antagonists. On the other hand, when effort-induced angina is a significant part of the symptomatology and when effort tolerance is markedly limited on treadmill testing even with vasodilator premedication, critical, organic coronary artery narrowing is usually present, and even complete paralysis of arterial smooth muscle could not be expected to abolish the stress-provoked angina. A trial of a beta-adrenergic antagonist *in conjunction with* arterial dilators might be appropriate.

I generally advise patients with spontaneous attacks of angina to have coronary arteriography as part of their evaluation. In conjunction with the results of exercise testing, this approach allows a better classification of patients for therapeutic and prognostic purposes,[10] allows selection of subjects in whom provocative testing for coronary artery spasm is appropriate and safe, and gives the physician a better feel for how far to push on with medical therapies before considering surgical treatment of the coronary obstruction. It also may allow detection of the rare case of transient recurrent coronary arterial occlusion not due to coronary spasm.[11,12]

Making observations on patients during their attacks is especially important in patients with a history of dizziness, lightheadedness, or syncope in conjunction with their angina. Patients with variant angina have a high incidence of serious, often life-threatening, arrhythmias with their attacks. The presence of such arrhythmias often dictates modification of therapy. Various types of tape systems for ambulatory, long-term recording of the ECG have aided the detection of transient ST segment shifts and these arrhythmias.

Difficulties in Evaluating Treatments for Vasospastic Angina

Little is known about the factors that control normal vasomotion of large coronary arteries and less about the causes of actual coronary artery spasm. Because the basic therapy for vasospastic angina involves interventions that dilate large coronary arteries and prevent their spontaneous contraction, much of what we know about this therapy is based on trial and error rather than on an understanding of the pathophysiology. This approach is complicated by the unpredictable natural course of coronary vasospasm. In a carefully controlled study of the effects of diltiazem in variant angina, there was a 30 percent incidence of complete absence of attacks during a period of placebo administration. [13] Many patients with vasospastic angina will have spontaneous remissions and not require long-term medication.[14,15] The clinical presentations of vasospastic angina are frequently dramatic and unstable, so that many physicians are unwilling to enroll such patients in double-blind, cross-over, placebo-controlled protocols for assessment of various treatments. Many of our present beliefs and practices in treating vasospastic angina are, therefore, based on anectodal experience in modest numbers of patients and on only a few well-constructed and well-executed drug trials in small groups of patients. Thus the reader is warned that the therapeutic concepts and practices summarized below will probably undergo considerable revision in the future with the advent of additional knowledge and new drugs.

ELIMINATION OF COMPLICATING ILLNESS AND ADVERSE ENVIRONMENTAL INFLUENCES

Coexisting Diseases

Conditions that might contribute to spontaneous angina and an unstable anginal syndrome should be sought out and treated. Anemia, hyperthyroidism, and uncontrolled hypertension are the most commonly encountered of these additional illnesses.

Illustrative Case No. 1

A 60-year-old man had been hospitalized in 1970 and again in 1976 for severe, single episodes of chest pain. No ECG or enzymatic abnormalities were found, and he remained otherwise free of cardiorespiratory symptoms. Mild hypertension, diagnosed in 1970, was being treated with 25 mg hydrochlorothiazide daily. In 1977, a treadmill test was negative, and the patient exhibited a good exercise capacity. Mycosis fungoides was diagnosed in 1973 and was controlled with local x-ray therapy, one course of chemotherapy, and immunotherapy.

In August 1980, an adenocarcinoma of the sigmoid colon was diagnosed by colonoscopy and biopsy. On August 20, 1980, he underwent a low anterior resection of his sigmoid colon with end-to-end anastomosis, with an estimated 900 ml operative blood loss. His preoperative hematocrit was 36 percent (hemoglobin 12.8 $g \cdot dl^{-1}$). There was some postoperative rectal bleeding, and by August 22 his hemotocrit had fallen to 29 percent. On August 23, at 3:00 AM, he awakened with severe, oppressive, retrosternal chest pain which was associated with a cold sweat and lasted 30 minutes before subsiding spontaneously. During the pain, in most ECG leads there was marked ST segment depression, which resolved with disappearance of the pain (Fig. 1). Similar episodes of chest pain occurred at 1:30 AM and 4:30 AM on August 25 and were relieved within a few minutes by sublingual nitroglycerin. At this time hematocrit was 28 percent (hemoglobin 9.6 $g \cdot dl^{-1}$). MB-creatine kinase blood levels remained

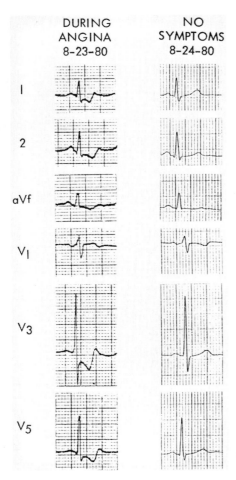

DURING
ANGINA
8-23-80

NO
SYMPTOMS
8-24-80

I

2

aVf

V₁

V₃

V₅

Figure 1. Electrocardiograms during (*left*) and after (*right*) spontaneous, nocturnal angina in a patient with an acute, euvolemic anemia due to subacute blood loss.

normal, as did the ECG between attacks. Between the 25th and 27th of August he received four units of packed red blood cells with stabilization of his hematocrit at 36 percent. He was also placed on nitroglycerin ointment at bedtime and 20 mg of propranolol four times daily. There were no further attacks of chest pain.

COMMENT. This patient illustrates one cause of unstable angina with attacks of myocardial ischemia at rest. Subclinical organic coronary arterial disease was unmasked by acute anemia. Correction of the anemia, along with other measures, abolished the spontaneous angina attacks. The early morning timing of attacks suggests the possibility that coronary vasoconstriction contributed to their genesis. It is interesting to speculate that with significant, pliable, organic coronary stenoses, normal circadian changes in vasomotor tone of large coronary arteries might induce, in the presence of anemia, a myocardial "ischemia" which would not have occurred with a normal hemoglobin level. If this were true, then treatment with transfusion alone, or organic nitrate vasodilators alone, might have abolished the angina, making propranolol therapy unnecessary. The subsequent finding of a normal ECG response to exercise or atrial pacing when hemoglobin levels were up would support this hypothesis, and would be helpful in planning rational long-term therapy for his ischemic heart disease.

Hyperthyroidism

Hyperthyroidism can provoke unstable angina merely by increasing the metabolic needs of the heart to the limit of the ability of a diseased coronary system to satisfy them. The patient then becomes the prisoner of minor changes in heart rate, blood pressure, sympathetic drive, or coronary artery tone. Moreover, some cases of vasospastic angina have been associated with hyperthyroidism, and some of these have even gone into remission upon resolution of the hyperthyroid state.[16,17]

Hypertension

Speculation that some vasospastic angina is part of a more general disorder of vascular smooth muscle reactivity has been encouraged by findings of some investigators of an unusually high incidence of associated Raynaud's phenomenon and migraine in patients with variant angina.[5,18] Although Waters and coworkers[18] could not show that the 40 percent incidence of hypertension in their variant angina group was significantly greater than that in their control population, the finding of the same high incidence in my own group of 75 patients with variant angina leads me to suspect some connection between the two conditions.

One possible connection is the effect of some antihypertensive medications on the coronary circulation. It is not rare in my experience for variant angina to begin shortly after a change in antihypertensive medication, especially after the institution of propranolol or other beta-adrenergic antagonists.[19] In this setting, the discontinuation of the beta-adrenergic blocking agent may result in control of anginal symptoms.

Severe hypertension can increase cardiac oxygen needs enough for angina at rest to occur in patients with preexisting stable coronary disease. Treatment of the hypertension with drug regimens that do not produce coronary artery constriction will usually stabilize symptoms again.

Environmental Influences

A careful search should be made for factors present in the external or internal environment of a patient that may be causing or aggravating the condition, and attempts should be made to eliminate any that are found. Some of these factors are listed in Table 1 and discussed below.

Vasoconstricting Substances

Tobacco smoking is so common in the general population that it is no wonder that many patients with vasospastic angina are afflicted with this habit. The vasoconstricting effects of nicotine are well known. Although tobacco smoking can rarely be a major cause of a patient's symptoms,[20,21] and even though it is *prudent* to get patients to stop this practice, I have not seen evidence in my own experience or in the published literature that convinces me that this is of definite therapeutic usefulness against vasospastic angina. For example, it is most

Table 1. Some vasoconstricting influences to which a patient might be exposed

---

Smoking

Parasympathomimetics (e.g., pilocarpine, methacholine)

Alpha-adrenergic agonists (e.g., phenylephrine, phenylopropanolamine, amphetamines, epinephrine in patients on propranolol)

Beta-adrenergic antagonists (e.g., propranolol, metoprolol)

Ergot alkaloids (e.g., ergotamine, ergonovine, methysergide)

Lysergic acid diethylamide (LSD)

Aspirin (particularly in high dose), indomethacin, and other cyclooxygenase inhibitors

Sudden withdrawal from organic nitrates (e.g., discontinuation of high dose isosorbide dinitrate; weekends for munitions workers)

Exercise (only in certain patients)

---

unusual for cessation of smoking to produce a definite change in the severity of variant angina attacks.

For other ailments or for recreation, individual patients may take various vasoactive drugs that have the potential for precipitating or aggravating vasospastic angina. These drugs should be discontinued in patients suffering from vasospastic angina and replaced with other agents if necessary.

PARASYMPATHOMIMETIC AGENTS. Provocation of attacks of variant angina has been reported following the use of pilocarpine[22] and methacholine, and the latter agent has been used as a diagnostic agent to bring on attacks of coronary artery spasm in patients with variant angina.[23] Although the mechanisms of this action are not known for sure, acetylcholine does produce contraction of in vitro coronary artery preparations from some animal species[24,25] and humans.[26]

ALPHA-ADRENERGIC AGONISTS. Drugs such as phenylephrine, ephedrine, and paredrine are present in many common over-the-counter remedies for colds, hay fever, and asthma. Stimulation of alpha-adrenergic receptors of coronary arteries, such as can occur with these agents, produces vasoconstriction.[26] Alpha-adrenergic stimulation has been used successfully as a provocative test for coronary artery spasm, in the form of epinephrine in patients premedicated with propranolol.[27]

BETA-ADRENERGIC ANTAGONISTS. Theoretically, by blocking the vasodilating influence of beta-adrenergic stimulation, these agents can be responsible for vasoconstriction by leaving alpha-adrenergic influences unopposed. Indeed, one does see modest constriction of coronary arteries angiographically following administration of propranolol.[7] There is clinical evidence that in some patients with vasospastic angina (particularly variant angina), beta-adrenergic blockers may aggravate symptoms (see section on beta-adrenergic blockers). The use of specific $beta_1$ antagonists (such as metoprolol) may not overcome this difficulty because coronary arterial beta-adrenergic receptors could be primarily $beta_1$ in nature.[28]

ERGOT ALKALOIDS. Ergotamine is commonly used for treatment of acute migraine attacks, and methysergide for the prevention of migraine and other vascular headaches. Ergonovine and methylergonovine are used in obstetrics and gynecology to produce uterine contraction. All these agents are potent arterial constrictors and should be avoided in patients suspected of vasospastic angina. Ergonovine and methylergonovine are being used increasingly and successfully in a diagnostic setting to provoke coronary artery spasm in susceptible persons[15,29] and presently are the agents of choice for this purpose.

PSYCHOMIMETIC DRUGS. Illegal, recreational use of psychoactive drugs is widespread in this country.

Amphetamine Abuse. Agents such as amphetamine, dextroamphetamine, and methamphetamine are used therapeutically as central nervous system stimulants to overcome fatigue, to treat narcolepsy, and to inhibit appetite. (It is of historical interest that Myron Prinzmetal first described the use of amphetamine for narcolepsy.[30]) These agents are sympathomimetic amines that have varying degrees of peripheral effects, including *vasoconstriction*. Their medical uses are perhaps overshadowed by their abuse for producing a euphoric "high." These drugs should be avoided by patients with vasospastic angina.

Cocaine. Illegal use of this central nervous system stimulant has grown markedly in recent years. Used clinically as a local anesthetic, cocaine can produce intense sympathetic stimulation by a combination of central and peripheral effects—one result of which may be vasoconstriction. It would seem prudent for patients with coronary vasospasm to avoid its use.

Lysergic Acid Diethylamide (LSD). This "hallucinogenic" drug has no recognized therapeutic use. It is structurally closely related to ergonovine and shares some of the latter drug's peripheral actions, including vasoconstriction. Patients with coronary vasospasm should be warned against its use.

CYCLOOXYGENASE INHIBITORS. The prostaglandins may play a role in the regulation of vascular smooth muscle tone and seem to be the only naturally occurring vasoactive agents capable of altering resting tone of human coronary artery segments in vitro.[26] Inhibition of formation of cyclic endoperoxides from arachidonic acid by cyclooxygenase inhibitors such as aspirin and indomethacin effectively prevents formation of both prostacyclin (a vasodilator) by the arterial wall and thromboxane A_2 (a vasoconstrictor) by platelets. The balance between the actions of these two substances is such that indomethacin administration to in vitro preparations of coronary arteries usually produces vasoconstriction,[26] raising the possibility that clinical use of this drug may aggravate vasospastic angina. Clinically, there is no evidence that low dose (0.3 gm daily) aspirin either improves or worsens vasospastic angina. However, a recent study from Japan demonstrated an aggravating effect of high dose aspirin (4 gm daily) on effort-provoked and spontaneous angina in patients with variant angina.[31] Until more is known about the role of prostaglandins and their antagonists on coronary vasomotion, it would be wise to ask patients with vasospastic angina to avoid the use of aspirin, indomethacin, and like drugs.

NITRATES. Although their direct action on blood vessels is vasodilation and they are important drugs in treatment of vasospastic angina, organic nitrate vasodilators such as nitroglycerin in chronic usage can condition arterial smooth muscle to develop tolerance to their action and, upon sudden withdrawal, leave behind a temporary state of *increased* tone. This "rebound" vasoconstriction produces a clinical syndrome of "weekend angina" in certain susceptible individuals working in munition plants where chronic, heavy nitrate exposure during the week followed by a sudden weekend withdrawal from exposure leads to manifestations of coronary vasospasm—angina pectoris or even myocardial infarction.[32] Such a rebound phenomenon from chronic nitrate exposure following therapeutic use of organic nitrate vasodilators for coronary heart disease has been encountered.[33] Sudden withdrawal of organic nitrates or other vasodilator therapy should be avoided in patients with coronary disease, but particularly in those with vasospastic angina.

Other Factors that May Influence Vasospasm

In individual cases, peculiar agents or circumstances may be responsible for provoking attacks of coronary artery spasm. These conditions should be meticulously sought out in taking the patient's history, and, if present, they should be eliminated whenever possible by changes in personal habits or daily routine.

EATING AND DRINKING. Occasional patients will note a provocation of their vasospastic angina following ingestion of alcoholic beverages[34] or cold drinks[35,36] or after eating.[36-38] In one case attacks seemed to occur only during hypoglycemia or after insulin was given.[39]

EXERCISE. Vasospastic angina can be provoked by effort in some patients.[40,41] This is particularly likely to occur in variant angina patients with the first effort of the day.[40,42] Symptoms from this provocation can be minimized by the liberal use of nitroglycerin or other coronary artery dilator immediately upon awakening and just before any exertion and by a gradual warm up before exercising.

DRUG THERAPY—GENERAL PRINCIPLES

The mainstay of treatment of vasospastic angina is a program of appropriate vasodilator medication carefully tailored to the patient's individual needs.

Goals of Drug Therapy

The ideal result of treatment would be a permanent cure of patient's symptoms and total freedom from attacks of myocardial ischemia without need for further medication. Although this not infrequently occurs spontaneously as the result of unknown factors, we cannot *predictably* achieve it with any *known* therapy.

135

Complete abolition of attacks can actually be attained with proper medication in up to 80 percent of patients, and significant reduction in frequency and severity of attacks occurs in most of the remaining cases. Because total prevention of attacks in many cases would require the use of frequent and high doses of two or more drugs (some still experimental) with trials of various drugs and titration of doses taking months to accomplish, what is a realistic therapeutic goal for the average patient? Because a cure is not always available, the relief of symptoms to the point that they no longer significantly interfere with a patient's desired life style and the minimization of chances of a life-threatening attack are reasonable ends to attain. It is apparent that the degree of control required for these ends will vary from case to case. The retired, sedentary patient may be satisfied if subject to only a few mild attacks per week—a situation possibly unacceptable to a high-rise construction worker, motorcycle racer, or trapeze artist. Physicians should diligently strive for absolute prevention of attacks, particularly in patients whose attacks are sometimes accompanied by life-threatening arrhythmias. Such patients can be identified often by a history of dizziness, faintness, or actual syncope during attacks, even if arrhythmias have not been documented during observation of some attacks not associated with such symptoms.

What Is an Effective Drug? An Effective Dose?

Vasodilator drugs of proven or potential use in vasospastic angina are listed in Table 2 and discussed below.

Timing of Doses

It must be remembered that even the most effective of these agents, nitrates and calcium channel blockers, will do no good if they are not present in effective concentrations in the body at times when the patient is susceptible to attacks. To achieve this goal in a patient whose attacks invariably occur at the same time of day, for example, between 2:00 AM and 4:00 AM, a single daily dose of medication at midnight or 1:00 AM may be sufficient; but a dose of medicine at 10:00 PM or 11:00 PM may not last long enough to cover the patient at 3:00 AM, because 4 to 6 hours is the effective duration of action of many of these agents. It may be necessary for the patient to use an alarm clock to awaken in the middle of the night for a dose to cover this period. Sometimes a double dose of drug at bedtime will keep the blood level high enough to achieve the same end. If the major attacks usually occur just after awakening in the morning or with the very first activity of the day (brushing teeth or dressing,

Table 2. Drugs for vasospastic angina

Of Proven Efficacy
    calcium channel blockers (e.g., nifedipine, verapamil, diltiazem)
    organic nitrates (e.g., nitroglycerin, isosorbide dinitrate)
Of Possible Use in Selected Cases, But Efficacy Not Proven
    alpha-adrenergic blockers (e.g., dibenzylene, phentolamine)
    beta-adrenergic blockers if used with organic nitrates
    atropine
    amiodarone
    beta-adrenergic agonists (e.g., nylidrin)
    specific thromboxane A_2 antagonists
Ineffective Drugs
    dipyridamole
    anticoagulants
Possibly Harmful Drugs
    beta-adrenergic blockers used alone
    cyclooxygenase inhibitors (e.g., aspirin, indomethacin)

for example), a rapidly acting drug such as sublingual nitroglycerin or isosorbide dinitrate should be taken immediately upon awakening.

The usual patient with vasospastic angina is subject to attacks that occur unpredictably at any time of day or night. In this case, drug therapy must cover the entire 24-hour daily cycle. To achieve this with available agents, whose effectiveness extends 6 to 8 hours *at most,* doses must be taken every 6 to 8 hours. In the case of some drugs and some patients, every 3 to 4 hours dosing is necessary; and in some very unstable and difficult-to-manage patients, a constant intravenous drug infusion is required to control attacks.

The efficacy of therapy is most easily gauged by relief of patients' symptoms, and having patients keep a written log of attacks helps in this regard. Ambulatory tape recording of the ECG may also be helpful in patients whose attacks are frequent. Because the majority of ischemic attacks may be unaccompanied by pain, this Holter-type ECG recording is the only way to be sure of actual disease control in patients rendered asymptomatic by drug therapy.[43,44] It is essential in the rare case of vasospastic myocardial ischemia without any angina.[45] The use of exercise testing as a guide to therapy may be useful in the selected case.[46]

Waters and colleagues[15] at the Montreal Heart Institute have studied the use of an ergonovine provocative test to determine if, on a specific treatment program, a patient is still subject to attacks of coronary artery spasm. The use of such a maneuver to guide therapy will have to be studied in larger groups of patients before its use in routine treatment can be recommended.

Titration of Doses

The treatment of vasospastic angina is not for those physicians who believe in "cookbook" medicine. There is such variability of attack rate, of patient drug requirement, of side effects from medication, and of patient compliance that the treatment of each case must be tailored to the patient's particular needs; and the minimum effective dose of medication must be found by a process of *titration,* which may take days, weeks, or even months. Starting with a low dose of drug that rarely causes side effects, the dose is gradually increased until one of several possible endpoints is achieved: abolition of symptoms, development of intolerable side effects, or reaching the maximum drug dose deemed safe. The importance of pursuing dose increases to a logical conclusion cannot be overemphasized. Many patients referred to me with "intractable" vasospastic angina have never before been given effective doses of organic nitrate vasodilators and respond nicely to an increase in dosage of their medicine.

I have found that requesting the patient to keep a written daily log of attacks is of great assistance during this titration phase. The patient records the time, severity, and any unusual circumstances of each attack; the number of nitroglycerin tablets used; and the time at which each dose of regular medication was actually taken. From this data it is easy to recognize patterns which assist in adjusting medication dose. If attacks cluster in periods just before the next dose of medicine, the interval between doses may need to be decreased. If there is a time of day that the patient is particularly symptomatic, the dose preceding that period may need to be increased. Because not all attacks of myocardial ischemia are symptomatic, it is wise to check a 24-hour ambulatory tape recording of the ECG at the beginning of therapy and again after symptomatic attacks are controlled in order to detect asymptomatic ischemia episodes.

In outpatients, much of the communication between doctor and patient needed to titrate the dose of medicine properly can be handled by phone to maximize patient convenience and use of physician's time. Patients need be seen only often enough to detect serious side effects (for example, postural hypotension) or to evaluate new or worsening symptoms.

Patient Compliance

Because medication usually has to be taken four to six times a day, every day, to prevent attacks of vasospastic angina, patient compliance with the prescribed program is sometimes a problem. No medicine will be effective if it never reaches the patient's body. Patients tend to forget doses when they come at inconvenient times of the day, particularly when the medication has completely abolished attacks or when they sense no improvement from a drug. The occasional patient who gets an attack each time the medicine has been forgotten has a built-in reminder and motivation. But the situation is not so simple in most cases. Continued efforts by the physician to educate the patient about the nature of the illness and the rationale for using specific medicines and dosages will maximize patient cooperation. Unfortunately, tests for blood or urine levels of the most useful drugs are not generally available but would be helpful in assessing compliance objectively in difficult cases (where absolute knowledge is essential to management).

Because of the possibility of rebound worsening of vasospastic attacks after sudden withdrawal of vasodilator medicine (particularly nitrates), patients should be warned to avoid doing this and advised of the reasons for this warning.

Combinations of Different Drug Types

Not every patient will have a completely adequate response to a single type of vasodilator. It is frequently necessary to combine two drugs with different modes of action. Nitrates and calcium channel blocking agents are the two most commonly combined classes of drugs, and their conjoint use is frequently successful in controlling symptoms for which either drug singly gives an insufficient response. Except in the most urgent and life-threatening cases (for example, where serious arrhythmias accompany attacks), it is preferable to start with only one type of drug and to increase its dose by titration. If no response is noted to maximum tolerable doses, then it is justifiable to stop this drug and to commence another type of agent. If definite but incomplete response is found with one drug class, then to the highest tolerable dose of the first drug can be added a low dose of a second drug type, with subsequent upward dose titration. If complete abolition of attacks is then achieved, in cases where attacks do not have life-threatening implications, the dose of the first drug can be gradually reduced, even to the point of discontinuance, to determine if the patient's symptoms remain controlled on the second drug alone. The calcium channel blocking drugs—diltiazem, verapamil, and nifedipine—cannot be considered as having identical modes of action, so patients unresponsive to one of these drugs may respond to another given alone or to a combination of two.[47]

Treatment of the Acute Attack Versus Long-Term Prophylaxis

For the abolition of an anginal attack that is already present, a vasodilator with very rapid onset of action is desired. Sublingual nitroglycerin is best for this because a therapeutic effect usually begins within 30 seconds. Many patients note that attacks are more rapidly and reliably aborted if they use this drug *at the first inkling* of an attack, whereas its efficacy is less if first taken after the attack becomes well established.[48] The attacks of some patients are so very brief and predictably self-limited that these patients elect to take no medication when the attack starts because, they claim, the attack will be over before any medicine can take effect. In general, I discourage this practice because one never knows ahead of time how severe an attack is going to be or how long it will last. Episodes of coronary artery spasm that result in myocardial infarction, sudden death, or at least a visit to the emergency room are usually indistinguishable from mild anginal attacks during their first 30 seconds. Therefore, I advise patients with vasospastic angina to carry sublingual nitroglycerin tablets with them at all times and to use them at the first suspicion that an attack is beginning.

The duration of effect of sublingual nitroglycerin is brief, and the *prevention* of attacks requires longer-acting medication because it is unrealistic to expect patients to take nitroglycerin every 15 minutes throughout the day. Long-acting organic nitrates and calcium channel blockers are primary drugs for this purpose.

138

How Long Should Therapy Be Continued?

Treatment is usually continued indefinitely in patients who continue to have symptoms. The natural history of vasospastic angina is varied and unpredictable. In many cases there is a tendency for spontaneous improvement with time,[1,10] and a stage is reached when drug therapy can be stopped without recurrence of symptoms.[14,15] For some patients, this stage may be reached after only a few weeks or months of treatment.[14] In patients who have remained free of symptoms for many months, the question arises of when it is safe to stop medication. A number of approaches are available. First, medication can be abruptly discontinued and the patient observed for recurrent attacks, with the admonition to resume previous medicines if any attack occurs. The possibility of rebound vasosconstriction exists in this setting,[49] with the patient unprotected by any medication with the first recurrence.

A variation of this technique has been used by Waters and his coworkers[15] in Montreal. They had their patients stop the medicines for a suitable period (usually 24 to 48 hours), and then they performed an inpatient ergonovine maleate provocative test. Of 22 patients with variant angina who had responded well to calcium channel blockers but who had had a positive ergonovine test before the institution of therapy, 12 had a negative ergonovine test following discontinuation of therapy, and none of these had a recurrence of angina without medication in the next 1 to 13 (average 4.2) months of followup. Ten patients had a positive, post-therapy ergonovine test and were placed back on drug treatment. This type of maneuver will need further study before it can be an accepted practice, but it is an ingenious attempt to get *quickly* an answer to a difficult therapeutic problem.

Another approach, which is available to every physician, is, after a suitably long time of freedom from attacks, to reduce gradually the dose of one drug at a time at intervals of 1 week to 1 month, until the patient is off all medication or until attacks resume. Again, the patient must be advised to resume the previously effective dose of medicine *at once* if an attack recurs and to let the doctor know immediately.

Yet another way to treat this question is to keep patients on the medication indefinitely. (Why change a winning game?) Aside from the inconvenience and not inconsiderable expense of chronic drug therapy, many patients do not feel *really well* as long as they have to take any medicine. And providing they can *safely* be withdrawn from dependence on drugs, it is desirable to do so. But there's the rub—safety. Patients whose attacks of vasospastic angina have resulted in one or more occasions of life-threatening arrhythmias can never be withdrawn safely from effective drug therapy, and there is little justification for attempting to do so, because a first recurrent attack has the potential to produce sudden death. I advise such patients that they should remain on effective drug therapy for the rest of their lives.

Illustrative Case No. 2

A 43-year-old woman was in apparent good health until November 1977, when hypertension was discovered during a brief hospitalization for removal of laryngeal polyps. She was started on 125 mg of alpha-methyldopa three times a day. About 2 weeks later she was awakened from sleep at 5:00 AM by her first attack of oppressive, retrosternal chest pain, which lasted about 3 minutes. She subsequently had frequent recurrences of this pain, which occurred usually between 3:00 AM and 7:00 AM or with the first effort of the day, but occasionally it occurred at other times of the day. A Holter ECG recording demonstrated marked ST segment elevation in an inferior lead during chest pains, sometimes complicated by asymptomatic Wenckebach-type second-degree atrioventricular block. ECG between attacks was normal. A treadmill stress test to heart rate of 180 per minute provoked neither symptoms nor ECG abnormalities. Coronary arteriograms revealed a 60 percent diameter stenosis of the right coronary artery just distal to the catheter tip, which dilated to a 30 percent stenosis after nitroglycerin. The rest of the right coronary artery and the left coronary arteries showed only a few minor luminal irregularities.

Treatment with propranolol, atropine, isosorbide dinitrate sublingually, Nitro-bid capsules, and nitroglycerin ointment at bedtime failed to improve her symptoms. She did not choose to use sublingual nitroglycerin for acute attacks because of their brief duration and the headache it caused. Her hypertension was treated with Dyazide and alpha-methyldopa. In May 1978, because of continued frequent anginal attacks (longest angina-free period in 6 months was 1 week), she was started on 80 mg of verapamil four times a day, and thereafter had no further attacks despite discontinuance of all organic nitrate vasodilators.

In August 1978, verapamil and alpha-methyldopa were stopped because of progressive rise in SGPT (to 755 units) and other liver enzymes. Over the next 6 weeks there was a fall in liver enzyme levels to nearly normal, but there was also a recurrence of anginal attacks with crescendoing frequency. Verapamil was restarted at 80 mg three times a day in September 1978, with complete disappearance of angina within 3 days. Progressive increase in levels of liver enzymes over the next month forced discontinuance of verapamil again in October 1978, followed within three days by recurrence of angina with increasing frequency up to nine attacks a day. At this time she was taking only Dyazide and, as needed, sublingual nitroglycerin. Ten days after stopping the verapamil, during an anginal attack at 7:30 AM, she suffered a cardiac arrest due to ventricular fibrillation. She was resuscitated by paramedics who were called by her daughter, and was immediately hospitalized. There were no permanent neurologic or cardiac sequelae, and the ECG remained normal. Three days after this event, she was started on 10 mg of nifedipine four times a day, with an increase in dose to 60 mg daily two weeks later because of a few mild attacks on the lower dose. She has had no further anginal episodes despite a reduction in dose to 50 mg daily in December 1980, because of a transient rise in levels of liver enzymes. After starting nifedipine she no longer had need for other antihypertensive medication.

COMMENT. This patient had a remarkable and complete response of her vasospastic angina to calcium channel blockers. Although she had not previously manifested serious arrhythmias with her attacks, following a second discontinuation of verapamil she sustained a cardiac arrest during a period of crescendoing angina while on no prophylactic vasodilator medication. This emphasizes the potential risks such patients face if withdrawn from effective medication, even after prolonged periods of freedom from symptoms. This patient should have been put on some other vasodilator as soon as her angina recurred, until arrangements could have been made to obtain nifedipine for her (it was still an investigational drug at the time). The importance of a patient notifying the physician of a recurrence of angina in these circumstances is obvious. This patient will probably be kept on effective vasodilator medication indefinitely.

INDIVIDUAL DRUGS

Organic Nitrate Vasodilators

These drugs were the mainstay of the treatment of vasospastic angina in the United States until the general availability of calcium channel blocking drugs, but even though the latter are now on the market, the organic nitrates will remain very important. Many drugs of this class are available in a variety of preparations. Table 3 presents some major pharmacologic characteristics of the preparations most commonly used. "Long-acting" compounds other than isosorbide dinitrate are available in sublingual or oral preparations (for example, erythrityl tetranitrate and pentaerythritol tetranitrate); and though there is little information on their efficacy for vasospastic angina, there is no reason to believe that what is true for equivalent isosorbide dinitrate preparations will not prove true also for them.

Table 3. Organic nitrate preparations

Drug	Preparations available	Dosage range	Onset of action	Duration of action
nitroglycerin	sublingual tablets 0.15, 0.3, 0.4, and 0.6 mg	0.15–0.6 mg	30–60 sec	15–20 min
	2% ointment (contains ~15 mg per inch)	¼–3 inches on the skin every 3–12 hr	15 min	up to 4 hr
	intravenous solution	50–300 μg IV bolus; 10–100 μg/min as constant infusion IV; 50–300 μg bolus intracoronary	within 10–20 sec	15–20 min after infusion stopped
isosorbide dinitrate	sublingual tablets 2.5, 5, and 10 mg	2.5–15 mg every 1–4 hr	2–5 min	1–2 hr
	chewable tablets 5 and 10 mg (scored)	2.5–15 mg every 1–4 hr	2–5 min	1–2 hr
	oral tablets 5, 10, 20, and 30 mg (scored)	2.5–80 mg every 6 hr	15–30 min	4–6 hr
	sustained release oral tablets and capsules 40 mg	40–80 mg every 6–12 hr	15–30 min	up to 12 hr
	intravenous solution*	1.25–15 mg/hr as constant infusion	30–60 sec	up to 2 hr after infusion stopped
	ointment*			

*Not commercially available in USA.

All drugs of this class have an identical mechanism of action, and their effects differ mainly by virtue of different modes and rates of absorption and elimination, different speeds of onset of action, and different duration of action.

Nitroglycerin and isosorbide dinitrate relax smooth muscle in general and vascular smooth muscle in particular. These agents have been shown angiographically to produce up to a 40 percent increase in diameter of large normal coronary arteries in unpremedicated humans.[7,8,9,50–53] Increase in luminal diameter of 30 to 60 percent at the sites of organic coronary stenosis is also produced by these drugs.[7,8,9,54] There is some controversy whether coronary arteries in patients with vasospastic angina are more responsive to nitrates than those of other patients.[7,9,53] Yasue[55] claims that in variant angina patients, nitroglycerin dilates the large coronary arteries more in the early morning (about 70 percent increase in diameter) than in the afternoon (about 10 percent increase in diameter). Nitroglycerin is also effective in overcoming the vasoconstriction and coronary artery spasm produced by ergonovine,[29,56–60] although occasionally it may have to be given directly into the coronary artery to be effective.[61,62] Organic nitrates also dilate capacitance veins, causing a shift of blood away from the heart, thus reducing cardiac preload, and to a lesser extent they dilate arterioles, reducing cardiac afterload. Until recently these extracoronary effects that result in reduced myocardial oxygen requirements were believed to be the sole reason for the efficacy of organic nitrates in angina pectoris.[63] It is, however, now realized that the direct effects of these agents on large coronary arteries may contribute significantly to their action in many patients with classic angina and are the major reason for their *particular* effectiveness in vasospastic angina.

The principal side effects of this class of drugs are headache and hypotension, both of which can be very severe on occasion. Fortunately, in most cases a dose can be found that is effective in treating or preventing vasospastic angina without producing intolerable side effects. A means of ensuring that a patient will become afraid or unwilling to take the medicine needed is to prescribe too high a dose to start with, producing severe, throbbing headache on the first few doses. I have seen such experiences make patients *permanently* unwilling to take nitrates. Some patients are exquisitely sensitive to nitrates, and syncope within minutes of their first exposure to an "average" dose of sublingual nitroglycerin or isosorbide dinitrate is a dramatic event that can be confusing diagnostically, particularly if it occurs during the course of a spontaneous anginal attack.

To minimize the chances of such adverse reactions, physicians should start patients on the smallest available dose, and titrate the dose upward thereafter, depending on the presence of side effects and therapeutic response. Patients differ so widely in their responses to nitrates that it is my practice to administer the first dose of sublingual or chewable nitrates with the patient under observation in the examining room. Occasional patients will be found who need to cut the smallest strength sublingual tablets into two to four approximately equal pieces in order to get a small enough dose to avoid side effects (a practice that causes pharmacists to pale visibly). Fortunately most patients will develop a partial tolerance to the nitrates with chronic usage, so that the tendency for headache disappears while a therapeutic antianginal effect remains.[64]

There are suggestions that a rebound increased tendency to coronary vasoconstriction can result from chronic administration of high doses of organic nitrate vasodilators.[49,65,66] Therefore, patients should be warned that such drugs should not be stopped abruptly, and physicians desiring to discontinue them should do so by *gradually* tapering down the dose.

Nitroglycerin

SUBLINGUAL NITROGLYCERIN. Its rapid onset of action and ease of administration make this the preparation of choice for treatment of acute attacks of vasospastic angina. The drug is absorbed directly into the bloodstream through the sublingual mucous membranes, and detectable levels are found in the blood within 30 seconds; peak blood levels occur at about 2 minutes, and levels are no longer detectable much after 20 minutes.[67] Thus the therapeutic activity of the drug parallels its blood level.

Up to 90 percent of patients with variant angina claim that their attacks of spontaneous angina are abbreviated or aborted by sublingual nitroglycerin.[43,48,68-73] The evidence for this claim is subjective because carefully controlled studies on this matter would be difficult and have not been done. My experience suggests that most patients with other types of vasospastic angina experience a similar efficacy from sublingual nitroglycerin for acute attacks. Paradoxical reactions to sublingual nitroglycerin, in which focal coronary artery spasm actually seemed to result from the drug at the time of coronary arteriography in patients without vasospastic angina, are extremely rare and may have been related to the unusual environment of the catheterization laboratory, because the two cases reported had good therapeutic responses to the drug both before and after the catheterization procedure.[74]

The doses of sublingual nitroglycerin needed to produce nearly maximum attainable dilation of large coronary arteries in vivo are smaller than doses generally prescribed for angina. Feldman and coworkers[52] found about 50 percent of peak response at a 75 μg dose and 80 percent of peak response at a 150 μg dose, with no significant effect on heart rate or blood pressure at these levels. Increase in dose to 450 μg produced a fall in blood pressure and only 20 percent further increase in coronary artery diameter. Experiments in conscious instrumented dogs confirm that the drug's action on large coronary arteries (and venous capacitance vessels) occurs at doses much smaller than that needed to detect effects on peripheral or coronary arterioles.[75] This evidence gives further support to the practice of using the smallest dose of nitroglycerin that is effective in vasospastic angina. This is particularly true for patients with variant angina in which attacks of angina frequently result in a fall in blood pressure which can be aggravated by unnecessarily high doses of nitroglycerin taken to break an attack.

Although most patients can tolerate a starting dose of 0.3 mg of sublingual nitroglycerin, many will need only 0.15 mg for a full therapeutic effect. Others, especially those who have been having frequent attacks and taking many nitroglycerin tablets daily, may develop a tolerance and require one or two 0.6-mg tablets at a time for relief.

Patients may have some strange ideas about this drug. Its very name implies a *powerful* medicine (It's dynamite!). Physicians need to counsel patients carefully about the benign nature of the drug and its great therapeutic usefulness so that they will not hesitate to use it for even minor distress. Since best results are obtained if it is taken at the very onset of an anginal attack, patients must keep some with them at all times. Nitroglycerin decomposes rapidly when exposed to light and heat and is quite soluble in many plastics and cardboard. To ensure that tablets retain their potency, they should be stored in airtight amber glass or metal containers. I suggest to my patients that they keep their large stock of tablets in the original container in the refrigerator and carry with them only what they might need for the day in a smaller bottle. Although some modern nitroglycerin preparations claim a shelf life of one year, it is prudent for patients dependent on nitroglycerin to get fresh tablets at least every 3 months (not a great expense because the tablets can be obtained for about $2.00 per hundred).

Because of its short duration of action, sublingual nitroglycerin is used prophylactically to prevent attacks of vasospastic angina only immediately before an activity or situation with a known potential for causing an attack (for example, exercise). It is quite effective in preventing effort-provoked vasospastic angina[76]—a reason for its avoidance before diagnostic exercise tests in patients being evaluated for chest pain.

NITROGLYCERIN OINTMENT. This preparation, which contains 2 percent nitroglycerin by weight, takes advantage of the fact that the drug is readily absorbed through the skin (an important route for industrial nitroglycerin exposure in munition workers). The ointment, which comes in a squeezable tube, is dispensed like toothpaste, measured out by the inch on preruled papers, and applied in a thin layer over a small area of skin anywhere on the body. Each inch of ointment contains about 15 mg of nitroglycerin. Slow, continuous absorption of nitroglycerin produces therapeutic blood levels for up to 4 hours after a single application, which makes it useful for prophylaxis against vasospastic angina. Blood levels achieved after application of three inches of this preparation (1.6 to 2.3 ng per ml) can equal those found with a sublingual dose of 0.6 mg nitroglycerin or with an intravenous infusion of nitroglycerin sufficient to lower blood pressure by 10 percent.[77]

Nitroglycerin ointment is effective in prevention of vasospastic angina.[78,79] In a randomized, single-blind, short-term study of 10 patients with vasospastic angina, ointment containing 15 mg of nitroglycerin applied every 6 hours completely prevented attacks in 7 patients and reduced attack frequency in the other 3.[80] In two of the latter cases, attacks while on nitroglycerin ointment tended to occur during the last 2 hours before the next dose, suggesting inadequate blood levels of drug at these times.

This preparation can be used by itself or in conjunction with other organic nitrates or with other classes of vasodilators to prevent vasospastic angina. The starting dose is ½ inch every 4 to 6 hours, with a titration up to 2 to 4 inches per dose if required for desired effect. The principal side effect is headache, which can be minimized by treatment with acetaminophen (Tylenol) until the patient develops tolerance, if for some reason a reduction in dose is not appropriate. Another side effect is mucking up of clothes by the ointment, which occurs even though the ointment is covered with the paper applicator. In some cases, because of this, patients prefer to use another form of long-acting organic nitrate during the day and put the ointment on when retiring for sleep at night. I have known patients whose attacks of spontaneous angina occurred exclusively during sleep to become completely free of angina with a single, bedtime application of nitroglycerin ointment, without need for any further medication during the day.

INTRAVENOUS OR INTRACORONARY NITROGLYCERIN. For the most *rapid* and *reliable* attainment of therapeutic blood levels of nitroglycerin, the drug can be given intravenously. Commercial, intravenous preparations have just become available. A solution safe for intravenous use can also be made up from sublingual nitroglycerin tablets by dissolving them in sterile isotonic saline in a syringe and then forcing the resulting solution through a 0.22 μm filter to remove particulate material and bacteria.[81,82] The resulting concentration of drug is imprecise because the *exact* amount in each tablet is unknown and because of the tendency of nitroglycerin to dissolve in most plastics. But if fresh tablets are used, it is close enough to theoretic concentration for most clinical uses. At UCLA Hospital, the pharmacy used to make up a batch of nitroglycerin for intravenous use as described about every 2 to 3 weeks and then chemically assayed each batch to determine actual drug concentration. The resulting stock solution, 0.6 to 0.8 mg per ml, was stored in 10 ml units in amber glass multidose vials capped with a Teflon-coated stopper. In this form, potency is maintained for over 4 weeks, especially if stored in the refrigerator. The drug is absorbed by plastic of intravenous infusion tubing, and the amount actually delivered to the patient via constant infusion is less than calculated from the nominal drug concentration in the infusion bottle.[83] To minimize this effect, the dilute solution for infusion can be kept in a glass rather than a plastic infusion bottle.[83] The solution should also be protected from direct light (for example, with a paper bag). Because the dose actually getting into the patient is unknown, titration of dose is important. The solution for infusion should be made up fresh at least every 12 hours.

Acute Use. Intravenous nitroglycerin is given acutely as 50 to 300 μg increments, each given over a period of 15 to 60 seconds to treat acute attacks of coronary artery spasm particularly in the catherization laboratory, in other circumstances when a rapid onset of action is essential, or in the operating room when sublingual use is inconvenient. Intracoronary administration of 50 to 200 μg is limited of necessity to the catheterization laboratory during coronary arteriography or to the operating room during coronary surgery. Side effects are limited mainly to transient headache and hypotension. Because there is no need to produce a profound drop in blood pressure for therapeutic effect in vasospastic angina, and because severe hypotension will aggravate myocardial ischemia in patients with organic coronary stenosis and may mask active coronary dilation by dropping the transmural distending pressure, great care must be used to avoid overdosing the patient.

These principles were demonstrated nicely in animal studies I performed in collaboration with Alexander Kolin, in which the actual response of large coronary arteries to intravenous nitroglycerin depended on the dose and the effect on blood pressure. Coronary dilation was seen with small doses which had little effect on blood pressure. Larger doses, which produce a modest fall in pressure, caused a biphasic response, with passive coronary arterial constriction seen early paralleling the fall in arterial pressure, followed by active vasodilation so that the arterial lumen increased despite a continued decreased distending pressure. Finally, with yet larger doses, a profound fall in blood pressure caused marked passive collapse of the vessels, so that subsequent active vasodilation was hidden, and only vasosconstriction was encountered unless blood pressure was artificially returned to normal by rapid infusion of volume expanders or occlusion of the descending aorta.[84] This latter reaction to nitroglycerin can be aggravated by the sympathetic vasoconstriction reflex activated by a marked fall in blood pressure.

For these reasons, I give nitroglycerin acutely in intravenous doses of only 50 to 100 μg over about 20 seconds and repeat the dose every minute or so until a desired response is seen. The nadir of the blood pressure will occur within 30 seconds following each dose; and I aim for a sustained fall in mean pressure of no more than 10 mm Hg or for relief of angina or coronary artery spasm. The same doses can be given directly into a coronary artery by catheter (or by needle during coronary surgery). The higher local concentrations achieved thereby in the coronary arteries relative to the peripheral hypotensive effect of the drug will sometimes relieve coronary artery spasm unresponsive to sublingual or intravenous nitroglycerin.[61,62,85] Therefore, parenteral nitroglycerin, diluted up and ready for immediate intravenous or intracoronary use, should be available whenever a pharmacologic provocative test is done for coronary artery spasm. Intravenously, it is highly effective for reversing ergonovine-induced coronary artery spasm.[86] Intracoronary nitroglycerin has also been used to test for vasospastic coronary artery occlusion in patients with acute myocardial infarction.[87–89]

Constant Infusion. Nitroglycerin is very effective in *preventing* acute attacks of vasospastic angina when given as a constant intravenous infusion to patients hospitalized because of the instability or severity of their angina.[66,90] It usually takes infusion of 10 to 100 μg per minute to achieve the desired effect. My experience indicates that this is a convenient means of obtaining rapid control of severe attacks for a short time (a few days), during which alternate therapy appropriate to eventual outpatient use can be figured out leisurely. The nitroglycerin infusion can be *gradually* tapered off as the drug is replaced by other organic nitrate preparations or a calcium channel blocking agent, or both. As with other organic nitrates, headache and hypotension are the main side effects, and the rate of the infusion should be accurately controlled by some type of constant rate infusion pump to minimize chances of the latter. The infusion rate will have to be adjusted frequently at the start of therapy and whenever the infusion tubing is changed.[83]

The reason intravenous nitroglycerin is perhaps the most predictably effective means for controlling vasospastic angina with organic nitrates is that it is the only mode of administration in which drug blood levels can be adjusted precisely and held absolutely constant hour after hour, day after day. Nitroglycerin blood levels necessary to reduce arterial pressure 10 percent (levels usually at least therapeutic for vasospasm) are 1.6 to 2.3 ng per ml.[77]

Patients should not be taken off their vasodilator therapy abruptly when they go for cardiac or noncardiac surgery. Yet it is usually necessary to interrupt their usual regimen at such a time. Intravenous nitroglycerin infusion is a convenient way to give medication and to prevent attacks in the perioperative period in patients with vasospastic angina. Although nitroglycerin ointment can be used for the same purpose, in difficult or unstable patients it does not offer the same degree of protection.

Isosorbide Dinitrate

This drug is used for long-term, prophylactic treatment to prevent attacks of vasospastic angina. Although the sublingual and chewable preparations have a relatively rapid onset of action, it is not nearly as rapidly active as sublingual nitroglycerin (see Table 3), and isosorbide dinitrate (or other "rapid" acting similar agents), therefore, is not the drug of choice in treatment of acute attacks.

Isosorbide dinitrate is well absorbed from the gut, but there is an extensive first pass conversion of the drug to inactive metabolites as portal blood passes through the liver, so that therapeutic concentrations are not easily nor reliably achieved by ingesting it. Several methods are used to overcome this problem.

SUBLINGUAL AND CHEWABLE PREPARATIONS. Like nitroglycerin, isosorbide dinitrate is well absorbed through the mucous membranes of the mouth, whence it can enter the systemic circulation without having to pass through the liver first. Sublingual and chewable tablets are available for this use, and which preparation is used depends on patient or physician preference because they are therapeutically equivalent. Following sublingual administration of 5 mg in humans, dilation of large coronary artery diameter by 8 to 26 percent is regularly seen by arteriography.[8,51,91] The duration of action of isosorbide dinitrate by this route can be increased slightly by increasing the dose; but keeping a constantly therapeutic level usually requires doses taken at least every 3 hours, which is particularly inconvenient during sleeping hours, when a longer-acting agent such as nitroglycerin ointment may be substituted.

Sublingual isosorbide dinitrate is effective in prevention of vasospastic angina in 20 to 70 percent of patients, depending on case selection and dose of drug used.[70,78,92-97] No controlled study has been published, however. Starting with 2.5 mg every 2 to 3 hours, the dose should be titrated up gradually until the desired therapeutic response or intolerable side effects are achieved. Doses as high as 15 mg every 3 hours are required in occasional patients. Failure to achieve control of attacks in some reported cases[98-104] may have been due to insufficient doses. It is a good practice to give the first dose with the patient under observation to see the acute response before sending the patient home on a regular schedule of drug. Occasional patients are exquisitely sensitive to organic nitrates and will have a splitting headache after a 2.5 mg tablet, the smallest one available. Most of these patients will be able to tolerate the drug by taking only ½ tablet or less (obtained by cutting it with a knife), and this may be all that such patients need for a therapeutic effect. Patients who experience *severe* vasodilator headache with their first few doses of isosorbide dinitrate often become quite resistant to any further use of the drug, because, unlike a nitroglycerin headache, that from isosorbide dinitrate may last for hours. Because the drug is so useful for vasospastic angina, special care should be used to minimize the chances of such a headache occurring at the outset of treatment. Patients should be reassured that most persons will develop tolerance for the drug and that their tendency for headache will decrease with chronic use of the drug.

ORAL PREPARATIONS. When isosorbide dinitrate is swallowed, therapeutic systemic blood levels of active drug can usually be achieved by giving doses high enough to saturate the enzyme system in the liver which inactivates the drug. Because individuals vary widely in their ability to metabolize the drug in the liver, the range of doses required is wide. It is often necessary to titrate the dose up to levels greatly in excess of those currently recommended by the drug manufacturers. Because drug absorption can be altered by changes in gut motility, and hepatic enzyme activity may not always be the same, oral administration of isosorbide dinitrate, even when done by careful titration, does not produce a therapeutic effect as reliable as when the drug is given sublingually. Thus this route of administration is seldom used as the *sole* means of getting the drug into the body in vasospastic angina. I know of no published studies of the use of this form of the drug for this purpose. It does have the theoretical advantage of a longer duration of action than sublingual preparations (because of gradual absorption from the gut—see Table 3) and, if used at all, is best employed to provide a background level of drug on which is superimposed the peaks and valleys of the briefly-acting sublingual drug.

I recommend starting with a dose of 5 to 10 mg orally every 6 hours and gradually increasing the dose until intolerable side effects or the desired therapeutic goal is attained. Rare patients may require doses exceeding 100 mg every 4 to 6 hours.

It should be remembered that patients on effective doses of long-acting organic nitrate vasodilators have their normal vascular reflexes blunted, and they are more than usually susceptible to develop severe hypotension from hypovolemia, as could result from aggressive use of diuretics or blood loss. Also, patients with severe liver disease may attain high and prolonged blood levels of isosorbide dinitrate after only modest doses.

An extended release form of isosorbide dinitrate for oral use is also marketed. It is my opinion that blood levels of the drug are even less predictable with this preparation than with the regular oral form and that it has little usefulness in vasospastic angina.

INTRAVENOUS PREPARATION. Isosorbide dinitrate can be given as a constant infusion intravenously, and when so administered it has been shown to be effective in preventing attacks of vasospastic angina in a well-controlled study.[65] Except for better chemical stability, it will probably offer little advantage over intravenous nitroglycerin.[66]

ISOSORBIDE DINITRATE OINTMENT. Just like nitroglycerin, this drug can be absorbed through the skin, and I understand an ointment preparation is being investigated.

Nitroprusside

Available exclusively as a solution for intravenous infusion, sodium nitroprusside can be used much like nitroglycerin as a constant infusion for short-term control of vasospastic angina in unstable hospitalized patients. When given either intravenously[105] at 20 to 150 μg per minute or as a 5 to 10 μg bolus directly into a coronary artery,[106,107] this drug produced dilation of normal and diseased segments of large coronary arteries of about the same magnitude as that obtained with nitroglycerin. Although there remains some debate about its relative activity on large and small coronary arteries,[108] anecdotal reports suggest that nitroprusside may be almost as effective as intravenous nitroglycerin in controlling vasospastic angina.[104,109,110] The possibility of a rebound vasoconstrictive state following abrupt withdrawal of this drug exists, just as with the organic nitrates.[111]

Calcium Channel Blockers

This exciting new class of agents causes vasodilation by a mechanism different from that of the organic nitrates or other vasodilators, and now that they are routinely available, they are the drugs of first choice for treatment of vasospastic angina. These agents inhibit the inward movement of calcium ions across the cell wall from the extracellular fluid by blocking the calcium channels in the cell membrane. This effect results in decreased levels of free calcium ions intracellularly, and because the latter are needed for contraction of vascular smooth muscle cells, vasodilation results. Movement of calcium ion into cells is important and basic to the function of many different types of cells in the body, so that these drugs have a variety of effects. Their most dramatic actions, however, are on vascular smooth muscle and myocardium. Fortunately, in inhibiting muscular contraction they are three to ten times more

Table 4. Pharmacokinetics of calcium channel blockers

Drug	Absorption from gut	Plasma protein binding	Terminal slow half-life in plasma (T½β)	Therapeutic plasma concentration	Metabolism	Excretion
Nifedipine (MW = 346)	>90% (also absorbed sublingually)	>90% mainly to albumin	4–5 hours	20–100 ng/ml	Rapidly metabolized to compounds that are pharmacologically inactive. Only 20–30% removed by liver on first pass.	50–80% via kidney, 20–40% via feces
Verapamil (MW = 491)	>90%	90%	3–7 hours	15–100 ng/ml	85% removed by liver in first pass metabolism. Some of metabolites are also vasoactive.	70% via kidney, 15% via feces
Diltiazem (MW = 451)	>90%	80%	4 hours	30–130 ng/ml	Extensively deacetylated.	35% via kidney, 60% via feces

MW = molecular weight.

Table 5. Some clinical effects of calcium channel blockers

Drug	Average dose	Rapidity of onset of action	Coronary and peripheral arterial dilation	Depression of AV conduction	Effect on fast inward Na^+ channel	Side effects
Nifedipine	10–20 mg q 4–8 hr orally and sublingually 3–15 μg/kg intravenously 1–2 μg/kg intracoronary	<20 min orally <3 min sublingually <1 min intravenously <30 sec intracoronary	++++	±		Dizziness, flushing, pedal edema, hypotension, headache, extremity dysesthesia
Verapamil	80–160 mg q 6–8 hr orally 75–150 μg/kg intravenously	~2 hrs orally <2 min intravenously	+++	+++	+++ Has local anesthetic actions	Constipation, leg edema, headaches, hypotension, AV conduction problems, bradycardia (interaction with beta-adrenergic blockers)
Diltiazem	60–90 mg q 6-8 hr orally 75–150 μg/kg intravenously	~15 min orally	+++	+++	++ Has local anesthetic actions	Dizziness, flushing, headache, AV conduction problems (interaction with beta-adrenergic blockers)

AV = atrioventricular.

potent in coronary artery smooth muscle than in myocardium, so that coronary artery dilation can be achieved with doses that do not measurably depress myocardial contractile function.[112] Moreover, their peripheral vasodilating effect results in a reduction of left ventricular afterload which, coupled with reflex sympathetic stimulation resulting from the vasodilation, tends to counterbalance any negative inotropic effect. A detailed discussion of the pharmacology of these drugs is beyond the scope of this chapter, and for a more comprehensive exposition, the reader is referred to several excellent recent reviews.[112-115]

There are a number of different calcium channel blocking agents, but the ones most studied and now approved for general use are verapamil, nifedipine, and diltiazem. Some pharmacologic properties of these drugs are summarized in Tables 4 and 5. Although currently lumped together into a single therapeutic class, these three drugs have little structural or chemical similarity and may affect intracellular calcium concentration in vascular smooth muscle by different mechanisms.[115,116]

Mechanism of Action

Nifedipine appears to diminish or to "block" the number of slow channels without affecting the function or kinetics of remaining channels. It has no local anesthetic properties and does not affect the fast sodium channel. Verapamil strongly affects the kinetics and reduces the rates of activation, inactivation, and recovery of the slow channels. Moreover, verapamil is a racemic mixture of two optical isomers. The (−) isomer produces the aforementioned effects on the slow channels, whereas the (+) isomer has local anesthetic properties and inhibits fast channel function.[115] The mode of action of diltiazem, although unclear, may be different. It seems to stimulate the sodium-potassium pump and may affect a reduction in intracellular calcium in part as a result of passive sodium-calcium exchange driven by reduced intracellular sodium and in part by stimulation of an energy-dependent mechanism of calcium extrusion.[116] Hence, though verapamil decreases smooth muscle oxygen consumption, diltiazem increases it.[116] Diltiazem also has local anesthetic properties and inhibits the fast channel in cardiac muscle.[115]

Differences in action at the cellular level cause some noticeable differences in clinical effects. Although in the isolated heart preparation all three drugs depress automaticity of the sinoatrial node and slow conduction through the atrioventricular node, this effect is clinically apparent in intact humans only with verapamil and diltiazem. The clinical effect on atrioventricular nodal tissue is the basis for the great utility of verapamil (and to a lesser extent diltiazem) in treatment of certain types of supraventricular tachyarrhythmias. Nifedipine has no similar antiarrhythmic efficacy. On the other hand, nifedipine can be administered relatively safely in conjunction with beta-adrenergic blocking drugs, whereas the latter must be used only with caution (particularly intravenously) in combination with verapamil or diltiazem because of additive depression of atrioventricular conduction and the risk of a high grade AV block. Though all three drugs possess negative inotropic effects, nifedipine seems to have less effect relative to its vasodilating potency than verapamil or diltiazem. Nifedipine can thus be used even in patients with moderately depressed left ventricular function because its arterial vasodilating action unloads the left ventricle; it has even been used as an afterload reducing agent in the treatment of heart failure.[117] These drugs appear to have their primary peripheral action on arterioles and arteries with little evidence of venodilating effect (in contrast with the effects of organic nitrates).

Vascular and Hemodynamic Effects

Acutely, nifedipine and verapamil produce peripheral and coronary arteriolar vasodilation resulting in an increase in coronary blood flow[118,119] and a drop in arterial pressure.[119-121] Cardiac output may increase or stay unchanged, but calculated peripheral resistance is reduced.[119–121] As a result, these drugs are useful antihypertensive agents. Nifedipine is more potent for this and is effective for treatment of acute hypertensive crises[122] as well as chronic hypertension.[123] The effectiveness of verapamil in chronic hypertension is only modest.[124] Heart rate is generally unchanged despite the fall in blood pressure. With nifedipine, left ventricular end-diastolic pressure usually changes little or may fall;[125] but with verapamil, it may increase slightly, and this is responsible for a slight rise in pulmonary artery wedge and pulmonary artery pressures.[119,121] Despite direct negative inotropic effects, which in the case of nifedipine have been unmasked by concomitant administration of beta-adrenergic blockers[126] or intracoronary injection of the drug,[125] these effects are not usually apparent clinically, and overall indices of left ventricular contractility are not measurably depressed after clinical oral or intravenous doses.[120,121,125] The hemodynamic effects of diltiazem have not been as well studied.

Diltiazem[127–129] and verapamil[119,130,131] dilate large coronary arteries in resting humans—an action apparently not shared by nifedipine.[132,133] Because all three drugs are of approximately equal efficacy in variant angina, modification of *basal* coronary arterial smooth muscle tone may not be essential to their clinical usefulness in this syndrome.

With chronic use of nifedipine and verapamil in oral doses effective in preventing variant angina attacks, heart rate at rest and heart rate and systolic blood pressure with exercise are depressed significantly with verapamil but not with nifedipine; using equilibrium gated blood pool scintigraphy, no differences were found in end-diastolic or end-systolic left ventricular volumes or ejection fraction at rest or in response to supine exercise.[134]

Other Cardiovascular Actions

These drugs by virtue of their peripheral vasodilation and negative intropic effects may reduce the oxygen requirements of ischemic myocardium and also may reduce the intracellular influx of calcium, which can result in irreversible structural damage in ischemically injured myocardium.[112,114,115] Thus they are effective in classic angina and may act to protect ischemic myocardium and to reduce myocardial necrosis following coronary occlusion by actions not possessed by organic nitrate vasodilators. Another property of these agents useful in coronary heart disease may be their ability to inhibit platelet aggregation induced by collagen[135] or epinephrine.[136]

Use in Vasospastic Angina

COMPARATIVE EFFICACY. No studies with completely adequate design have been performed to establish the *relative* effectiveness of these three calcium channel blockers in vasospastic angina. Open label, uncontrolled drug studies have shown equal efficacy of nifedipine and diltiazem in variant angina patients, with 60 to 80 percent achieving complete prevention of spontaneous attacks and an additional 10 to 20 percent obtaining at least a halving of their attack frequency.[95,137] An apparent lesser efficacy of verapamil in a study from Japan may have been due to the low dose of the drug used (average dose 228 mg per day).[137] In a single blind cross-over study of nifedipine, verapamil, and placebo, utilizing verapamil in average dosages of 400 mg per day, both drugs showed essentially equal efficacy[138]—a result similar to my own open label, non-placebo-controlled experience with the same two drugs (Table 6). In an unblinded, randomized cross-over study of the ability of these drugs to prevent attacks of coronary artery spasm induced by ergonovine in 31 patients with variant angina, Waters and colleagues[139] showed complete prevention of attacks in 41 percent, 30 percent, and 41 percent, and increase in dose of ergonovine needed to produce spasm in an additional 41 percent, 37 percent, and 41 percent of patients with nifedipine 20 mg every 6 hours, verapamil 160 mg every 8 hours, and diltiazem 120 mg every 8 hours, respectively. The differences between drugs were not statistically significant.

Table 6. Experience with nifedipine and verapamil in variant angina*

	Verapamil† (N = 11)	Nifedipine†† (N = 11)
Angina completely prevented	4	2
>50% reduction in angina frequency	3	5
Angina unchanged	4	4

*Open label study without cross-over or placebo control. Organic nitrate vasodilators given concurrently in 9 of 11 cases. All patients unsatisfactorily responsive to maximum tolerable doses of organic nitrates. In 5 cases tested with each drug sequentially, identical results were achieved with both drugs (angina prevented completely by both in one case, and angina unaffected by both drugs in four cases).

†Average dose 480 mg/day (range 240–640 mg). Verapamil made available through the courtesy of Knoll Pharmaceutical Company of Whippany, New Jersey.

††Average dose 80 mg/day (range 40–120 mg). Nifedipine made available through the courtesy of Delbay Pharmaceuticals, Bloomfield, New Jersey, and Pfizer Pharmaceuticals of New York City, New York.

With present knowledge, it seems that for variant angina at least these three drugs are of approximately equal efficacy. Therefore, selection of a drug for a patient will be determined by associated problems such as paroxysmal supraventricular tachycardia, ventricular arrhythmias, sinus node dysfunction, slow atrioventricular nodal conduction, need for concurrent beta-adrenergic antagonists, severe ventricular dysfunction, and severe hypertension. Of course, in a given patient one drug may be more effective than another,[140-142] so that failure with one should prompt a trial with another.[139]

Waters and his colleagues[139] have found a good correlation between the ability of a calcium channel blocker to prevent a positive response to ergonovine and subsequent ability of that drug to prevent spontaneous variant anginal attacks over a long term. Of 15 patients taking the particular drug that produced a negative ergonovine test, 14 were maintained free of attacks and the other patient was improved; whereas of 12 patients taking a drug that did *not* prevent a positive ergonovine test, only 4 remained free of attacks and another 4 were improved. The use of such testing to determine which drug to use is seldom clinically necessary but may be useful in special cases.

For other syndromes of vasospastic angina, there is insufficient information to assess comparative drug efficacy.

USE OF TWO CALCIUM CHANNEL BLOCKERS IN COMBINATION. Because these agents all affect intracellular calcium by a different mechanism, it is possible that the combined action of two or more drugs would be more efficacious than any drug singly or combined just with organic nitrate. This appears to be true in some cases for nifedipine and dilitazem,[47,137] but more studies will be needed before the true therapeutic role of such combinations can be determined.

COMBINED USE WITH ORGANIC NITRATES. The different modes of action of the calcium channel blockers and organic nitrates raise the possibility that their combined effects may be more efficacious than when either drug class is used alone. In my own experience this seems to be true. Most studies suggest that when used alone, calcium channel blockers are more effective than organic nitrates against variant angina. But cases resistant to organic nitrates alone can frequently be found in which an incomplete or insufficient response to calcium channel blockers is converted to an excellent response with the addition of organic nitrates.[143] Although this point has received little study, I consider it to be of the *greatest* clinical importance.

NIFEDIPINE. This dihydropyridine derivative is packaged as units of 10 mg in a gelatin capsule which is suitable for oral use, or for sublingual administration when the capsule is broken by chewing. The oily contents of the capsule have a powerful taste, making placebo studies difficult when the capsule is chewed. The drug is rapidly and nearly completely absorbed from the gut and has little first pass hepatic metabolism. Even more rapid onset of action is obtained with sublingual administration, but not fast enough to treat acute attacks, for which nitroglycerin is still the drug of choice (see Table 5). For prophylaxis of vasospastic angina the capsule is usually swallowed whole, although I have encountered one patient who failed to achieve a therapeutic result until he started chewing the capsules. The drug is usually begun at a dose of 10 mg orally every 6 to 8 hours with titration up to 20 mg every 4 to 6 hours until a therapeutic response or intolerable side effects occur. Occasionally a patient will need and tolerate a total daily dose in excess of 120 mg.

Nifedipine is also prepared as a solution for parenteral administration. The use of the drug intravenously as a constant infusion is rarely necessary because therapeutic blood levels can be rapidly and reliably achieved with the sublingual or oral routes. Acute intravenous doses of 0.2 to 1.0 mg can be used to initiate treatment in patients with severe life-threatening attacks[144] or for hemodynamic investigations.[125] It can also be given directly into a coronary artery in doses of 100 to 200 μg to treat acute, spontaneous, or ergonovine-induced coronary artery spasm at the time of arteriography;[125,145] but its onset of action is slower than that of nitroglycerin, which is the preferred drug both for this use and to prevent coronary artery spasm resulting from transluminal balloon angioplasty. Intracoronary nifedipine causes a profound transient local depression of myocardial contractility[125] and should be avoided in patients with severe chronic impairment of ventricular function.

Effectiveness. Most studies of nifedipine for vasospastic angina have dealt with variant angina, and in that subset of patients nifedipine was quite effective. Most published studies of a sizable group of patients involve uncontrolled, open label protocols.[86,137,145–154] Although the percent of patients becoming completely free of variant angina attacks after being started on nifedipine varied from a low of 0[149] to 100 percent,[148] the average was 72 percent—which is similar to the 78 percent found in a well-controlled, cross-over study of 13 patients by Previtali and coworkers.[155] An additional approximately 20 percent of patients from the uncontrolled studies had a 50 percent or greater reduction in frequency of attacks with nifedipine, so that about 92 percent of all patients seemed to derive some benefit from the drug—which is impressive, considering that most of these patients had *not* previously obtained adequate symptomatic relief from organic nitrate vasodilators. In many cases, these results were obtained with the concomitant use of organic nitrates, which in my experience may produce better control of attacks than either drug alone.[156] The true efficacy of nifedipine was proven in many patients, even in uncontrolled trials, by the recurrence of attacks, after their successful suppression, by temporary discontinuance of the drug,[86,145,149,150] or by substituting a placebo.[137]

Not all patients will have recurrence of symptoms when an apparently effective drug (for example, nifedipine) is stopped. The tendency in variant angina is for spontaneous amelioration of attacks with time,[10,42] and some patients require effective drug therapy only for a few months, after which an attack-free state is maintained without medication.[14,15]

The likelihood of a good therapeutic response to nifedipine in variant angina does not seem related to the presence or absence of severe underlying coronary disease.[137,155] There is, in my experience and in that of others,[150] a tendency for patients with acutely unstable symptoms to have a more favorable response of their symptoms to any calcium channel blocker, including nifedipine, than patients with chronic, stable symptoms.

Prevention of Provoked Attacks. As already mentioned, nifedipine is very effective in preventing ergonovine-induced coronary artery spasm, or at least in making it necessary to use higher ergonovine doses to induce a positive response.[139,145,157] It is also able in most cases to prevent exercise-induced variant angina, which is usually due to coronary artery spasm.[14,158,159] Although experience is small, it also can be effective in preventing coronary artery spasm provoked by the cold pressor test.[150,160]

In Other Vasospastic Anginal Syndromes. Patients hospitalized with spontaneous (rest) angina associated with ST segment depression or T wave changes (but not ST segment elevation) have a form of unstable angina that in most instances is probably related to coronary artery spasm superimposed on underlying organic coronary obstructive disease.[1] In such patients, nifedipine can be effective. Freedom from spontaneous angina was achieved in about 80 percent of reported cases.[125,148,154,161,162] In two recent studies, patients whose attacks of angina at rest were unresponsive to organic nitrates and propranolol combined in therapeutic doses (current "standard" medical treatment) had nifedipine (30 to 120 mg daily in divided doses) *added* to the former drugs.[125,154] A "good" therapeutic response was obtained in 50 percent of cases in one study,[154] and complete freedom from spontaneous angina was achieved in 87 percent of cases in the other.[125] Improvement was maintained in a long-term followup in most cases. Temporary withdrawal from nifedipine after leaving the hospital resulted in recurrence of rest angina in most but not all the patients on whom it was tried.

Further studies are needed on this type of patient, but it appears that nifedipine is a useful addition to the drugs available in treating this form of unstable angina.

Myocardial Infarction While on Nifedipine. An initial control of attacks of coronary artery spasm with nifedipine does not guarantee freedom from risk of myocardial infarction while taking the drug. Acute myocardial infarction unexpectedly interrupting apparently successful treatment of variant angina is not a rarity[95,152,155,156] and occurred in two of seven of my own patients who seemed to be responding well to nifedipine at doses of 80 mg and 100 mg per day in the two cases respectively. It also occurs in other vasospastic anginal syndromes, such as severe spontaneous angina with ST depression or T wave changes only during attacks (one form of unstable angina).[125] This unsettling event is fortunately usually not fatal and probably reflects the severity and instability of the underlying coronary disease in these patients.

Side Effects. Side effects are noted in about 39 percent of patients taking nifedipine chronically. Most of these reactions are not severe, but they frequently limit the dose of drug a patient can take, and in about 5 percent of cases may be severe enough to necessitate discontinuing the drug entirely.[152] The most common side effects noted are dizziness (13 percent), muscle cramps (2 percent), nausea (2 percent), palpitations (2 percent), rash (1 percent).[152] It is worth noting that headache, the bane of so many patients taking organic nitrates, is an uncommon side effect of nifedipine (or of other calcium channel blockers). Noncardiac leg edema is not a complication unique to nifedipine; it is a nonspecific result of therapy with many types of vasodilators in some patients. Important side effects—those requiring reduction of dose or discontinuance of the drug—seem more common with nifedipine than with verapamil in my experience and in that of others.[138]

Nifedipine causes an increase in plasma digoxin concentration in patients on chronic therapy with the latter drug,[163] and such patients' digoxin dose should be watched carefully.

About 40 percent of my own patients taking nifedipine chronically have developed and maintained a slight elevation of their serum creatine kinase. Analysis has shown this to be 100 percent MM-CK (skeletal muscle origin presumably), whereas MB-CK (cardiac) levels are not elevated. None of these patients has any muscular symptoms or signs of elevation of other muscle enzymes, and therapy has not been stopped for this laboratory abnormality which has not been reported by any other investigator studying nifedipine. Its real significance is presently unknown.

VERAPAMIL. This drug is a papavarine derivative. It is available in this country as a solution for intravenous use, packaged as 5 mg of drug in a 2 ml ampule, for which the only FDA-approved use is the acute treatment of certain supraventricular tachyarrhythmias, and as coated 80 mg and 120 mg tablets for oral use. The drug is nearly completely absorbed from the gut, but about 85 percent is metabolized on first passage through the liver so that bioavailability of unchanged drug is only 10–22 percent.[115] Its metabolites may retain some vasodilator activity and have a much longer half-life in the plasma than does verapamil itself, but their contribution to the clinical effects of the drug is unknown.[115] Therapeutic blood levels

153

are, therefore, not as easily nor as predictably achieved as with nifedipine, and the optimal dose in a given patient is usually determined empirically. Laboratory assays of blood levels of verapamil and its major metabolite are available to the clinician.

For prophylaxis of vasospastic angina, the drug is usually started at 80 mg orally every 8 hours and the dose titrated up to 160 mg every 6 to 8 hours. Occasional patients will require larger doses. The use of a constant intravenous infusion of verapamil for vasospastic angina has received little attention. It might be of use in the hospitalized patient with severe attacks of spontaneous angina, but I have seen only one report of this being done.[164] In that study the drug was infused into 45 patients at rates equivalent to between 7 and 175 μg per minute, using the blood pressure and patients' symptoms as a guide. In one other study, the drug was successfully used as a 5 mg intravenous bolus to relieve severe spontaneous anginal attacks associated with symptoms and signs of left heart failure.[131] I have found only one study in which the drug in doses of 0.25 to 0.5 mg was given directly into the coronary artery in an attempt to produce vasodilation or successfully to treat ergonovine-induced coronary artery spasm.[131]

Effectiveness. Verapamil is quite effective in variant angina. In one short-term double-blind, cross-over study with placebo control, a marked reduction in frequency of ischemic attacks occurred during verapamil administration, although only one of eight patients had *complete* prevention of attacks (the remaining seven had a reduction in frequency).[165] In many of these patients, a beneficial therapeutic effect was maintained with long-term verapamil treatment. Another well-designed and well-controlled study of long-term therapy with verapamil in 16 patients noted an average reduction in weekly attack rate while on the drug to about one seventh of that present when on placebo; moreover, there were seven instances of clinical instability during placebo periods, but none with verapamil.[43] In yet another blind, cross-over study with placebo, verapamil was compared to nifedipine.[138] A 71 percent reduction in frequency of attacks with verapamil and a 65 percent reduction with nifedipine were not significantly different.

In basically uncontrolled clinical trials, about 35 percent of patients with variant angina were rendered completely free of attacks (range 10 percent to 65 percent), whereas another 53 percent had a 50 percent or greater reduction in frequency of attacks.[137,140,142,166,167] Though the percent of patients becoming free from attacks with verapamil in these trials is less than found in other uncontrolled trials with nifedipine or diltiazem, it should be noted that approximately equal efficacy of these drugs has been shown in controlled studies comparing the drugs.[138,139] The aforementioned discrepancy can be explained in various ways. First, patient selection may have been different in studies of the two drugs. More important perhaps is the dose of verapamil used. The result achieved is critically dependent on the dose of verapamil.[168] The largest single series reported was from Japan[137] and used doses of verapamil (120 to 320 mg per day) that are now known to be inadequate for many patients. Moreover, the concomitant use of organic nitrate vasodilators was not controlled in many of these studies, but it is of crucial importance in the results. In one study of ten patients with variant angina refractory to organic nitrates used alone, only one patient became free of attacks when switched to verapamil alone, whereas seven patients became attack free (and two others improved) when organic nitrate therapy was *added* to verapamil.[143]

As with nifedipine, improvement with verapamil may be most marked in patients with the most frequent attacks.[43]

Prevention of Provoked Attacks. Verapamil is effective in preventing or ameliorating ergonovine-induced coronary artery spasm but may not be quite as successful in this regard as nifedipine or diltiazem.[139] It also protects against effort-provoked coronary artery spasm in most patients subject to this problem,[46,169,170] but not in all.[76] As with prevention of spontaneous attacks, the blood level of the drug may be very important in successful prophylaxis of exercise-induced attacks.[46]

In Other Vasospastic Anginal Syndromes. In the majority of patients with spontaneous angina associated with ST segment depression, verapamil is effective, although the numbers

154

of patients in published reports is small.[164,165,171] It is a valuable adjunct to treatment of this group of patients, although further, controlled studies are needed to assay the degree of its effectiveness.

Special Effectiveness in Ischemia-Related Arrhythmias. Because of its unique properties, verapamil may protect against some ectopic ventricular arrhythmias resulting from acute, severe myocardial ischemia. In anesthetized dogs, verapamil inhibited development of ventricular tachycardia and fibrillation resulting from coronary artery ligation or subsequent reperfusion, and increased the threshold for ventricular fibrillation in the ischemic myocardium.[172-175] Nifedipine does not have this activity.[175] Because such arrhythmias are a common result of acute vasospastic coronary artery occlusion in man,[1] verapamil may have a special usefulness in this setting. In acute myocardial infarction, verapamil intravenously was reported to have abolished the frequent premature ventricular beats arising in the first few post-infarct hours in 24 of 28 cases,[176] but this result needs to be confirmed.

Myocardial Infarction While on Verapamil. Just as with nifedipine, apparently successful treatment with verapamil does not always guarantee against subsequent development of acute myocardial infarction.[164,165]

Precautions and Side Effects. Because of their additive depression of sinoatrial node activity and conduction through the atrioventricular node, verapamil and beta-adrenergic antagonists are not generally given together.[114,115,177] *Particular* caution should be used with the intravenous preparations of one of these drugs when the patient is already on the other drug.[112] Propranolol and verapamil administered orally can be successfully given together in selected patients who do not have preexisting sinoatrial or atrioventricular node disease, with attentive monitoring of the ECG to detect toxicity early.[178] Prior digitalization is not a contraindication to the use of verapamil, provided preexisting disease of the AV node is absent.[179] Because its negative inotropic actions are greater at clinical doses than those of nifedipine, verapamil is usually not given to patients with very severe depression of left ventricular function. However, because of its afterload-reducing properties, it may be tolerated surprisingly well in patients without heart failure who have markedly reduced ejection fractions.[134] Because of its inherent negative inotropic action, and effects on the fast sodium channel, it should not be used in conjunction with disopyramide except in special instances, and its use with quinidine or procainamide should be carefully monitored.

An increase in plasma digoxin levels has been reported in patients taking verapamil,[163] and digoxin dose should be reviewed carefully in patients starting verapamil.

Adverse effects of verapamil occur in only about 9 percent of patients and are serious enough to require discontinuance of the drug in only about 1 percent.[179] When given orally, the drug is well tolerated, and the incidence of constipation, pedal edema, nausea, vertigo, headaches, and other symptoms is very low.[43,142,165,171,179] In my own experience, about 40 percent of patients on long-term therapy developed a mild elevation of serum creatine kinase activity, which has been maintained as long as the drug has been given. As discussed in the preceding section on nifedipine, only CK of skeletal muscle type is elevated, with no apparent clinical signs or symptoms; it has not required discontinuance of therapy. One of my patients developed laboratory evidence of hepatic toxicity from verapamil, with marked reversible elevation of liver enzymes each time the drug was given; this is apparently a very rare reaction.

DILTIAZEM. This drug is a 1,5-benzothiazepine derivative. It is currently available in this country as 30 and 60 mg tablets. It is nearly completely absorbed from the gut and does not undergo extensive hepatic first-pass degradation, although eventually about 60 percent is metabolized in the liver and excreted via the feces. It is given in doses of 30 to 90 mg every 6 to 8 hours for vasospastic angina, although the upper limit of safe and effective dosage is as yet undetermined. It is also prepared in a solution for intravenous administration,[129,180] but this is available only for investigational uses in this country.

Effectiveness. There is less experience with diltiazem in vasospastic angina than with nifedipine and verapamil because of its more recent development. It was approximately as effective as nifedipine in preventing attacks of variant angina in 81 percent of cases in an uncon-

155

trolled study from Japan,[137] with freedom from attacks of variant angina achieved in between 60 and 100 percent of patients on long-term treatment in other reports.[139,180–182] In two double-blind, randomized cross-over, placebo-controlled studies, complete freedom from attacks of variant angina was achieved in about 50 percent of patients (none concurrently on long-acting organic nitrates) at a dosage of 60 mg four times a day, with improvement in symptoms in another 20 percent.[183,184] In these two studies, less benefit was obtained at dosage of 30 mg four times a day. There was no evidence of rebound exacerbation of coronary artery spasm on abrupt withdrawal of the drug. A combination of diltiazem and nifedipine may be effective when neither drug works sufficiently well alone.[47]

Prevention of Provoked Attacks. Against ergonovine-induced coronary artery spasm, diltiazem has the same efficacy as nifedipine and may be slightly superior to verapamil, and there is a correlation between this ability and its clinical efficacy.[139]

Diltiazem also is effective in most cases in preventing the angina associated with either ST segment elevation[14] or depression[6] resulting from exercise-induced vasospastic angina. It can also prevent coronary vasospasm induced by hyperventilation and alkalinization with Tris buffer.[185]

Spontaneous Angina with ST Segment Depression. In this form of unstable angina, there is little experience with diltiazem. Excellent results in one study[180] were not duplicated in another.[181] Clearly, additional controlled studies are needed.

Precautions and Side Effects. Because diltiazem has actions similar to verapamil on the atrioventricular node, it should be used cautiously in patients taking beta-adrenergic blocking drugs or with preexisting disease of the atrioventricular node. Until more is known about its clinical effects and drug interactions, caution should be exercised in giving it to patients taking disopyramide, quinidine, or procainamide, or to those with markedly depressed left ventricular function, although studies in conscious dogs suggest that diltiazem produces less depression of myocardial contractile function than does verapamil.[186]

Adverse effects from oral diltiazem are apparently very infrequent,[183,184] but the number of patients studied is still small.

PERHEXILINE MALEATE. Although classified by some as a calcium channel blocker, the action of this coronary vasodilator in this regard is weaker than verapamil, nifedipine, or diltiazem. In this country it remains an investigational drug. In long-term use it does appear quite effective in preventing attacks of variant angina; between 76 and 100 percent of patients have had their attacks completely or partially controlled by 200 to 1000 mg of this drug per day in the few studies reported.[110,187,188] In short-term use, it is not as effective as nifedipine, verapamil, or diltiazem in preventing ergonovine-induced coronary artery spasm.[189] In 16 patients with apparent complete suppression of variant angina symptoms, 3 developed myocardial infarction, and 2 died suddenly while on the drug.[188] Perhexiline caused a very high incidence of side effects during chronic use (in up to 76 percent of patients),[187,188,190] which necessitated discontinuing the drug in about 25 percent.[188] Most frequent adverse effects were elevated liver enzymes (in 39 percent of cases) and dizziness. These very frequent side effects will severely limit the usefulness of this drug.

Other Possibly Effective Drugs

AMIODARONE. This agent was introduced as an antianginal drug in 1967, but more recently it has been under study for its potent antiarrhythmic properties. It is an effective dilator of peripheral and coronary arterioles and lowers blood pressure and peripheral and coronary vascular resistances.[191] It is still investigational in this country. It has been useful acutely in controlling variant angina attacks in some patients,[192,193] but not in others.[159,194] Its usefulness for chronic prophylactic treatment of vasospastic angina is unknown and might be limited by a significant incidence of side effects.[179]

SPECIFIC INHIBITORS OF THROMBOXANE A_2. Prostaglandins have been suggested as substances that might play a role in vasospastic angina. Thromboxane A_2 is a potent coronary

156

artery constrictor; and elevated levels of its metabolite, thromboxane B_2, have been found in peripheral and coronary sinus blood in relation to attacks of vasospastic angina.[4,195] In the only published clinical study I could find, the thromboxane A_2 antagonist, phthalazinol, abolished variant angina attacks in all eight patients to whom 0.6 mg was given daily.[196] Such drugs deserve further study, but as of this writing none is available in this country for investigational use.

Controversial Drugs

BETA-ADRENERGIC BLOCKERS. Reasoning physiologically, one would not expect these drugs to dilate coronary arteries or to prevent vasospasm inasmuch as blockade of beta-adrenergic, vasodilator effects would leave unopposed alpha-adrenergic vasoconstrictor influences. The result might be constriction of coronary arteries, which is what is actually observed in humans when the drug is given in the absence of vasodilator drugs.[7] Why, then, has this class of drugs generated so much interest in vasospastic angina? Its great effectiveness in classic angina was probably the initial, naive reason. However, an early, reasonably well-controlled study by Guazzi and his colleagues[197] showed abolition of variant angina attacks in 73 percent of 15 cases of variant angina, not on organic nitrates, with doses of propranolol averaging 368 mg per day; practolol was ineffective. Both propranolol *and* practolol were effective in about 40 percent of cases of spontaneous angina with ST segment depression. These authors commented that the effect was dose dependent, that doses greater than needed for nearly complete pharmacologic beta-adrenergic blockade were frequently required, that the efficacy might not rely on beta-blocking properties of the drug, and that other investigators had not obtained similar results possibly because they used smaller doses of drugs. Another more recent study of 42 patients with variant angina associated with severe coronary obstructive disease reported that most of these patients' symptoms were stabilized with propranolol and organic nitrates combined, with results the same as those obtained with patients having similar symptoms and coronary disease but with ST segment depression during attacks.[198]

On the other hand, contemporaneous, alarming reports appeared of actual aggravation of attacks of variant angina by beta-adrenergic blockers in significant numbers of cases.[27,40,199,202] Most studies demonstrated no evidence of efficacy of propranolol and other beta-blockers,[10,70,73,137,151,152,180,200–202] but doses used in many cases were less than those employed by Guazzi's group.[197]

My own experience is that when patients are on *maximum tolerable* doses of organic nitrate vasodilators, the addition of propranolol does not usually aggravate variant angina symptoms. This finding is consistent with the observation that in humans, nitroglycerin completely abolishes the coronary vasoconstrictive effect of propranolol.[7] However, I have not found propranolol effective in any variant angina patient.

In talking recently with experts on coronary artery spasm from many parts of the world, I have found little current enthusiasm for use of beta-adrenergic blockers in patients whose angina is mainly the result of coronary artery spasm without *severe* organic coronary disease. Indeed, most consider these drugs *contraindicated* in such cases because of their potential for aggravating attacks and because of availability of other clearly efficacious drugs. Thus, there is presently neither rationale nor justification for using beta-adrenergic antagonists as primary or secondary drugs for angina due mainly to coronary spasm. In rare cases, where usually more effective drugs have failed, beta-adrenergic blockers may be worth a try, provided that the patient is kept on full doses of organic nitrate vasodilators concurrently.

This leaves an interesting paradox. If beta-adrenergic blockers are contraindicated or no good in vasospastic angina, and if angina at rest with ST segment depression is frequently due to coronary artery spasm in patients with significant organic coronary disease,[1] then why do the majority of such unstable angina patients actually get better on propranolol with organic nitrates, which is currently standard treatment for this syndrome? I can only guess at the answer to this question. In these patients there may be a relatively greater role of organic obstruction and a relatively lesser role of spasm, so that the oxygen-sparing effects of the beta-blockers are more important than in the average case of variant angina. Also, beta-blockers are almost always used in patients already receiving organic nitrates, which are very effective for coronary artery spasm. Some institutions have almost abandoned the use of beta-blocking drugs in unstable angina. I think that is going a bit too far. I do recommend, however, that their use should *not* be routine in such cases, but, rather, each case should be carefully analyzed for evidence of critical organic obstruction and vasospasm, and beta-blockers should be utilized fully in conjunction with organic nitrates when the former condition is present. Remember, not all these patients will have severe organic coronary obstruction.

ALPHA-ADRENERGIC BLOCKERS. Because alpha-adrenergic receptor stimulation is a built-in mechanism for vasoconstriction and is one important determinant of basal coronary arterial smooth muscle tone,[203] and because coronary artery spasm can be provoked in susceptible patients with alpha-adrenergic agonists,[7,27] an abnormality of alpha-adrenergic regulation has been postulated as a cause of variant angina.[27] These findings prompted therapeutic trials with alpha-adrenergic blocking drugs, but none of these studies has been adequately controlled. Despite a few reports of successful prevention of spontaneous attacks of variant angina with phenoxybenzamine,[204,205] most patients studied have not responded to these agents[168,180,206-208]—a finding that agrees with my own experience. In some cases, phenoxybenzamine[40,207,209] and phentolamine[14,40] were successful in preventing effort-induced angina of probable vasospastic origin, but this efficacy was not always seen.[76] Interestingly, intravenous phentolamine has been shown effective in blocking an inappropriate increase in coronary vascular resistance resulting from a cold pressor test in patients with classic angina.[210]

At present, nonselective alpha-adrenergic blockers must be relegated to the category of rarely effective for vasospastic angina. Moreover, frequent and significant side effects limit their use.[205,211]

There are no published reports of trials in vasospastic angina with prazosin, a selective alpha-adrenergic antagonist.

NYLIDRIN. This beta-adrenergic agonist is used as a peripheral arterial dilator for patients with occlusive vascular disease. It was originally suggested for use in variant angina by Prinzmetal and his coworkers,[48] who claimed improvement in three of four patients with this drug. There have subsequently been practically no further cases of efficacy reported,[212] and the drug has never had a controlled trial for vasospastic angina.

ATROPINE. This parasympathetic antagonist was tried in vasospastic angina because in some patients methacholine, a parasympathetic agonist, could provoke attacks of variant angina, and atropine premedication could prevent this.[23,213] Although in some cases with frequent attacks the drug appeared helpful,[22,23,214] in general, results have been disappointing,[70,101,180,215-217] and its efficacy must be considered equivocal.

PROSTACYCLIN (PGI$_2$). This prostaglandin, synthesized from arachidonic acid by the vascular endothelium, is a potent dilator of coronary arteries, an inhibitor of platelet aggregation, and a natural antagonist of the effects of platelet-derived thromboxane A$_2$.[218] Production of prostacyclin by atherosclerotic arteries may be depressed.[219] These facts have led to preliminary trials of prostacyclin (intravenously) in vasospastic angina. Maseri and his coworkers[220] infused prostacyclin 10-20 ng per kg per minute into six patients with vasospastic angina in a cross-over study with placebo. Although the drug produced obvious systemic vasodilation and reduction in platelet aggregation in vitro, it had no effect on ischemic episodes of five patients. In one case, however, it consistently abolished attacks. In an uncontrolled study, Szczeklik and colleagues[221] infused 5 to 10 ng per kg per minute for 72 hours in seven patients with spontaneous anginal attacks. A reduction in frequency of anginal attacks seemed to result, and the reduction lasted at least two to three months. The same infusion of prostacyclin failed to protect from angina and ST depression provoked by atrial pacing in another seven patients with classic stable angina. Further trials with this agent are warranted; but even if it is found effective, its usefulness for long-term prophylaxis of vasospasm would be limited by the need for intravenous infusion.

Ineffective Drugs

Platelet and Nonselective Prostaglandin Inhibitors

The evidence suggesting increased thromboxane A$_2$ generation in vasospastic angina[4,195] and deficient prostacyclin production in atherosclerotic vessels[219] has been mentioned already. Unfortunately, these drugs, exemplified by aspirin and indomethacin, inhibit prostacyclin as well as thromboxane A$_2$ production and may actually result in an increased tendency for vasoconstriction.[217]

CYCLOOXYGENASE INHIBITORS. Therapeutic trials with low dose aspirin[221-223] and with indomethacin[4,224] have failed to demonstrate efficacy, with one exception.[225] Moreover, a recent study of the effects of giving 4 gm aspirin per day to patients with variant angina revealed that the drug turned repeatedly negative afternoon exercise tests positive (seven of seven cases) and aggravated spontaneous attacks in six of eight cases.[31] I conclude that these drugs have no role in treatment of vasospastic angina and should be avoided by such patients.

DIPYRIDAMOLE. This drug is a potent dilator of arterioles, especially in the coronary artery bed. It does not dilate large coronary arteries. Although originally marketed for use in chronic stable angina pectoris, evidence for its efficacy is highly questionable. More recently it has been shown predictably to *provoke* myocardial ischemia in patients with severe coronary obstructive disease by diverting blood away from the subendocardium distal to a stenosis.[226] Dipyridamole also has antiplatelet activity, part of which may be due to stimulation of vascular prostacyclin production. There is no evidence that this agent is of any use in vasospastic angina.[180]

Other Drugs

RESERPINE. There are two reports (three patients) of improvement in variant angina following the use of reserpine (0.25 mg two to three times daily).[227,228]

ANTICOAGULANTS. There has been no controlled trial of anticoagulants for vasospastic angina, and no efficacy has been claimed for them. It is of interest that in experience collected from a number of institutions in Japan, treatment of variant angina with anticoagulants resulted in a greater percentage of patients with freedom from attacks than did treatment with beta-adrenergic blockers (40 percent versus 11 percent).[137] One interpretation of this finding is that the rate of symptomatic improvement with anticoagulants represents the effect one can get with a placebo, and the worse results with beta-blockers reflect the tendency of these drugs to aggravate symptoms.

TREATMENT OF ARRHYTHMIAS DUE TO CORONARY ARTERY SPASM

Arrhythmias during spontaneous angina resulting from acute, severe myocardial ischemia are common in variant angina, being observed in up to 60 percent of cases;[1,42,95,229,230] and about one third of these arrhythmias are life-threatening.[1] Of my own series of 73 patients, 8 required resuscitation from ventricular fibrillation at least once during some part of their course, and another 4 with known arrhythmias complicating their attacks died suddenly and unexpectedly during an attack outside the hospital. Serious arrhythmias encountered acutely with anginal attacks are not as common in other anginal syndromes of coronary vasospasm, presumably because of less severe and extensive ischemia.

Such severe arrhythmias can be a major problem in management of variant angina and in some cases dominate the patient's clinical presentation. They are the most common cause of death in variant angina patients.[231] The most common serious arrhythmias encountered are complex premature ventricular beats, ventricular tachycardia, ventricular fibrillation, and high-grade atrioventricular block.[1,231,232] Even when none of these arrhythmias has been observed during monitored attacks, their occurrence can be suspected if the patient gives a history of syncope with attacks—which occurs in roughly one third of variant angina patients.[200,231] Syncope, however, is not synonymous with arrhythmia because it may result from the hypotension of severe, acute myocardial insufficiency without arrhythmia.[95,202]

Management

The best treatment for these arrhythmias is to prevent them, and this requires the *absolute* prevention of coronary artery spasm attacks and hence of the myocardial ischemia that generates the arrhythmia. If this result can be achieved, the patient can be guaranteed that there will no longer be spontaneous angina or arrhythmia. When a life-threatening arrhythmia is suspected or documented during attacks, the patient should be kept monitored in the hospital *as long as needed* to devise treatment that achieves this goal. It is admittedly impossible to know when one has found a regimen that will completely prevent future attacks (this requires a crystal ball); and because a patient's first post-discharge attack could be fatal, the initial therapy chosen should be the one most likely to be successful, namely, the *combined* use of maximum tolerable doses of an organic nitrate and a calcium channel blocker. No reliance should be placed on standard antiarrhythmic drugs, which are usually ineffective in this setting. In difficult cases where an *extremely* high-grade organic stenosis is present in the vessel involved with spasm, consideration can be given to surgical treatment for that obstruction (or balloon angioplasty) *combined* with pre-operative and post-operative drug therapy mentioned above; but this approach should be considered a last resort only, because enhanced irritability of the vessel following manipulation has been known to convert tolerable arrhythmia problems into fatal ones.

The problem of how long apparently completely effective therapy should be continued in these patients is insoluble. My present belief is that such patients should be treated indefinitely, provided they are tolerating the drugs reasonably well. If for some reason therapy must be stopped eventually, it might be wise to hospitalize the patient at the time and perform a provocative test under optimum conditions while off the drugs to determine if the patient is still susceptible to coronary vasospasm.[15] Patients must always be warned to report recurrence of symptoms at once, even if they are still on drug therapy.

When absolute prevention of attacks cannot be achieved, additional antiarrhythmic therapy requires documentation of the nature of the rhythm disorder involved.

PREMATURE VENTRICULAR BEATS, VENTRICULAR TACHYCARDIA AND FIBRILLATION. The ventricular arryhythmias of acute mycardial ischemia due to brief coronary occlusion are probably due to re-entry mechanisms.[233] Animal experiments have not yielded evidence that quinidine, procainamide, or lidocaine pretreatment *reliably* prevents these arrhythmias. Most reports of cases with variant angina complicated by ventricular tachycardia and ventricular fibrillation, in which these drugs have been tried, show failure to prevent the arrhythmia,[70,98,100,101,144,234-238] although exceptions occurred. This has also been my experience. Nevertheless, one is sometimes forced to use these drugs while trying to achieve control of the vasospasm.

Verapamil may have some effectiveness in this setting unrelated to its vasodilator properties[172,173,175,176,182] and might be preferable to nifedipine as a calcium channel blocker in patients whose attacks are associated with such ventricular arrhythmias.

There is not enough information yet about newer agents such as bretylium and amiodarone to know if they will be useful for these problems.

TRANSIENT ATRIOVENTRICULAR (AV) BLOCK. This disorder occurs as the result of acute ischemia of the atrioventricular node when its main arterial supply comes from an artery undergoing severe vasospasm. It is thus more common with spasm of the right coronary artery than with spasm of the left coronary artery and is almost always associated with ST segment elevation in inferior leads. First degree AV block requires no treatment. Minor degrees of second degree AV block, such as Wenckebach periods, may also be asymptomatic. Higher grade AV block that impairs cardiac performance can be the cause of acute symptoms, with impairment or loss of consciousness. When the latter occurs, a temporary lead can be placed perivenously for demand ventricular pacing until vasospastic attacks are controlled. If long-term prevention of coronary artery spasm and resulting AV block episodes cannot be achieved, the implantation of a permanent pacemaker system will ensure an adequate ventricular rate and usually will prevent syncope, even though anginal attacks continue.[151,239–243] Unfortunately, in some cases the loss of a properly timed atrial contraction and acute depression of ventricular function by ischemia can result in persistence of syncopal attacks during angina from hypotension, despite a normally functioning artificial ventricular pacemaker.[93,95,243,244]

EXERCISE THERAPY

My colleague, Albert Kattus, has for many years been an advocate of exercise therapy for vasospastic angina. He has reasoned that in many patients attacks occur primarily at rest and rarely during effort, that exercise is a potent vasodilator stimulus for the coronary arteries which may by suitable training be carried over into periods of rest, and that such therapy can be safely carried out, especially with premedication with organic nitrate vasodilators, to minimize the chances of vasospasm during or just after exercise—to which a minority of patients are subject. He has pointed out also that the practice of putting patients at bed rest in the hospital, if their angina at rest is due to coronary artery spasm and not to critical organic coronary obstruction, merely ensures the patient will be in a state most susceptible to spontaneous angina 24 hours a day rather than only the 8 to 12 hours a day in that condition before hospitalization. Patients occasionally even volunteer that they feel better when physically active and actually obtain relief from acute spontaneous anginal attacks by getting up and moving around the room briskly.[21,245–247]

No controlled study has been done to evaluate efficacy of exercise therapy in vasospastic angina, and one which could actually be carried out would be difficult to design. Nevertheless, we[42] have regularly prescribed individualized, endurance-type exercise programs to most of our patients with vasospastic angina as *one part* of a comprehensive plan of management. We also try to overcome the contrary biases of CCU nurses and physicians and request our hospitalized patients, while monitored, to walk about their beds and the wards as much as possible rather than allow them to lie in bed, if their coronary anatomy and clinical state allow this approach. Such therapy seems to accelerate improvement in symptoms in some patients, and we have had no evidence of its harming anyone.

SURGERY IN VASOSPASTIC ANGINA

The purpose of this section is not to describe the surgical therapy of vasospastic angina but, rather, to mention those special precautions which should be taken when a patient with vasospastic angina has to undergo cardiac or major noncardiac surgery.

The risk of anesthesia and surgery is particularly increased by concurrent clinical instability of anginal symptoms, by severe underlying organic coronary disease, and by chronic left ventricular dysfunction. Elective procedures should be deferred until symptoms have been stabilized for several months. In patients who urgently require nonelective surgery, what time is available should be used efficiently to optimize the patient's medical treatment and to discuss perioperative management with anesthesiologist and surgeon. Patients who have had stable or no symptoms for at least several months can be gotten through needed surgery with acceptable risk.

Presurgical Conference

It is wise to have an unhurried conference with the surgeon and anesthesiologist to agree on details of management and to give them special instruction for perioperative monitoring and drug therapy. Surgeons and anesthesiologists may be hesitant to operate on these patients until reassured by an experienced cardiologist.

Perioperative Therapy

A major principle is that *effective coronary vasodilator therapy must not be interrupted;* it must continue right through the period in the operating room. If this means that surgeons and anesthesiologists will face using drugs with which they are unfamiliar, then someone acquainted with their use should follow the patient through the procedure. In some cases, all that is needed is an application of nitroglycerin ointment just before the patient goes to the operating room. In other cases, continuous intravenous infusions of nitroglycerin, nifedipine, or verapamil might be required. Special thought and care must be given to this problem in each case because the autonomic instability surrounding the operative period may encourage coronary vasoconstriction, which could be aggravated by a state of rebound vasoconstriction when the vasodilator effect wears off.

Physiologic Monitoring

All these patients should have *ECG monitoring for rhythm and ST-T changes,* starting before induction of anesthesia and continuing for variable times into the postoperative period. The cardiologist should tell the anesthesiologist, surgeon, and intensive care unit nurses which lead or leads to use and what to look for.[248] In patients still having significant angina preoperatively, in those with severe obstructive coronary disease or markedly impaired ventricular function, and in those going for cardiac surgery or major vascular procedures, the pulmonary artery wedge, pulmonary artery, and right atrial pressures and cardiac output should be monitored with a Swan-Ganz-type catheter, and the systemic pressure should be monitored with a radial artery catheter. This approach will allow early detection and treatment of myocardial ischemia, prompt diagnosis and management of causes of hypotension, and proper supervision of any vasodilator infusions.

Choice of Anesthetic

For a number of reasons, I usually recommend *general anesthesia.* In my experience, most general anesthetics are depressants of vascular smooth muscle activity and hence are "antispasmodics." Once the period of induction is over, there is little autonomic instability, when the anesthetic is managed skillfully, until it wears off. Spinal or epidural anesthesia is associated with vasodilation below the anesthetic level but with *compensatory vasoconstriction above this level,* which includes the region of the heart and coronary arteries. Any blood loss or hypotension can further enhance constrictor stimuli on the coronary arteries, which may result in enough coronary artery spasm to cause myocardial ischemia.[249]

There may be an interaction between intravenous nitroglycerin infusion and pancuronium. In animal experiments, the recovery from pancuronium-induced neuromuscular blockade was prolonged when the drug was given to animals already on a nitroglycerin infusion. This effect did not occur if nitroglycerin was started *after* the pancuronium was given and was not seen with succinylcholine or tubocurarine.[250] This interaction should be taken into account in selecting a neuromuscular blocking agent in vasospastic angina patients going for surgery.

Recognition and Treatment of Intraoperative Myocardial Ischemia

During surgery under general anesthesia, patients cannot complain of angina. Acute myocardial ischemia can manifest as changes in the ST segments or T waves of the ECG, arrhythmia, an unexplained rise in pulmonary artery or pulmonary capillary wedge pressure, hypotension, or any combination of these findings. A careful watch must be kept for any of these. Any sign of myocardial ischemia not easily explained by a gross rise in determinants of myocardial oxygen consumption or flagrant hypovolemia should be assumed to be due to coronary artery spasm and should be treated with a rapid intravenous infusion of nitroglycerin (50 to 200 μg repeated at 2- to 3-minute intervals, depending on response). If the patient is already on a vasodilator infusion, also check to make sure it has not become accidentally interrupted or disconnected. This means that some hypotensive patients will have to be given nitroglycerin. But if the hypotension is due to coronary artery spasm, it may respond to nothing else. Once the acute attack has been broken, it might be worthwhile to start a constant infusion of nitroglycerin in order to prevent further attacks or to increase the rate of an infusion of vasodilator if one is already being administered. Other basic principles of treating coronary patients under anesthesia should be followed also.

Postoperatively, the patient should be placed back on the usual program of drugs as soon as possible, with alterations if instability of attacks develop.

Published data is small for noncardiac surgery.[249,251–255] My own experience with six operations in five patients with variant angina has been good. Only one of these developed attacks perioperatively, and he was not receiving any vasodilator medication at the time; his attacks were completely suppressed with verapamil. None developed evidence of ischemia during the operative procedure.

ACKNOWLEDGMENTS

Thanks are due to Miss Toshi Yamada and Mrs. Jeanne Yamaguchi for their assistance in preparing this manuscript.

REFERENCES

1. MASERI, A, SEVERI, S, NES, MD, ET AL: *"Variant" angina: one aspect of a continuous spectrum of vasospastic myocardial ischemia.* Am J Cardiol 42:1019, 1978.
2. MACALPIN, RN: *Contribution of dynamic vascular wall thickening to luminal narrowing during coronary arterial constriction.* Circulation 61:296, 1980.
3. BROWN, BG: *Coronary vasospasm. Observations linking the clinical spectrum of ischemic heart disease to the dynamic pathology of coronary arteriosclerosis.* Arch Intern Med 141:716, 1981.
4. ROBERTSON, RM, ROBERTSON, D, ROBERTS, LJ, ET AL: *Thromboxane A2 in vasotonic angina pectoris. Evidence from direct measurements and inhibitor trials.* N Engl J Med 304:988, 1981.
5. HEUPLER, FA, JR: *Syndrome of symptomatic coronary arterial spasm with nearly normal coronary arteriograms.* Am J Cardiol 45:873, 1980.
6. YASUE, H, OMOTE, S, TAKIZAWA, A, ET AL: *Exertional angina pectoris caused by coronary arterial spasm: Effects of various drugs.* Am J Cardiol 43:647, 1979.
7. BROWN, BG, BOLSON, E, FRIMER, M, ET AL: *Angiographic distinction between variant angina and non-vasospastic chest pain.* Circulation 58 (Suppl 2):122, 1978.
8. RAFFLENBEUL, W, URTHALER, F, RUSSELL, RO, ET AL: *Dilatation of coronary artery stenoses after isosorbide dinitrate in man.* Br Heart J 43:546, 1980.
9. RAIZNER, AE, CHAHINE, RA, ISHIMORI, T, ET AL: *Provocation of coronary artery spasm by the cold pressor test. Hemodynamic, arteriographic and quantitative angiographic observations.* Circulation 62:925, 1980.
10. SEVERI, S, DAIRES, G, MASERI, A. ET AL: *Long-term prognosis of "variant" angina with medical treatment.* Am J Cardiol 46:226, 1980.
11. SMITHEN, C, WILNER, G, BALTAXE, H, ET AL: *Variant angina pectoris.* Am Heart J 89:87, 1975.
12. DIMATTÉO, J, DELAGE, B, CACHERA, JP, ET AL: *Dissection primitive isolée de l'artère coronaire droite.* Arch Mal Coeur 70:1137, 1977.

13. SCHROEDER, JS: Personal communication, 1981.

14. YASUE, H: *Pathophysiology and treatment of coronary arterial spasm.* Chest 78:216, 1980.

15. WATERS, DD, SZLACHCIC, J. THÉROUX, P, ET AL: *Ergonovine testing to detect spontaneous remissions of variant angina during long-term treatment with calcium antagonist drugs.* Am J Cardiol 47:179, 1981.

16. OLIVA, PB, POTTS, DE, AND PLUSS, RG: *Coronary arterial spasm in Prinzmetal angina. Documentation by coronary arteriography.* N Engl J Med 288:745, 1973.

17. WEI, JY, GENECIN, A, GREENE, HL, ET AL: *Coronary spasm with ventricular fibrillation during thyrotoxicosis: Response to attaining euthyroid state.* Am J Cardiol 43:335, 1979.

18. MILLER, D, WATERS, DD, WARNICA, W, ET AL: *Is variant angina the coronary manifestation of a generalized vasospastic disorder?* N Engl J Med 304:763, 1981.

19. RUGGEROLI, CW, COHN, K, AND LANGSTON, M: *Prinzmetal's variant angina: A pathophysiological and clinical kaleidoscope.* Am J Cardiol 33:167, 1974.

20. MOSCHOWITZ, E: *Tobacco angina pectoris.* JAMA. 90:733, 1928.

21. WILSON, FN, AND JOHNSTON, FD: *The occurrence in angina pectoris of electrocardiographic changes similar in magnitude and in kind to those produced by myocardial infarction.* Am Heart J 22:64, 1941.

22. YAMAMOTO, M, AND KATAYAMA, S: *Angina pectoris induced by marked vagotonic state.* Jap Circ J 32:1856, 1968.

23. YASUE, H. TOUYAMA, M, SHIMAMOTO, M, ET AL: *Role of autonomic nervous system in the pathogenesis of Prinzmetal's variant form of angina.* Circulation 50:534, 1974.

24. KOVALČÍK, V: *Effect of bradykinin on isolated coronary arteries.* Nature 196:174, 1962.

25. NAKAYAMA, K, FLECKENSTEIN, A, BYON, YK, ET AL: *Fundamental physiology of coronary smooth musculature from extramural stem arteries of pigs and rabbits.* Europ J Cardiol 8:319, 1978.

26. GINSBERG, R, BRISTOW, MR, HARRISON, DC, ET AL: *Studies with isolated human coronary arteries. Some general observations, potential mediators of spasm, role of calcium antagonists.* Chest 78:180, 1980.

27. YASUE, H, TOUYAMA, M, KATO, H, ET AL: *Prinzmetal's variant form of angina as a manifestation of alpha-adrenergic receptor-mediated coronary artery spasm: Documentation by coronary arteriography.* Am Heart J 91:148, 1976.

28. ROSS, G: *Adrenergic responses of the coronary vessels.* Circ Res 39:461, 1976.

29. HEUPLER, FA, PROUDFIT, WL, RAZAIR, M, ET AL: *Ergonovine maleate provocative test for coronary artery spasm.* Am J Cardiol 41:631, 1978.

30. PRINZMETAL, M, AND BLOOMBERG, W: *The use of benzedrine for the treatment of narcolepsy.* JAMA 105:2051, 1935.

31. MIWA, K, KAMBARA, H, AND KAWAI, C: *Exercise-induced angina provoked by aspirin administration in patients with variant angina.* Am J Cardiol 47:1210, 1981.

32. LANGE, RL, REID, MS, TRESCH, DD, ET AL: *Nonatheromatous ischemic heart disease following withdrawal from chronic industrial nitroglycerin exposure.* Circulation 46:666, 1972.

33. DISTANTE, A, SEVERI, S, BIAGINI, A, ET AL: *Clinical results with nitrates in patients with "primary" angina at rest.* In MASERI, A, KLASSEN, GA, AND LESCH, M (EDS): *Primary and Secondary Angina Pectoris.* Grune & Stratton, New York, 1978, p 389.

34. FERNANDEZ, D, ROSENTHAL, JE, COHEN, LS, ET AL: *Alcohol-induced Prinzmetal variant angina.* Am J Cardiol 32:238, 1973.

35. HILAL, H, AND MASSUMI, R: *Variant angina pectoris.* Am J Cardiol 19:607, 1967.

36. CHERRIER, F, CUILLIERE, M, NEIMANN, JL, ET AL: *L'angor de Prinzmetal.* Ann Med Nancy 14:11, 1975.

37. SILVERMAN, ME, AND FLAMM, MD: *Variant angina pectoris. Anatomic findings and prognostic implications.* Ann Intern Med 75:339, 1971.

38. RIZZON, P, BRINDICCI, G, BIASCO, G., ET AL: *Sul problema della vasoconstrizione coronary parossistica.* Mal Cardiovasc 9:635, 1968.

39. HARRISON, TR: *Clinical aspects of pain in the chest. I. Angina pectoris.* Am J Med Sci 207:56l, 1944.

40. YASUE, H, OMOTE, S, TAKIZAWA, A, ET AL: *Circadian variation of exercise capacity in patients with Prinzmetal's variant angina: Role of exercise-induced coronary arterial spasm.* Circulation 59:938, 1979.

41. SPECCHIA, G, DE SERVI, S, FALCONE, C, ET AL: *Coronary arterial spasm as a cause of exercise-induced ST-segment elevation in patients with variant angina.* Circulation 59:948, 1979.

42. MACALPIN, RN, KATTUS, AA, AND ALVARO, AB: *Angina pectoris at rest with preservation of exercise capacity. Prinzmetal's variant angina.* Circulation 47:946, 1973.

43. JOHNSON, SM, MAURITSON, DR, WILLERSON, JT, ET AL: *A controlled trial of varapamil for Prinzmetal's variant angina.* N Engl J Med 304:862, 1981.

44. CURRY, RC, JR, PEPINE, CJ, AND CONTI, R: *Ambulatory monitoring to evaluate therapy results in variant angina patients.* Circulation 60 (Suppl 2):190, 1979.

45. GORFINKEL, JH, INGLESBY, TV, LANSING, AM, ET AL: *ST-segment elevation, transient left posterior hemiblock, and recurrent ventricular arrhythmias unassociated with pain. A variant of Prinzmetal's anginal syndrome.* Ann Intern Med 79:795, 1973.

46. FREEDMAN, B, DUNN, RF, RICHMOND, DR, ET AL: *Coronary artery spasm during exercise: Treatment with verapamil.* Circulation 64:68, 1981.

47. PHANEUF, DC, WATERS, DD, DAUWE, F, ET AL: *Refractory variant angina controlled with combined drug therapy in a patient with a single coronary artery.* Cath Cardiovasc Diag 6:413, 1980.

48. PRINZMETAL, M, KENNAMER, R, MERLISS, R, ET AL: *Angina pectoris I. A variant form of angina pectoris.* Am J Med 27:375, 1959.

49. GERBER, JG, AND NIES, AS: *Abrupt withdrawal of cardiovascular drugs.* N Engl J Med 301:1234, 1979.

50. LIKOFF, W, KASPARIAN, H, LEHMAN, JS, ET AL: *Evaluation of "coronary vasodilators" by coronary arteriography.* Am J Cardiol 13:7, 1964.

51. GENSINI, GG, KELLY, AE, DACOSTA, BC, ET AL: *Quantitative angiography: The measurement of coronary vasomobility in the intact animal and man.* Chest 60:522, 1971.

52. FELDMAN, RL, PEPINE, CJ, CURRY, RC, JR, ET AL: *Coronary arterial responses to graded doses of nitroglycerin.* Am J Cardiol 43:91, 1979.

53. HILL, J, FELDMAN, RL, PEPINE, CJ, ET AL: *Altered regional coronary vasodilator responses to nitroglycerin in variant angina patients.* Clin Res 27:736A, 1979.

54. ORAVETZ, R, LEE, G, BAKER, L, ET AL: *Prominent dilation of stenotic coronary artery lesions following sublingual nitroglycerin by quantitative arteriography.* Circulation 58 (Suppl 2):25, 1978.

55. YASUE, H: *Management of variant angina.* Arch Inst Cardiol Mex 50:249, 1980.

56. CASTILLO FENOY, A, BENACERRAF, A, TONNELIER, M, ET AL: *Le test au maléate de méthyl-ergométrine dans l'etude du spasme coronarien.* Nouve Presse Med 8:2339, 1979.

57. CATTELL, M, STONE, D, BALCON, R, ET AL: *Induction of coronary artery spasm with ergometrine.* Br Heart J 39:927, 1977.

58. BERTRAND, ME, ROUSSEAU, MF, LABLANCHE, JM, ET AL: *La détection du spasme des artères coronaires par le test à la méthylergométrine.* Arch Mal Coeur 72:123, 1979.

59. SPECCHIA, G, VALSECCHI, O, DE SERVI, S, ET AL: *Spasmo coronarico indotto neli' uomo de ergonovina maleato.* Bol Soc Ital Biol Sper 53:1452, 1977.

60. WATERS, DD: *Rationale for ergonovine testing in the CCU.* Cath Cardiovasc Diag 6:428, 1980.

61. BUXTON, A, GOLDBERG, S, HIRSHFELD, JW, ET AL: *Refractory ergonovine-induced coronary vasospasm: Importance of intracoronary nitroglycerin.* Am J Cardiol 46:329, 1980.

62. PEPINE, CJ: *Recommendations for use of ergonovine to provoke coronary artery spasm.* Cath Cardiovasc Diag 6:423, 1980.

63. EPSTEIN, SE, REDWOOD, DR, GOLDSTEIN, RE, ET AL: *Angina pectoris: Pathophysiology, evaluation, and treatment.* Ann Intern Med 75:263, 1971.

64. ABRAMS, J: *Nitrate tolerance and dependence.* Am Heart J 99:113, 1980.

65. DISTANTE, A, MASERI, A, SEVERI, S, ET AL: *Management of vasospastic angina at rest with continuous infusion of isosorbide dinitrate.* Am J Cardiol 44:533, 1979.

66. WILKINSON, CJ, AND SANDERS, JH, JR: *Massive doses of nitroglycerin in a patient with variant angina.* Anesth Analg 59:707, 1980.

67. ARMSTRONG, PW, ARMSTRONG, JA, AND MARKS, GS: *Blood levels after sublingual nitroglycerin.* Circulation 59:585, 1979

68. DONSKY, MS, HARRIS, MD, CURRY, GC, ET AL: *Variant angina pectoris: A clinical and coronary arteriographic spectrum.* Am Heart J 89:571, 1975.

69. MASERI, A, MIMMO, R, CHIERCHIA, S, ET AL: *Coronary artery spasm as a cause of acute myocardial ischemia in man.* Chest 68:625, 1975.

70. ENDO, M, KANDA, I, HOSODA, S, ET AL: *Prinzmetal's variant form of angina pectoris. Re-evaluation of mechanisms.* Circulation 52:33, 1975.

71. DELAHAYE, JP, TOUBOUL, P, PORTE, J, ET AL: *L'angine de Prinzmetal et ses indications thérapeutiques.* Actual Cardiovasc Med-Chir 7:143, 1975.

72. AMIEL, M, DELAYE, J, DELAHAYE, JP, ET AL: *Prinzmetal et spasme coronarien concomitants.* J Radiol Electrol 58:27, 1977.

73. PASTERNALS, RC, HUTTER, AM, DESANCTIS, RW, ET AL: *Variant angina. Clinical spectrum and results of medical and surgical therapy.* J Thorac Cardiovasc Surg 78:614, 1979.

74. FELDMAN, RL, PEPINE, CJ, AND CONTI, CR: *Unusual vasomotor coronary arterial responses after nitroglycerin.* Am J Cardiol 42:517, 1978.

75. BASSENGE, E: Personal communication, 1981.

76. FULLER, CM, RAIZNER, AE, CHAHINE, RA, ET AL: *Exercise-induced coronary arterial spasm: Angiographic demonstration, documentation of ischemia by myocardial scintigraphy and results of pharmacologic intervention.* Am J Cardiol 46:500, 1980.

77. WEI, JY, AND REID, PR: *Quantitative determination of trinitroglycerin in human plasma.* Circulation 59:588, 1979.

78. ROBERTSON, D, ROBERTSON, RM, NIES, AS, ET AL: *Variant angina pectoris: Investigation of indexes of sympathetic nervous system function.* Am J Cardiol 43:1080, 1979.

79. PREVITALI, M, SALERNO, JA, MEDICI, A, ET AL: *Poor reliability of ergonovine maleate test in predicting response to treatment in angina at rest.* Circulation 60 (Suppl 2):249, 1979.

80. SALERNO, JA, PREVITALI, M, MEDICI, A, ET AL: *Treatment of vasospastic angina pectoris at rest with nitroglycerin ointment: A short-term controlled study in the coronary care unit.* Am J Cardiol 47:1129, 1981.

81. KAPLAN, JA, AND TREASURE, RL: *Intravenous nitroglycerin during coronary artery surgery.* Military Med 142:152, 1977.

82. McNIFF, BL, McNIFF, EF, AND FUNG, HL: *Potency and stability of extemporaneous nitroglycerin infusions.* Am J Hosp Pharm 36:173, 1979.

83. ROBERTS, MS, COSSUM, PA, GALBRAITH, AJ, ET AL: *The availability of nitroglycerin from parenteral solutions.* J Pharm Pharmacol 32:237, 1980.

84. MACALPIN, RN, AND KOLIN, A: Unpublished observations, 1980.

85. STOLZENBERG, J, AND POLLAK, RH: *Rapid redistribution of thallium 201 post stress testing in a patient with variant angina.* Clin Nucl Med 4:283, 1979.

86. THÉROUX, P, WATERS, DD, AFFAKI, GS, ET AL: *Provocative testing with ergonovine to evaluate the efficacy of treatment with calcium antagonists in variant angina.* Circulation 60:504, 1979.

87. OLIVA, PB, AND BRECKINRIDGE, JC: *Arteriographic evidence of coronary arterial spasm in acute myocardial infarction.* Circulation 56:366, 1977.

88. GOLD, HK, AND LEINBACH, RC: *Acute angiography during anterior myocardial infarction: Analysis of nitroglycerin and propranolol therapy.* Circulation 60 (Suppl 2):69, 1979.

89. RENTROP, P, BLANKE, H, KARSCH, KR, ET AL: *Selective intracoronary thrombolysis in acute myocardial infarction and unstable angina pectoris.* Circulation 63:307, 1981.

90. HIGGINS, CB, WEXLER, L, SILVERMAN, JF, ET AL: *Clinical and arteriographic features of Prinzmetal's variant angina: Documentation of etiologic factors.* Am J Cardiol 37:831, 1976.

91. CATTELL, MR, STONE, DL, BROOKS, N, ET AL: *Ergometrine-induced spasm in normal or minimally diseased coronary arteries.* In KALTENBACH, M, LICHTLEN, P, BALCON, R, ET AL: (EDS): *Coronary Heart Disease.* Georg Thieme, Stuttgart, 1978, p 147.

92. ROZANSKI, JJ, MELLER, J, KLEINFELD, M, ET AL: *Nonmechanical ST-segment alternans in Prinzmetal's angina.* Ann Intern Med 89:76, 1978.

93. HARPER, R, PETER, T, AND HUNT, D: *Syncope in association with Prinzmetal variant angina.* Br Heart J 37:771, 1975.

94. HUCKELL, VF, ADELMAN, AG, DOUGLAS, BC, ET AL: *Prinzmetal's angina: Ischemia due to spasm.* Circulation 54 (Suppl 2):173, 1976.

95. KIMURA, E, HOSODA, S, KATOH, K, ET AL: *Panel discussion on the variant form of angina pectoris.* Jpn Circ J 42:455, 1978.

96. KING, MJ, ZIR, LM, KALTMAN, AJ, ET AL: *Variant angina associated with angiographically demonstrated coronary artery spasm and REM sleep.* Am J Med Sci 265:419, 1973.

97. HANAZONO, N, ODA, H, ISHIDA, H, ET AL: *Prinzmetal's angina pectoris with normal coronary arteriograms.* Jpn Heart J 17:43, 1976.

98. RIZZON, P, ROSSI, L, CALABRESE, P, ET AL: *Angiographic and pathologic correlations in Prinzmetal variant angina.* Angiology 29:486, 1978.

99. ETTINGER, PO, MOORE, RJ, CALABRO, J, ET AL: *Temporal course of progressive potassium induced coronary vasoconstriction.* Clin Res 25:220A, 1977.

100. PRCHKOV, VK, MOOKHERJEE, S, SCHIESS, W, ET AL: *Variant anginal syndrome, coronary artery spasm, and ventricular fibrillation in absence of chest pain.* Ann Intern Med 81:858, 1974.

101. NORDSTROM, LA, LILLIHEI, JP, ADICOFF, A, ET AL: *Coronary artery surgery for recurrent ventricular arrhythmias in patients with variant angina.* Am Heart J 89:236, 1975.

102. BERMAN, ND, McLAUGHLIN, PR, HUCKELL, VF, ET AL: *Prinzmetal's angina with coronary artery spasm. Angiographic, pharmacologic, metabolic and radionuclide perfusion studies.* Am J Med 60:727, 1976.

166

103. KATTENBACH, M, KREHAN, L, KOBER, G, ET AL: *Coronarographic findings in patients with ST elevation in the exercise ECG and Prinzmetal angina.* In LICHTLEN, PR (ED): *Coronary Angiography and Angina Pectoris.* George Thieme, Stuttgart, 1976, p 76.

104. PAOLILLO, V, MARRA, S, AND AQUARO, G: *Sodium nitroprusside in the treatment of Prinzmetal's variant angina.* Chest 77:807, 1980.

105. DOERNER, TC, BROWN, BG, BOLSON, E, ET AL: *Vasodilatory effects of nitroglycerin and nitroprusside in coronary arteries—a comparative analysis.* Am J Cardiol 43:416, 1979.

106. YEH, BK, GOSSELIN, AJ, SWAYE, PS, ET AL: *Sodium nitroprusside as a coronary vasodilator in man. I. Effect of intracoronary sodium nitroprusside on coronary arteries, angina pectoris, and coronary blood flow.* Am Heart J 93:610, 1977.

107. SWAYE, PS, SHIEH, SM, GOSSELINE, AJ, ET AL: *Nitroprusside induces coronary vasodilation in man.* Clin Res 23:210, 1975.

108. MANN, T, HOLMAN, BL, GREEN, LH, ET AL: *Effect of nitroprusside on regional myocardial blood flow, and comparison with nitroglycerin, in patients with coronary artery disease.* Circulation 56 (Suppl 3):33, 1977.

109. MUKHERJEE, D, FELDMAN, MS, AND HELFANT, RH: *The use of nitroprusside in patients with recurrent chest pain, ST elevations and ventricular arrhythmias.* Circulation 52 (Suppl 3):221, 1975.

110. RAABE, DS, JR: *Treatment of variant angina pectoris with perhexiline maleate.* Chest 75:152, 1979.

111. PACKER, M, MELLER, J, MEDINA, N, ET AL: *Rebound hemodynamic events after the abrupt withdrawal of nitroprusside in patients with severe chronic heart failure.* N Engl J Med 301:1193, 1979.

112. STONE, PH, ANTMAN, EM, MULLER, JE, ET AL: *Calcium channel blocking agents in the treatment of cardiovascular disorders. Part II: Hemodynamic effects and clinical applications.* Ann Intern Med 93:886, 1980.

113. ANTMAN, EM, STONE, PH, MULLER, JE, ET AL: *Calcium channel blocking agents in the treatment of cardiovascular disorders. Part I: Basic and clinical electrophysiologic effects.* Ann Intern Med 93:875, 1980.

114. ELBRODT, G, CHEW, CYC, AND SINGH, BN: *Therapeutic implications of slow-channel blockade in cardiocirculatory disorders.* Circulation 62:669, 1980.

115. HENRY, PD: *Comparative pharmacology of calcium antagonists: Nifedipine, verapamil, diltiazem.* Am J Cardiol 46:1047, 1980.

116. ZELIS, R, AND FLAIM, SF: *"Calcium influx blockers" and vascular smooth muscle: Do we really understand the mechanisms?* Ann Intern Med 94:124, 1981.

117. POLESE, A, FIORENTINI, C, OLIVARI, MT, ET AL: *Clinical use of a calcium antagonistic agent (nifedipine) in acute pulmonary edema.* Am J Med 66:825, 1979.

118. LICHTLEN, P, ENGEL, HJ, AMENDE, I, ET AL: *Mechanisms of various antianginal drugs. Relationship between regional flow behavior and contractility.* In JATENE, AD, AND LICHTLEN, PR (EDS): *3rd International Adalat Symposium. New Therapy of Ischemic Heart Disease.* International Congress Series No. 388, Excerpta Medica, Amsterdam, 1976, p 14.

119. CHEW, CYC, BROWN, BG, WONG, M, ET AL: *The effects of verapamil on coronary hemodynamics and vasomobility in patients with coronary artery disease.* Am J Cardiol 45:389, 1980.

120. LYDTIN, H, LOHMÖLLER, G, LOHMÖLLER, R, ET AL: *Hemodynamic studies on Adalat in healthy volunteers and in patients.* In LOCHNER, W, BRAASCH, W, AND KRONEBERG, G (EDS): *Second International Adalat Symposium.* Springer-Verlag, New York, 1975, p 112.

121. FERLINZ, J, EASTHOPE, JL, AND ARONOW, WS: *Effects of verapamil on myocardial performance in coronary disease.* Circulation 59:313, 1958.

122. KUWAJIAMA, I, UEDA, K, KAMATA, C, ET AL: *A study of the effects of nifedipine in hypertensive crises and severe hypertension.* Jpn Heart J 19:455, 1978.

123. OLIVARI, MT, BARTORELLI, C, POLESE, A, ET AL: *Treatment of hypertension with nifedipine, a calcium antagonistic agent.* Circulation 59:1056, 1979.

124. PEDERSEN, OL: *Does verapamil have a clinically significant antihypertensive effect?* Eur J Pharmocol 13:21, 1978.

125. HUGENHOLTZ, PG, MICHELS, HR, SERRUYS, PW, ET AL: *Nifedipine in the treatment of unstable angina, coronary spasm and myocardial ischemia.* Am J Cardiol 47:163, 1981.

126. JOSHI, PI, DALAL, JJ, RUTTLEY, MSJ, ET AL: *Nifedipine and left ventricular function in beta-blocked patients.* Br Heart J 45:457, 1981.

127. TAKEDA, K, NAKAGAWA, Y, KATANO, Y, ET AL: *Effects of coronary vasodilators on large and small coronary arteries of dogs.* Jpn Heart J 18:92, 1977.

128. YASUE, H, OMOTE, S, NAGAO, M, ET AL: *Angina decubitus. Responses of angina at rest to various drugs.* Modern Medicine 31:2201, 1976.

129. YABE, Y, ABE, H, YOSHIMURA, S, ET AL: *Effect of diltiazem on coronary hemodynamics and its clinical significance.* Jpn Heart J 20:83, 1979.

130. MIGNAULT, SH: *Coronary cineangiographic study of intravenously adminstered Isoptin.* Can Med Ass J 95:1252, 1966.

131. PARODI, O, AND SIMONETTI, I: *Vasospastic angina.* Clin Invest Med 3:119, 1980.

132. PIEGAS, LS, PAES NETO, F, KONSTANDINIDIS, T, ET AL: *Hemodynamic evaluation of a new antianginal drug: nifedipine.* In JATENE, AD, AND LICHTLEN, PR (EDS): *3rd International Adalat Symposium. New Therapy of Ischemic Heart Disease.* International Congress Series No. 388, Excerpta Medica, Amsterdam, 1976, p 76.

133. MOSTBECK, A, PARTSCH, H, AND PESCHL, L: *Investigations on peripheral blood distribution.* In JATENE, AD, AND LICHTLEN, PR (EDS): *3rd International Adalat Symposium. New Therapy of Ischemic Heart Disease.* International Congress Series No. 388, Excerpta Medica, Amsterdam, 1976, p 91.

134. JOHNSON, SM, MAURITSON, DR, CORBETT, J, ET AL: *Effects of verapamil and nifedipine on left ventricular function at rest and during exercise in patients with Prinzmetal's variant angina pectoris.* Am J Cardiol 47:1289, 1981.

135. SHINJO, A, SASAKI, Y, INAMASU, M, ET AL: *In vitro effect of the coronary vasodilator diltiazem on human and rabbit platelets.* Thrombosis Research 13:941, 1978.

136. OWEN, NE, AND LEBRETON, GC: *Potentiation of human platelet aggregation by epinephrine or ADP: A calcium mediated process.* Circulation 58 (Suppl 2):228, 1978.

137. KIMURA, E, AND KISHIDA, H: *Treatment of variant angina with drugs: A survey of 11 cardiology institutes in Japan.* Circulation 63:844, 1981.

138. JOHNSON, SM, MAURITSON, DR, WILLERSON, JT, ET AL: *Comparison of verapamil and nifedipine in the treatment of variant angina pectoris: Preliminary observations in 10 patients.* Am J Cardiol 47:1295, 1981.

139. WATERS, DD, THÉROUX, P, SZLACHCIC, J, ET AL: *Provocative testing with ergonovine to assess the efficacy of treatment with nifedipine, diltiazem and verapamil in variant angina.* Am J Cardiol 48:123, 1981.

140. TAURINO, L, STORELLI, A, AND ROMA, F: *I farmici Ca^{++} antagonisti nell' angina di Prinzmetal.* Boll Soc Ital Cardiol 21:111, 1976.

141. DUNN, RF, KELLY, DT, SADICK, N, ET AL: *Multivessel coronary artery spasm.* Circulation 60:451, 1979.

142. FREEDMAN, B, RICHMOND, DR, AND KELLEY, DT: *Coronary spasm management with verapamil (Isoptin).* Med J Austral 2:22, 1980.

143. RAIZNER, AE, GASTON, W, CHAHINE, RA, ET AL: *The effectiveness of combined verapamil and nitrate therapy in Prinzmetal's variant angina.* Am J Cardiol 45:439, 1980.

144. KIMURA, E, TANAKA, K, MIZUNO, K, ET AL: *Suppression of repeatedly occurring ventricular fibrillation with nifedipine in variant form of angina pectoris.* Jpn Heart J 18:736, 1977.

145. BERTRAND, ME, LABLANCHE, JM, AND TILMANT, PY: *Treatment of Prinzmetal's variant angina. Role of medical treatment with nifedipine and surgical coronary revascularization combined with plexectomy.* Am J Cardiol 47:174, 1981.

146. KODAMA, K, OHGITANI, N, AND MINAMINO, T: *Clinical-therapeutic and hemodynamic studies with Adalat, a new coronary active substance.* In LOCHNER, W, BRAASCH, W, AND KRONENBERG, G (EDS): *2nd International Adalat Symposium. New Therapy of Ischemic Heart Disease.* Springer-Verlag, New York, 1975, p 260.

147. FUKUZAKI, H, OKAMOTO, R, YOKOYAMA, M, ET AL: *Clinical study on nifedipine.* In HASHIMOTO, K, KIMURA, E, AND KOBAYASHI, T (EDS): *1st International Nifedipine "Adalat" Symposium. New Therapy of Ischemic Heart Disease.* University of Tokyo Press, Tokyo, 1975, p 205.

148. ITOH, Y, TAWARA, I, AND ITOH, T: *Clinical experience with nifedipine.* In HASHIMOTO, K, KIMURA, E, AND KOBAYASHI, T (EDS): *1st International Nifedipine "Adalat" Symposium. New Therapy of Ischemic Heart Disease.* University of Tokyo Press, Tokyo, 1975, p 251.

149. HEUPLER, FA, JR, AND PROUDFIT, WL: *Nifedipine therapy for refractory coronary arterial spasm.* Am J Cardiol 44:798, 1979.

150. GOLDBERG, S, REICHEK, N, WILSON, J, ET AL: *Nifedipine in the treatment of Prinzmetal's (variant) angina.* Am J Cardiol 44:804, 1979.

151. CORTADELLAS ANGEL, J, VALLE TUDELA, V, MUR FRANCO, J, ET AL: *Angor de Prinzmetal. Estudio clínico y evidencia de espasmo coronaria.* Rev Esp Cardiol 32:133, 1979.

152. ANTMAN, E, MULLER, J, GOLDBERG, S, ET AL: *Nifedipine therapy for coronary artery spasm: Experience in 127 patients.* N Engl J Med 302:1269, 1980.

153. DELAHAYE, JP, AND GASPARD, P: *Le spasme coronarien. Revue général et étude critique à propos de 87 observations personnelles d' angene de Prinzmetal.* Lyon Médical 245:123, 1981.

154. MOSES, JW, WERTHEIMER, JH, BODENHEIMER, MM, ET AL: *Efficacy of nifedipine in rest angina refractory to propranolol and nitrates in patients with obstructive coronary artery disease.* Ann Intern Med 94:425, 1981.

168

155. Previtali, M, Salerno, JA, Tavazzi, L, et al: *Treatment of angina at rest with nifedipine: A short-term controlled study.* Am J Cardiol 45:825, 1980.

156. Muller, JE, and Gunther, SJ: *Nifedipine therapy for Prinzmetal's angina.* Circulation 57:137, 1978.

157. Tiefenbrunn, AJ, Sobel, BE, Siddhesh, G, et al: *Nifedipine blockade of ergonovine-induced coronary arterial spasm: Angiographic documentation.* Am J Cardiol 48:184, 1981.

158. Waters, DD, Chaitman, BR, Bourassa, MG, et al: *Clinical and angiographic correlates of exercise-induced ST-segment elevation. Increased detection and multiple ECG leads.* Circulation 61:286, 1980.

159. Broustet, JP, Griffo, R, Seriès, E, et al: *Angor de Prinzmetal declencé par l'arrêt de l'effort. Cinq cas à coronarographie normale.* Arch Mal Coeur 72:391, 1979.

160. Gunther, S, Green, L, Muller, JE, et al: *Prevention by nifedipine of abnormal coronary vasoconstriction in patients with coronary artery disease.* Circulation 63:849, 1981.

161. Niitani, H, and Jujimaki, T: *Clinical experience with nifedipine for ischemic heart disease.* In Hashimoto, K, Kimura, E, and Kobayashi, T (eds): *1st International Nifedipine "Adalat" Symposium. New Therapy of Ischemic Heart Disease,* University of Tokyo Press, Tokyo, 1975, p 268.

162. Moses, J, Feldman, MS, and Helfant, RH: *Efficacy of nifedipine in the intermediate syndrome refractory to propranolol and nitrate therapy.* Am J Cardiol 45:390, 1980.

163. Belz, GG, Aust, PE, and Munkes, R: *Digoxin plasma concentrations and nifedipine.* Lancet 1:844, 1981.

164. Piccolo, E, Furlanello, F, Treir, GP, et al: *Il verapamil per infusione venosa nel trattamento dell 'angor refrattario e delle aritmie da instabilita elettrica associate.* Min Med 66:1865, 1975.

165. Parodi, O, Maseri, A, and Simonetti, I: *Management of unstable angina at rest by verapamil. A double-blind cross-over study in coronary care unit.* Br Heart J 41:167, 1979.

166. Hansen, JF, and Sandoe, E: *Treatment of Prinzmetal's angina due to coronary artery spasm using verapamil: A report of three cases.* Europ J Cardiol 7:327, 1978.

167. Hansen, JF, and Sandoe, E: *The spectrum from adverse effect to efficacy of beta-adrenergic blockade in Prinzmetal's variant angina.* In Sandoe, E, Julian, DG, and Bell, JW (eds): *Management of Ventricular Tachycardia—Role of Mexiletine.* Proceedings of a Symposium held in Copenhagen, 25–27 May 1978. Excerpta Medica, Amsterdam-Oxford, 1978, p 311.

168. Solberg, LE, Nissen, RG, Vliestra, RE, et al: *Prinzmetal's variant angina—response to verapamil.* Mayo Clin Proc 53:256, 1978.

169. Lahiri, A, Subramanian, B, Millar-Craig, M, et al: *Exercise-induced S-T segment elevation in variant angina.* Am J Cardiol 45:887, 1980.

170. Freedman, B, Dunn, RF, and Kelly, DT: *Exercise-induced coronary spasm: Alpha-adrenergic mechanism?* Circulation (Suppl 2):265, 1979.

171. Freedman, B, Dunn, RF, and Richmond, DR, et al: *Coronary artery spasm—treatment with verapamil.* Circulation 60 (Suppl 2):249, 1979.

172. Kaufman, AJ, and Aramendía, P: *Prevention of ventricular fibrillation induced by coronary ligation.* J Pharmacol Exper Ther 164:326, 1968.

173. Brooks, WW, Verrier, RL, and Lown, B: *Protective effect of verapamil on vulnerability to ventricular fibrillation during myocardial ischemia and reperfusion.* Cardiovasc Res 14: 295, 1980.

174. Sugiyama, S, Ozawa, T, Suzuki, S, et al: *Effects of verapamil and propranolol on ventricular vulnerability after coronary reperfusion.* J Electrocardiol 13:49, 1981.

175. Rebeiro, LGT, Brandon, TA, Debauche, TL, et al: *Antiarrhythmic and hemodynamic effects of calcium channel blocking agents during coronary arterial reperfusion. Comparative effects of verapamil and nifedipine.* Am J Cardiol 48:69, 1981.

176. Fazzini, PF, Marchi, F, and Pucci, P: *Effects of verapamil on ventricular premature beats of acute myocardial infarction.* Am Heart J 98:816, 1979.

177. Marriot, HJL, and Castillo, HT: *Radiotransparent electrodes for recording precordial electrocardiographic leads during catheterization.* J Electrocardiol 7:281, 1974.

178. Balasubramanian, V, Bowles, M, Davies, AB, et al: *Combined treatment with verapamil and propranolol in chronic stable angina.* Br Heart J 45:349, 1981.

179. Singh, BN, Collett, JT, and Chew, CYC: *New perspectives in the pharmacologic therapy of cardiac arrhythmias.* Prog Cardiovasc Dis 22:243, 1980.

180. Yasue, H, Omote, S, Takizawa, A, et al: *Pathogenesis and treatment of angina pectoris at rest as seen from its response to various drugs.* Jpn Circ J 42:1, 1978.

181. Bardet, J, Baudet, M, Rigand, M, et al: *Diltiazem, a new calcium antagonist, versus propranolol in treatment of spontaneous angina pectoris.* Am J Cardiol 43:416, 1979.

182. NAKAMURA, M, AND KOIWAYA, Y: *Beneficial effect of diltiazem, a new antianginal drug, on angina pectoris at rest.* Jpn Heart J 20:613, 1979.

183. ROSENTHAL, SJ, GINZBURG, R, LAMB, IH, ET AL: *Efficacy of diltiazem for control of symptoms of coronary arterial spasm.* Am J Cardiol 46:1027, 1980.

184. PEPINE, CJ, FELDMAN, RL, WHITTLE, J, ET AL: *Effect of diltiazem in patients with variant angina: A randomized double-blind trial.* Am Heart J 101:719, 1981.

185. YASUE, H, NAGAO, M, OMOTE, S, ET AL: *Coronary arterial spasm and Prinzmetal's variant form of angina induced by hyperventilation and Tris-buffer infusion.* Circulation 58:56, 1978.

186. WALSH, R, BADKE, F, AND O'ROURKE, R: *Differential effects of diltiazem and verapamil on left ventricular performance in conscious dogs.* Circulation 60 (Suppl 2):15, 1979.

187. CURRY, RC, JR: *Prinzmetal's angina. Provocative test and current therapy.* JAMA 240:677, 1978.

188. MIZGALA, HF, CRITTIN, J, WATERS, DD, ET AL: *Results of immediate and long term treatment of variant angina (VA) with perhexiline maleate.* Circulation 60 (Suppl 2):181, 1979.

189. WATERS, DD, THÉROUX, P, SZLACHCIC, J, ET AL: *A comparative study of calcium-ion antagonists in patients with variant angina.* Clin Invest Med 3:129, 1980.

190. MIZGALA, HF, THÉROUX, P, AND CONVERT, G: *Preliminary results of the use of perhexiline maleate in unstable and variant angina.* In *Perhexiline Maleate—Proceedings of a Symposium.* International Congress Series No. 424, Excerpta Medica, Amsterdam, 1978, p 169.

191. CÔTÉ, P, BOURASSA, MG, DELAYE, J, ET AL: *Effects of amiodarone on cardiac and coronary hemodynamics and myocardial metabolism in patients with coronary disease.* Circulation 59:1165, 1979.

192. FAUCHIER, JP, CHARBONNIER, F, BROCHIER, M, ET AL: *L'amiodarone injectable et par voie orale dans le traitement de l'angor de Prinzmetal sévère et syncopal.* Ann Cardiol Angéiol 27:193, 1978.

193. COURTADON, M, JOURDE, M, ALIX, B, ET AL: *Modifications électrocardiographiques de type "Prinzmetal" provoquées par épreuve d'effort. A propos de 2 cas.* Coeur 4:729, 1973.

194. BERTRAND, ME, LaBLANCHE, JM, TILMANT, JM, ET AL: *Complete denervation of the heart (autotransplantation) for treatment of severe, refractory coronary spasm.* Am J Cardiol 47:1375, 1981.

195. HIRSH, PD, HILLIS, LD, CAMPBELL, WB, ET AL: *Release of prostaglandins and thromboxane into the coronary circulation in patients with ischemic heart disease.* N Engl J Med 304:685, 1981.

196. SHIMAMOTO, T, NUMANO, F, AND MOTOMIYA, T: *Myocardial ischemic attacks induced experimentally by thromboxane A_2 and their prevention by thromboxane A_2 antagonist, EG626, and its clinical trial.* Jpn Circ J 41:785, 1977.

197. GUAZZI, M, FIORENTINI, C, POLESE, A, ET AL: *Treatment of spontaneous angina pectoris with beta blocking agents. A clinical, electrocardiographic and hemodynamic appraisal.* Br Heart J 37:1235, 1975.

198. RUSSELL, RO, JR, RESNEKOV, L, WOLK, M, ET AL: *Unstable angina pectoris: National Cooperative Study Group to Compare Surgical and Medical Therapy. III. Results in patients with ST segment elevation during pain.* Am J Cardiol 45:819, 1980.

199. YASUE, H: *Beta-adrenergic blockade and coronary arterial spasm.* In SANDOE, E, JULIAN, DG, AND BELL, JW (EDS): *Management of Ventricular Tachycardia—Role of Mexiletine.* Proceedings of a Symposium held in Copenhagen, 25–27 May 1978. Excerpta Medica, Amsterdam, Oxford, 1978, p 305.

200. DELAHAYE, JP, TOUBOUL, P, PORTE, J, ET AL: *Discussion de l'attitude thérapeutique dans l'angine de Prinzmetal. A propos de 46 observations.* Arch Mal Coeur 68:1133, 1975.

201. VIGANÒ, M, BALDRIGHI, V, RIGOLETTI, L, ET AL: *Angina di Prinzmetal. Studio coronariografico e terapia chirurgica.* Boll Soc Ital Cardiol 17:842, 1972.

202. CHERRIER, F, NEIMANN, JL, GROUSSIN, P, ET AL: *Prinzmetal angina: A study of 100 cases.* In KALTENBACH, M, LICHTLEN, P, BALCON, R, ET AL: *Coronary Heart Disease.* Georg Thieme, Stuttgart, 1978, p 191.

203. BASSENGE, E, HOLTZ, J, AND KOLIN, A: *Sympathetic control of coronary vasomotion in conscious dogs: Comparison of conductance and resistance vessels.* Internation Union of Physiological Sci 14:315, 1980.

204. RICCI, DR, ORLICK, AE, CIPRIANO, PR, ET AL: *Altered adrenergic activity in coronary arterial spasm: Insight into mechanism based on study of coronary hemodynamics and the electrocardiogram.* Am J Cardiol 43:1073, 1979.

205. THANAVARO, S, KRONE, RJ, KLEIGER, RE, ET AL: *Phenoxybenzamine therapy for variant angina: Successful treatment of a patient with normal coronary arteries.* Southern Med J 72:221, 1979.

206. LIPTON, SA, MARKIS, JE, PINE, MB, ET AL: *Cessation of smoking followed by Prinzmetal's variant angina and diffuse esophageal spasm.* N Engl J Med 299:775, 1978.

207. LEVENE, DL, AND FREEMAN, MR: *Alpha-adrenoreceptor-mediated coronary artery spasm.* JAMA 236:1018, 1976.

208. DUNN, RF, KELLY, DT, SADICK, N, ET AL: *Multivessel coronary artery spasm.* Circulation 60:451, 1979.

170

209. YOKOYAMA, M, AND HENRY, PD: *Supersensitivity of atherosclerotic arteries to ergonovine partially mediated by a serotonergic mechanism.* Circulation 60 (Suppl 2):100, 1979.

210. GUNTHER, S, MULLER, JE, MUDGE, GH, JR, ET AL: *Therapy of coronary vasoconstriction in patients with coronary artery disease.* Am J Cardiol 47:157, 1981.

211. NEVINS, MA, LYON, LJ, AND PANTAZOPOULOS, J: *Pharmacotherapy of variant angina.* Cardiovasc Med 3:445, 1978.

212. MAUTNER, R, KANADE, A, AND PHILLIPS, J: *Coronary artery spasm in a patient with unstable angina pectoris.* Southern Med J 71:729, 1978.

213. STANG, JM, KOLIBASH, AJ, AND BUSH, CA: *Methacholine provocation of Prinzmetal's variant angina pectoris (coronary artery spasm).* Am J Cardiol 39:326, 1977.

214. YASUE, H, TOUYAMA, M, TANAKA, S, ET AL: *Prinzmetal's angina: Atropine suppression.* Ann Intern Med 80:553, 1974.

215. MASERI, A, SEVERI, S, CHIERCHIA, S, ET AL: *Characteristics, incidence and pathogenetic mechanism of "primary" angina at rest.* In MASERI, A, KLASSEN, GA, AND LESCH, M (EDS): *Primary and Secondary Angina Pectoris.* Grune & Stratton, New York, 1978, p 265.

216. MCLAUGHLIN, PR, DOHERTY, PW, MARTIN, RP, ET AL: *Myocardial imaging in a patient with reproducible variant angina.* Am J Cardiol 39:126, 1977.

217. SCHROEDER, JS, ROSENTHAL, S, GINSBERG, R, ET AL: *Medical therapy of Prinzmetal's variant angina.* Chest 78:231, 1980.

218. FAM, WM, AND MCGREGOR, M: *Pressure-flow relationships in the coronary circulation.* Circ Res 25:293, 1969.

219. SINZINGER, H, FEIGL, W, AND SILBERBAUER, K: *Prostacyclin generation in atherosclerotic arteries.* Lancet 2:469, 1979.

220. MASERI, A, CHIERCHIA, S, AND L'ABBATE, AL: *Pathogenetic mechanisms underlying the clinical events associated with atherosclerotic heart disease.* Circulation 62 (Suppl 5):3, 1980.

221. SZCZEKLIK, A, SZCZEKLIK, J, NIZAMKOWSKI, R, ET AL: *Prostacyclin for acute coronary insufficiency.* Artery 8:7, 1980.

222. SERNERI, GGN, MASOTTI, G, GENSINI, GF, ET AL: *Prostacyclin and thromboxane A_2 formation in response to adrenergic stimulation in humans: A mechanism for local control of vascular response to sympathetic activation.* Cardiovasc Res 12:287, 1981.

223. ARRIGO, F, COGLITORE, S, VIRGA, T, ET AL: *Angina di Prinzmetal. Considerazioni a proposito di un caso clinico.* Boll Soc Ital Cardiol 22:283, 1977.

224. FULLER, C, RAIZNER, AE, CHAHINE, RA, ET AL: *Exercise-induced coronary artery spasm: Pharmacological interventions.* Clin Res 27:727A, 1979.

225. LEWY, RI, SMITH, JB, SILVER, MJ, ET AL: *Detection of thromboxane B_1 (TB_2) in peripheral blood of patients with Prinzmetal's angina.* Clin Res 27:462A, 1979.

226. BOBBA, F, ANTONINI, M, LEONE, G, ET AL: *Il test al dipiridamolo nella diagnosi di insufficienza coronarica. (Raffronti con il test all' isoproterenolo e le prove da sforzo al cicloergometro).* Bol Soc Ital Cardiol 22:755, 1977.

227. HERNANDEZ-CASAS, G, DEAR, W, AND LEACHMAN, RD: *Prinzmetal's variant angina pectoris with normal coronary arteriograms: Effect of long-term reserpine treatment.* Cardiovasc Dis 1:194, 1974.

228. GUADALAJARA, JF, HORWITZ, S, AND TREVETHAN, S: *Angina de Prinzmetal. La respuesta al tratamiento con reserpina. Revisión de sus mecanismos fisiopatológicos.* Arch Inst Cardiol Mex 47:101, 1977.

229. BUONANNO, C, DANDER, B, TREVI, GP, ET AL: *Angina "variante." Aspetti clinici, elettrocardiografici e coronariografici in 40 casi. Considerazioni terapeutiche.* G Ital Cardiol 6:762, 1976.

230. BAEDECKER, W, SEBENING, H, WIRTZFELD, A. ET AL: *Die "Prinzmetal-Angina-pectoris."* Dtsch med Wschr 99:2008, 1974.

231. BESSE, P, PRIBAT, P, SICART, M, ET AL: *Aspects actuels de l'angor de Prinzmetal.* Ann Cardiol Angéiol 25:421, 1976.

232. PEREZ-GOMEZ, F, MARTIN DEDIOS, R, REY, J, ET AL: *Prinzmetal's angina: Reflex cardiovascular response during episode of pain.* Br Heart J 42:81, 1979.

233. LAZZARA, R, EL-SHERIF, N, HOPE, RR, ET AL: *Ventricular arrhythmias and electrophysiological consequences of myocardial ischemia and infarction.* Circ Res 42:740, 1978.

234. MADIAS, JE: *The syndrome of variant angina culminating in myocardial infarction.* Circulation 59:297, 1979.

235. BOGART, DB, LEWIS, HD, JR, HINTHORN, DR, ET AL: *Prinzmetal angina. Long-term follow-up after recurrent ventricular arrhythmias.* J Kan Med Soc 79:14, 1978.

236. CAMPBELL, TJ, HICKIE, JB, MICHELL, G, ET AL: *Nifedipine in the treatment of life threatening Prinzmetal angina.* Aust NZ J Med 9:293, 1979.

237. SUSSMAN, EJ, GOLDBERG, S, POLL, DS, ET AL: *Surgical therapy of variant angina associated with nonobstructive coronary disease.* Ann Intern Med 94:771, 1981.

238. KLEIBER, GE, SCHATZ, IJ, KIRSH, MM, ET AL: *Variant angina: Clinical, laboratory and operative study of eight cases.* J Am Osteop Ass 76:880, 1977.

239. WHITING, RB, KLEIN, MD, VANDERVEER, J, ET AL: *Variant angina pectoris.* N Engl J Med 282:709, 1970.

240. GIANELLY, R, MUGLER, F, AND HARRISON, DC: *Prinzmetal's variant of angina pectoris with only slight coronary atherosclerosis.* California Med 108:129, 1968.

241. KERINE, N, AND SCHWARTZ, A: *Prinzmetal angina with transient complete heart block.* Arch Intern Med 134:542, 1974.

242. BLACK, M, BLACK, A, AND HUNTINGTON, P: *Prinzmetal's variant angina with syncope.* New York State J Med 76:255, 1976.

243. ROY, G, SELINGER, H, AND CARTER, WH: *Stokes-Adams attack in Prinzmetal variant angina.* West Virg Med J 73:5, 1977.

244. CHERRIER, F, CUILLIÉRE, M, DODINOT, B, ET AL: *Angor de Prinzmetal; aspects coronarographiques; considérations thérapeutiques. A propos de 7 observations.* Arch Mal Coeur 66:579, 1973.

245. MACMILLAN, RM, ROSE, FD, KLINGHOFFER, JF, ET AL: *Variant angina pectoris.* Cardiology 58:306, 1973.

246. SAWAYAMA, T, SHIOZU, N, NIKI, I, ET AL: *Unusual form of impending myocardial infarction in a premenopausal woman.* Jpn Circ J 29:943, 1965.

247. AMICHOT, JL, AND JOUVE, A: *Une forme inhabituelle d'angor spontané. L'angor dit de Prinzmetal.* Méd Hygiene 29:984, 1970.

248. MACALPIN, RN: *Correlation of the location of coronary arterial spasm with the lead distribution of ST segment elevation during variant angina.* Am Heart J 99:555, 1980.

249. KRANTZ, EM, VILJOEN, JF, AND GILBERT, MS: *Prinzmetal's variant angina during extradural anaesthesia.* Br J Anaesth 52:945, 1980.

250. GLISSON, N, EL-ETR, AA, AND LIM, R: *Prolongation of pancuronium-induced neuromuscular blockade by intravenous infusion of nitroglycerin.* Anesthesiology 51:47, 1979.

251. DUCHOSAL, PW, AND HENNY, G: *Angine de portrine et hyperthyroïdisme.* Cardiologia 5:371, 1942.

252. BALAGOT, RC, SELIM, H, BANDELIN, VR, ET AL: *Prinzmetal's variant angina in the immediate post anesthetic state.* Anesthesiology 46:355, 1977.

253. HASHIMOTO, R, KUBOTA, S, SHIMIZU, T, ET AL: *A case of suprasellar tumor associated with so-called atypical angina pectoris.* (In Japanese) Noshinkei Geka 4:979, 1976.

254. WATSON, GK, AND MARSHALL, RJ: *Atypical angina pectoris.* Irish J Med Sci 6:35, 1966.

255. SALHADIN, P, LEBEDELLE, M, VANTHIEL, E, ET AL: *L'apparition à l'effort de l'image de lésion sous-épicardique en l'absence de signes de nécrose myocardique.* Acta Cardiol 32:401, 1977.

Role of Platelet-Active Drugs in Coronary Artery Disease

Sol Sherry, M.D.

Acute "heart attacks" represent the single largest cause of mortality in the United States. Approximately one third of all deaths annually are due to fatal acute coronary events, and such events are almost always associated with underlying coronary artery disease, usually arteriosclerosis.

The rationale for testing platelet-active drugs in coronary artery disease is that the two major immediate causes of "coronary death," that is, sudden cardiac death (presumably due to an acute fatal arrhythmia) and the more classical myocardial infarction, may, in large part, be due to controllable platelet phenomena.

Platelet thrombi readily form on the injured intima of coronary vessels, an event that frequently occurs in coronary artery disease; such thrombi also are likely to shed platelet emboli. These thrombi and emboli could readily produce areas of transient ischemia both by physical obstruction and by the powerful vasoconstrictive properties of serotonin and thromboxane A_2, which are released from aggregating platelets; the resulting ischemia could precipitate an arrhythmia sufficient to cause sudden death.

Alternatively, in areas of more extensive injury to a coronary artery—such as a sudden crack, fissure, or ulcer in an atheromatous plaque—a plug of platelets rapidly fills the lesion, activates the clotting mechanisms, and initiates a large coagulation thrombus often sufficient in size to occlude the entire vessel and to cause an extensive transmural infarction.

Sulfinpyrazone, aspirin, and dipyridamole will be the only drugs under consideration in this chapter. All three have undergone and continue to be under extensive investigation for their antithrombotic effects in coronary artery disease. Each of them, despite differences in their pharmacologic actions, influences prostaglandin-mediated pathways, which regulate the ability of platelets to aggregate in response to vascular injury. Other drugs, for example, clofibrate and beta blockers, have also demonstrated platelet-inhibitory activity, but they will be excluded from consideration because either their mechanism of action is unclear, or they have not undergone extensive testing, or the rationale for their use in various trials was unrelated to their platelet effects.

BACKGROUND CLINICAL DATA

Interest in the possible role of aspirin in preventing acute coronary events can be traced to the report of Craven in the early 1950s that in 1465 sedentary, overweight men, aged 45 to 65 years, placed on a daily regimen of 300 mg of aspirin over a 7-year period, no coronary occlusion or insufficiency occurred.[1] While Cobb and coworkers[2] did not speculate on the association of aspirin therapy and the unexpectedly low incidence of myocardial infarction as

173

the cause of death in the autopsy findings of a large series of patients dying with rheumatoid arthritis at the Massachusetts General Hospital, their observations, in retrospect, could be interpreted as providing evidence for Craven's view. However, it is only in the last decade or since the discovery of the effect of aspirin on platelet function that Craven's remarkable claims, albeit in an uncontrolled study, have led to subsequent studies.

In an epidemiologic survey reported in 1974,[3] the Boston Collaborative Drug Surveillance Group found that the percentage of patients who had regularly (usually daily, but of undetermined dosage) taken aspirin during the month before hospitalization was significantly lower in 325 patients hospitalized with acute myocardial infarction than in 3807 patients hospitalized for other causes (0.09 percent versus 4.9 percent). In an update of their retrospective data published two years later in 1976,[4] the group reported that this negative association between aspirin use and risk of myocardial infarction was maintained with the accumulation of approximately twice the original data. However, a similar finding could not be confirmed in an American Cancer Study survey of records of over 1,000,000 men and women maintained during a 5-year period;[5] the rate of death from coronary heart disease was no lower for those who took aspirin "often" than for those who took the drug "seldom" or "never." Unfortunately, the use of aspirin and the cause of deaths were loosely defined in the records surveyed.

Perhaps the greatest stimulus for undertaking major prospective trials with aspirin or other platelet-acting drugs came from the Coronary Drug Project Aspirin Study. This study, completed in 1975, evaluated total mortality, cause-specific mortality, nonfatal events, and combinations of fatal and nonfatal events in aspirin-treated and control (placebo) groups.[6] The study population was selected from groups who had been receiving dextrothyroxine or estrogen therapy in another Coronary Drug Project Study but who had terminated treatment. The 1529 patients, all male, had had at least one documented myocardial infarction; one third had had serious complications or more than one infarction. Five or more years had elapsed since the last infarction for approximately 75 percent of the patients, and more than 60 percent of them were over 55 years of age. The patients were randomly assigned, on a double-blind basis, to daily treatment with 972 mg of aspirin (324 mg three times per day) or placebo for periods ranging from 10 to 28 months. Patients were evaluated at 4-month intervals, and compliance was monitored. Overall mortality was 5.8 percent in the aspirin group and 8.3 percent in the placebo group (an observed difference of 30 percent). In regard to cause-specific mortality, the aspirin group had a reduction relative to the placebo group of 27 percent for coronary deaths and 19 percent for sudden cardiovascular deaths (that is, deaths occurring within 60 minutes after onset of symptoms). The incidence of definite nonfatal myocardial infarction was only slightly lower in the aspirin group (3.7 percent) than in the placebo group (4.2 percent). The largest clinical difference in definite or suspect nonfatal cardiovascular events was for the development of hypertension since entry, which occurred in 12.2 and 9.6 percent of the aspirin and placebo groups, respectively—an incidence that was 27 percent higher in the aspirin group.

Considering that this study represented a prospective evaluation, it deserves a special comment. Inasmuch as 75 percent or more of the patients had had their myocardial infarctions 5 or more years earlier, the placebo group mortality was low, approximately 4 percent per year. Therefore, the number of patients in the trial was never adequate to provide a statistically significant difference even if mortality in the aspirin group was reduced by 30 percent or so. Also, the study was complicated through the admission into the trial of three cohorts of patients from the Coronary Drug Project (those previously on high-dose estrogen, dextrothyroxine, and low-dose estrogen, with the last group being entered more than a year later than the others). Mortality in the placebo group of each of these cohorts differed; and the effect of aspirin, while positive in two, was negative in the other. Though the data have been interpreted as providing highly suggestive evidence that aspirin benefited patients whose infarcts occurred many years earlier, the data supporting this conclusion are far from impressive.

CLINICAL CONSIDERATIONS PERTINENT TO THE DESIGN OF PROSPECTIVE TRIALS WITH PLATELET-ACTIVE DRUGS

Many factors need to be taken into consideration in planning and designing prospective trials aimed at evaluating platelet active drugs in the prevention of acute coronary events; probably none are more important than the following clinical considerations.

Primary versus Secondary Prevention Trials

To provide convincing data on the efficacy of an agent in preventing acute coronary events, a mortality study will usually be required; here the endpoints are hard, objective, and unequivocal. Because in a mortality study only the deaths in the two groups count, a large number of endpoints are required to establish a significant difference. Thus the trial size, that is, the number of patients under observation, is dependent on the mortality rate: when mortality rates are very low, enormous numbers of patients are required; alternatively, when mortality rates are high, fewer patients are necessary. Accordingly, from a logistical standpoint, it would be best to select a group at significant risk of dying of an acute coronary event. It is for this reason that only one major primary prevention trial has been undertaken so far, for the trial size would have to be very large and the duration of observation very long to establish a significant difference in mortality.

The single primary prevention study is a large trial of aspirin in the prevention of death and cardiovascular events (stroke, heart attack) being conducted in 4200 healthy subjects (all physicians) in England.[7] Patients have been randomly allocated to a control (untreated) group or treatment with aspirin, 500 mg daily, and will be observed for many years.

Other than for this single instance, all major trials conducted so far have been secondary intervention trials, that is, the patient population is composed of individuals with a previous myocardial infarction because the latter provides evidence of underlying coronary artery disease and an increased risk of dying from a subsequent acute coronary event.

Special Problems in the Clinical Design of Secondary Intervention Trials

"Intent to Treat" versus "Clinical Efficacy" Studies

The type of prospective, double-blind, long-term intervention trials to be undertaken is currently an area of considerable controversy.[8,9] In general, such trials can be divided into two types: "intent to treat" trials and "clinical efficacy" studies. In the former, all patients are randomized into the study on the basis of an intent to treat with either the active drug or an appropriate control (usually a placebo). Once randomized, regardless of whether the patient is subsequently shown never to have met the eligibility criteria or never to have taken the assigned medication or to have withdrawn from the trial, any event of the type to be analyzed is forever counted as being related to the drug group to which the patient was assigned. In the past, this approach has dominated the methodology of biometricians, because it is highly protective against bias; however, in this type of trial, the results are so diluted (by inclusion in the analysis of significant numbers of ineligible patients, drop-ins, and drop-outs) that, at best, only a qualitative effect of the true efficacy of the drug is possible. Furthermore, with current sample sizes and a high dilution factor, a significant result is demonstrated only when the drug's effect is very striking. Alternatively, a modest effect, although real, is unlikely to reach statistical significance unless the number of endpoints measured is very large.

On the other hand, "clinical efficacy" studies, in which only those events among eligible patients being actively treated with adequate amounts of the drug (active agent or control) are analyzed, have the advantage of allowing for a quantitative assessment of the drug's true effect and allow for conclusions to be reached with a smaller trial size. However, such studies may not effectively control against bias, as do "intent to treat" studies; and the interpretation

175

of the results from such trials is, therefore, likely to be more suspect. Nevertheless, this approach, because of its several practical advantages, is becoming more popular and recently has been employed in several important studies.[10-12]

Analysis of Mortality

The hypothesis underlying the use of platelet-active drugs is that platelets may play a significant role in the pathogenesis of sudden death and fatal myocardial infarction. Yet most trials have used total deaths, regardless of cause, as the analyzable endpoint. The inclusion of deaths from other causes only serves to dilute any benefit that could be attributed to these agents. Even when cardiac mortality is the primary endpoint, deaths from other cardiac causes (congestive heart failure, cardiac surgery, and so forth) for which myocardial infarction patients are also at risk can weaken the analysis of the benefit. Thus the more the primary analysis is restricted to the specific causes of death most likely to be affected, the better the chance of demonstrating a significant benefit from an effective drug.

However, even more important to the specific topic of this chapter is the question of the contribution of platelet-mediated phenomena to sudden death and fatal acute myocardial infarction. It is unlikely that all these fatalities always occur through a similar pathogenetic mechanism, that is, there may well be multiple causes for the initiation of these lethal events, and platelet-mediated phenomena may be an important, but not exclusive, trigger. If so, only a percentage of such deaths can be prevented by platelet-active drugs; and if that percentage is a modest one, trials of the size currently being undertaken, regardless of all other previously noted considerations, would be unlikely to demonstrate a significant benefit even if the drugs were effective. The argument may be made that the demonstration of a modest benefit should not be the goal of this type of research; however, from the perspective of the magnitude of the public health problem posed (fatal acute coronary events are the single largest cause of death in the Western world, and the annual number of deaths from this cause is enormous— 600,000 in the United States alone), even a modest benefit, if proven, would represent an important advance.

Natural History of Cardiac Mortality Following an Acute Myocardial Infarction

Mortality following an acute myocardial infarction is not linear with time, an observation originally stressed by Zumoff and associates,[13] nor are the causes of death similar during different periods; such considerations also complicate the evaluation of a drug's effect in patients with this disorder. In describing mortality following an acute myocardial infarction, three periods with different rates and with different primary causes of death can be readily identified.

NATURAL HISTORY OF CARDIAC MORTALITY FOLLOWING AN ACUTE MYOCARDIAL INFARCTION: BY PERIOD. *In-Hospital or "Recovery" Period.* This is generally recognized as a very high mortality period. In-hospital mortality is not linear with time but is highest during the first day and progressively decreases on a daily basis during the entire period of hospitalization, as is well documented in the literature.[14-19] Illustrative of this point is the study by Beard and coworkers[14] of patients admitted to US Veterans Administration hospitals who were 50 years of age or older; they observed annualized mortality rates of 438.9 percent for 0 to 7 days, 248.6 percent for 8 to 14 days, and 84 percent for 15 to 28 days.

The mortality during this in-hospital or recovery period (the latter usually refers to the first 30 days) varies considerably among reported studies because there are differences among the patient groups in length of hospitalization, age, sex, smoking habits, geographic areas, ethnic backgrounds, types of therapy, hospital facilities (coronary care units, and so forth), and various other aspects. Ibrahim and colleagues,[20] after a careful review of an extensive literature, concluded that mortality from the first hour to 30 days following hospitalization for an acute myocardial infarction averages 14.5 percent (the annualized rate would be approximately 174 percent).

"Early" Post-Recovery Period. Following the recovery period, the mortality among survivors of a recent myocardial infarction, while initially high, progressively declines over approximately the next 6 months and then reaches a steady and much lower level. The break in the survival curve, which is noted at approximately 6 months after hospital discharge and first described by Zumoff and associates,[13] has received adequate confirmation in the recent literature.[18,19,21,22] This break serves to separate the entire post-recovery period into two periods: an "early" post-recovery period and a "late" post-recovery period, based on different mortality rates. The early post-recovery period is still a high mortality period but one during which mortality progressively decreases. The late post-recovery period is characterized by a low and constant mortality that extends for 5 or more years after the early period.

The differences in mortality between the first 6 months post-discharge (early post-recovery period) and subsequent periods is quite striking, as noted in the literature. Cannom and colleagues[22] found an 11.7 percent mortality during the first 6 months post-discharge and 5.5 percent during the following 6 months. Weinblatt and coworkers[19] observed a cardiac mortality of 8.5 percent for the 5-month period ending 6 months after the index infarction. The cardiac mortality for the periods 7 to 30 months and 31 to 54 months after the index infarction was 3.7 and 2.9 percent, respectively. Helmers and associates[16] described a 17.9 percent mortality during the first year after hospital discharge. Mortality during the first 6 months was 11.2 percent and during the second 6 months, 7.6 percent. In another study involving 12 different Swedish hospitals, Helmers and Lundman[23] reported an 8.5 percent cardiac mortality during the first 6 months post-discharge (mortality during the first 2 months was double that during the last 2 months), and this accounted for 25 percent of all the deaths encountered over a 4- to 5-year followup. Beard and coworkers[14] in their study observed a 28-day to 6-month (5-month period) mortality of 6.4 percent, but the mortality for the next 6 months was 4.6 percent. A Cooperative Study[15] observed a 29- to 90-day mortality of 4.52 percent (2.26 percent per month), a 91- to 120-day mortality of 4.56 percent (1.52 percent per month), and a 120- to 360-day mortality of 6.05 percent (0.76 percent per month). Bigger and colleagues[24] followed 100 patients discharged from the Presbyterian Hospital in New York City. Of the 19 cardiac deaths that occurred during the 1-year observation period, 15, or 79 percent, occurred during the first 6 months.

Estimates of the mortality during the early post-recovery period have varied widely, undoubtedly because of the many differences among the patient groups. However, a reasonable approximation for an average group would be that 6 to 10 percent of the survivors of the recovery period will die during the early post-recovery period (that is, an annualized mortality of 12 to 20 percent).

"Late" Post-Recovery Period. As noted previously, this period, which follows the early post-recovery period, is characterized by a constant and low mortality extending for several years after the index infarction. The mortality during the late post-recovery period has been estimated at about 3 to 4 percent per year.[18,19]

This description of the natural history of mortality following acute myocardial infarction from a temporal standpoint emphasizes certain aspects essential to the proper interpretation of any therapeutic intervention: (1) Unless the periods of observation are exactly similar in both groups, errors in interpretation may arise. Thus it is most desirable to have all patients enter the study at the same time after the infarct and to have them followed serially against the natural history of the disease. (2) As Bigger and associates[24] have stated, "Because the excess influence on mortality exerted by infarction is almost dissipated by six months, any therapeutic intervention, such as antiarrhythmic prophylaxis or a cardiac surgical procedure, designed to alter favorably the post-hospital course of high risk patients should be applied early after acute myocardial infarction." (3) A proper interpretation of the effect of any therapeutic intervention must take into account the disparate mortalities during each period, and the effect of any intervention should be analyzed separately for each period of different mortality.

THE NATURAL HISTORY OF CARDIAC MORTALITY FOLLOWING AN ACUTE MYOCARDIAL INFARCTION: BY CAUSE. Though it is generally recognized that many different causes exist for cardiac mortality among survivors of myocardial infarction (recurrent myocardial infarction, sudden death, congestive heart failure, and so forth), it is less well appreciated that the contribution of each of these causes of death varies during different periods, and these periods coincide well with the three distinct mortality periods described above.

Mortality during the Recovery Period. Aggressive monitoring of patients and prompt antiarrhythmic therapy, as practiced in hospitals today, has largely eliminated electrical instability as a prominent cause of in-hospital mortality among infarcted patients. Currently, probably 90 percent of the deaths are mechanical, that is, pump failure arising from the infarct itself or from one of its direct complications. Fairly typical are the observations reported of the in-hospital mortality at the Montreal Cardiological Institute:[25] shock, 64 percent; congestive heart failure, 11 percent; cardiac rupture, 14 percent; renal failure, 3 percent; thromboembolism, 5 percent; sudden death, 3 percent. The most important prognostic indicator for survival during the recovery period appears to be the effect of the infarct itself on the mechanical efficiency of the heart as a pump.

Mortality during the "Early" Post-Recovery Period. By the end of the recovery period, the mechanical aspects are no longer very prominent; either they have improved or they are under control, or the patient has succumbed. However, the electrical instability of the heart, which accompanies the infarct, only slowly subsides over the next several months, and it and its lethal counterpart, sudden death, dominate mortality during the early post-recovery period. Bigger and coworkers[24] reported that 80 percent of the deaths during the first 6 months post-discharge were sudden deaths, and a similar incidence was reported by Schulze and associates[26] from their study at Johns Hopkins Hospital. Helmers and colleagues[16] reported that a third of all the sudden deaths observed in a 5-year followup of a group of 475 patients occurred within the first 6 months. Others have commented that the first 2- to 3-month period following discharge from the hospital is remarkable for its high incidence of sudden death. Since electrical instability is the main factor determining mortality during this period, it is not surprising that the presence of complex ventricular arrhythmias on Holter monitoring has proven to be a useful indicator for prognosis.[26–28]

Mortality during the "Late" Post-Recovery Period. The cardiac death rate during this period (3 to 4 percent per year) is similar to that described for chronic ischemic heart disease in general[18,19] and the major causes of mortality are the same, that is, recurrent myocardial infarction, congestive heart failure, sudden death, and so forth. However, in contrast to earlier periods, no one cause predominates. The enhanced risk of mortality associated with the acute infarction itself has essentially disappeared at the end of the early post-recovery period, and the patient entering the low-mortality late post-recovery period now has the same probability for survival as any patient with chronic ischemic heart disease and similar risk factors. Therefore, it is not surprising that the most important prognostic factor for patients in the late post-recovery period appears to be the nature and distribution of the underlying coronary vascular disease, as demonstrated by coronary angiography. Mechanical and electrical phenomena continue to play a contributory, but less important, role.

Based on these considerations, two additional points may be made concerning the interpretation of the results of long-term intervention trials of the effects of a drug on mortality following an acute myocardial infarction: (1) Cognizance must be taken of the fact that cardiac mortality varies by cause during different periods. (2) Drugs used in long-term intervention trials are not likely to influence the various causes of mortality to the same degree; consequently, the effect may be expected to be more prominent at one time than another. Therefore, a proper interpretation of a drug's effect (assuming great care has been taken in properly classifying the deaths by cause) requires an independent evaluation by cause as well as by period. This may be particularly important for sudden death, because the electrical instability of the heart during the early post-recovery period appears to be related to the acute infarct, whereas during the late post-recovery period it no longer appears to be related to the previous infarct. Since the pathogenesis of a lethal re-entry arrhythmia during each of these two periods may be different, the drug's effect should be considered independently by period, as well as *in toto*.

This latter information on the causes of death during each of the three fairly distinct mortality periods following a myocardial infarction has been reviewed to emphasize that a drug with a specific pharmacologic action that has the ability to prevent one of the specific causes of death following a myocardial infarction is unlikely to show a beneficial effect statistically in modern trials if only total mortality is the endpoint independent of any separation according to cause and time-frame. Accordingly, if we are to make progress in drug evaluations, we must begin to design trials that overcome these handicaps. For example, reduction of in-hospital mortality should have as its major therapeutic objective the use of agents or procedures that can reduce infarct size; and a separate primary analysis should be conducted on this period independent of what happens to these patients subsequently. As far as the early post-recovery period, with its high incidence of sudden death, the major therapeutic objective should be to prevent lethal ventricular arrythmias, and a primary analysis on the effect of an agent that may do this should be carried out for this period and for sudden death, independent of any other observations made. Finally, determining the efficacy of any agent or procedure during the late post-recovery period will prove to be the most difficult because of the low mortality rate and because no one cause of death predominates. Nevertheless, in testing any agent during this period, a primary analysis should be conducted on the specific cause of death that the agent is most likely to affect.

As will be evident, few of the trials with platelet acting drugs have taken any of these factors into consideration, but they will be the subject of comments in the following review of the trial results.

CLINICAL TRIALS

Aspirin Alone

Medical Research Council Studies

The results of a prospective, randomized, controlled Medical Research Council Study conducted in England by Elwood and associates were reported in 1974.[29] In a double-blind trial, the investigators compared the effects on mortality of daily treatment with 300 mg of aspirin for 2 years with those of placebo in 1239 men who had a confirmed diagnosis of myocardial infarction. The low dosage of aspirin was chosen on the basis that it was well above the level needed to inhibit collagen- or ADP-induced platelet aggregation. In the aspirin-treated group, reductions in total mortality of 12 percent and 25 percent over that in the placebo group were found at 6 and 21 months, respectively. These reductions were not statistically significant. However, when the results were analyzed in respect to the interval between myocardial infarction and admission to the study, a stronger difference was found. Approximately half the patients entered the study less than 6 weeks after myocardial infarction. The mortality rate for the aspirin-treated group that entered the study within 6 weeks after myocardial infarction was 7.8 percent, compared with a 13.5 percent rate in the placebo group, or a 42 percent reduction.

The same investigators completed another Medical Research Council Study of a similar multicenter, randomized, double-blind design.[30] For this study, however, a higher daily dosage of aspirin, 900 mg (300 mg three times daily), was used for a period of just 1 year. Moreover, women were included in the study and comprised 15 percent of the total 1682 patients in the study. In addition to total mortality, mortality from ischemic heart disease and rehospitalization resulting from myocardial infarction, ischemic heart disease without myocardial infarction, or other causes were measured.

The total mortality in patients given aspirin was 12.3 percent, compared with 14.8 percent in those receiving placebo. The 17.3 percent reduction in mortality attributable to aspirin was not statistically significant. However, these data may have been influenced by the fact that two factors strongly prognostic of death, pulmonary congestion and cardiac enlargement, were more common in the aspirin-treated group. The analysis of specific mortality resulting from ischemic heart disease suggested a greater, statistically significant reduction in the aspirin-treated group, but when this rate was adjusted for slight age differences between the groups, it was no longer significant. There were only slight differences between the treatment groups in numbers of rehospitalizations for ischemic heart disease without myocardial infarction or for other causes. However, 7.1 percent of the aspirin-treated group was readmitted for infarction, compared with 10.9 percent for the placebo group—a 34 percent reduction that was statistically significant. The total mortality combined with the nonfatal ischemic heart disease morbidity increased with age in men but not consistently so in women;* the combined rate was significantly reduced in the aspirin-treated group by 28 percent (p less than 0.05) in all patients.

The investigators noted that their data "suggested that the mortality difference between the treatments emerges very early, and about three months after infarction little further difference developed." Again, their findings in this respect could not be considered conclusive.

COMMENT. The Elwood trials illustrate many of the problems previously discussed. In the first trial, the intent was to admit all patients within the first 6 weeks after their infarction and to follow them for a period of 2 years. Later, so that the number of patients in the trial could be increased, patients were admitted who had had an infarct at any time during the previous 6 months. Thus, although there was equal randomization between the patients in terms of their trial entry, each group now contained patients in whom not only the mortality risk but also possibly the preventable causes of death had been markedly reduced. Consequently, the initial trend based on the early entry group, which was markedly in favor of aspirin, was soon blunted, and the benefit achieved never reached significance. Therefore, the second trial was designed to admit all patients early. However, the original design was not followed, and patients were admitted much earlier, that is, during the in-hospital period and as early as 3 days post-infarct, the dose was changed from 0.3 to 0.9 gm daily, and women were included. Furthermore, in this "intent to treat" trial, a large number of dropouts were included in the analysis. As with the first trial, a difference between the treatment groups favoring aspirin appeared to emerge early after the infarction, but after 3 months little further difference developed. It is unfortunate that both trials were not run similarly, except for the entry point, and that the trial size was not large enough to allow an analysis of the early post-recovery period independent of the late post-recovery period. Nevertheless, these inconclusive studies still leave one with the impression that aspirin did reduce mortality during the early post-recovery period.

German-Austrian Multicenter Study

In this study, completed in 1977, aspirin was compared with phenprocoumon or placebo for the secondary prevention of myocardial infarction or sudden death.[33,34] The 946 patients admitted to the study 4 to 6 weeks after their qualifying infarction were randomly allocated to one of three treatment groups: aspirin, 1.5 gm daily; placebo; or phenprocoumon. Phen-

---

*The inclusion of women in these drug trials raises a special problem because the risk of subsequent mortality following an acute myocardial infarction is probably different than for men, that is, the course of the former may be more benign. It also has been claimed that women may respond differently to aspirin than men.[31,32]

procoumon, an anticoagulant widely used in Germany and Austria for the prevention of rein-farction, was given at a dosage adjusted individually to maintain prothrombin time values between 15 and 25 percent or thrombotest values around 10 percent. The trial was double-blind regarding treatment with placebo or aspirin but open regarding treatment with phen-procoumon. Randomization was within strata, including hospital, age, sex, secondary infarc-tion, cardiac failure, and hyperlipidemia or cholesterolemia. Over a 2-year observation period, patients received clinical and laboratory evaluations at 2- to 4-week intervals. Nonfatal myo-cardial infarction and sudden death, as well as total and cardiac mortality, were selected as endpoints for the trial, and patients experiencing a nonfatal event were not enrolled as par-ticipants in the trial thereafter.

A final analysis of the data has not yet been published. However, some results have been reported.[34] A total of 61 patients died of verified myocardial infarction or sudden death during the trial. Most of these died during the first half year. The highest numbers of coronary deaths occurred in the phenprocoumon group, with 26, and in the placebo group, with 22; only 13 such deaths occurred in the aspirin group. This reduction reaches a level of significance close to a p value of 0.05. When compared with the placebo, the benefit from aspirin was restricted to the first 6 months, although, because of the smaller numbers of deaths during this partic-ular time, a statistically significant benefit could not be established.

COMMENT. The trial, while not conclusive because of the relatively small numbers of patients studied (309 placebo, 317 aspirin, and 320 phenprocoumon), is, like the Elwood stud-ies, highly suggestive that aspirin reduces mortality from acute coronary events during the early post-recovery period but not thereafter. The dose of aspirin (1.5 gm daily) is the largest used in any of the aspirin trials and is at a level likely to interfere with prostacyclin produc-tion; yet the beneficial effects claimed (42 percent reduction in deaths as compared with pla-cebo group) are as great, if not greater, than those observed in Elwood's study utilizing 0.3 gm daily.

Aspirin Myocardial Infarction Study (AMIS)

By far the largest prospective trial of aspirin for the secondary prevention of death from myocardial infarction has been the recently completed Aspirin Myocardial Infarction Study.[35] This double-blind, controlled study, sponsored by the National Heart, Lung, and Blood Institute and conducted at 30 clinical centers in the United States, was designed to test whether the regular administration of aspirin to patients who had experienced at least one documented myocardial infarction would result in a significant reduction of total mortality over a 3-year period. Secondary objectives, such as cause-specific mortality and nonfatal car-diovascular events, were also evaluated. Over a 13-month period, 4524 patients with a pre-vious, documented myocardial infarction were entered into the study. Of these, 4021 (89 percent) were men. The patients were between the ages of 30 and 69 years, with a mean age of 54.8 years. In a double-blind fashion, patients were randomly assigned to treatment with aspirin or placebo. Based on the experience of the Coronary Drug Project Aspirin Study,[6] a total daily dosage of 1 gm (0.5 gm twice daily) of aspirin was selected. The time of entrance into the study after the qualifying myocardial infarction ranged anywhere from 8 weeks to as long as 5 years, with a mean of 25 months. Results were further compromised by the fact that, as a happenstance of the randomization process, seven baseline characteristics were dis-tributed unevenly enough between the two groups to make the discrepancies statistically sig-nificant. These risk factors included previous heart failure, angina pectoris, cardiomegaly, and histories of using digitalis, nitroglycerin, propranolol, or "other drugs." For all seven, the inferred risk fell more heavily on the aspirin group.

Fatal events were analyzed with the Cox statistical procedure (based on a proportional hazard model). For nonfatal events, such as recurrent myocardial infarction, angina pectoris, stroke, intermittent cerebral ischemic attacks, and cardiovascular surgery, a 2 × 2 table analysis was employed. All randomized patients were included in the analysis.

In terms of the study's primary endpoint, total mortality, no significant benefit from aspirin was found. The total mortality after 38 months of followup was 10.8 percent in the aspirin group and 9.7 percent in the placebo group. On the other hand, the cardiovascular-morbidity tallies favored the aspirin-treated group. The percentage of nonfatal myocardial infarction was 6.3 percent in the aspirin group and 8.1 percent in the placebo group. Only "unimpressive" differences were found between men's and women's responses to aspirin, although, as expected, the women had a lower overall mortality. On the basis of their findings, the investigators stated that "aspirin is not recommended for routine use in patients who have survived an MI."

COMMENT. This study, involving a very large number of patients followed for a 3-year period, was designed to be the "definitive" study on aspirin. Unfortunately, it was based on the findings of the Coronary Drug Project Aspirin study but did not take into account the findings of the first Elwood study nor the natural history of mortality following an acute myocardial infarction. Consequently, it was primarily a study of a dose of 1 gm of aspirin given daily during the late post-recovery period only. The findings are not dissimilar from those reported in the two Elwood trials or the German-Austrian multicenter study for this particular period. It is sad that the study was not designed as a study of the effect of aspirin on the natural history of mortality following an acute infarction, with all patients entering during a rather narrow window shortly after survival from an acute infarct. Consequently, the trial offers no useful data for the period during which others claim that aspirin may have a beneficial effect.

Other Studies in Progress or Unpublished

An open, randomized study of the effects of aspirin (1.5 gm daily) versus those of oral anticoagulants on reinfarction and cardiac death in patients with myocardial infarction has been conducted in 15 hospitals in France under the Institut National de la Sante et de la Recherche Medicale (INSERM), but details of the study have not yet been published. An enrollment of 1500 patients to be followed by 2 years is called for.[36]

No other studies are presently in progress for the investigation of treatment with aspirin alone for the *secondary* prevention of death in patients with ischemic heart disease, as indicated by prior myocardial infarction. However, two studies have been started to study the effects of aspirin on myocardial infarction and death in patients with unstable angina pectoris.

One double-blind, randomized study, being conducted in 10 Veterans Administration hospitals in the United States, compares the effects of low doses of aspirin (324 mg) with those of placebo given daily for 12 weeks.[7] Patients are men who have been admitted to a coronary care unit for new or worsening angina and have evidence of coronary artery disease but not acute myocardial infarction.

The other double-blind, randomized study, sponsored by the Medical Research Council of Canada and designed to cover a 2-year followup period, will measure the effects of aspirin (1.3 gm daily) and sulfinpyrazone (800 mg daily), singly and in combination, versus those of placebo in 700 patients admitted to a coronary care unit with unstable angina pectoris. The study, scheduled for completion in 1984, will have acute myocardial infarction and death as its endpoints.[37]

General Comment on Studies with Aspirin Alone

The results of the various prospective studies with aspirin alone in reducing cardiac mortality following an acute myocardial infarction remain inconclusive. In those trials in which aspirin was tested early after an infarction, there is a beneficial effect in reducing the high mortality observed during the early post-recovery period. In general, the findings are reminiscent of those more clearly established with sulfinpyrazone in the Anturane Reinfarction Trial (see below).

When beneficial results have been claimed, they have been observed with doses of aspirin varying from 0.3 to 1.5 gm daily; this suggests that the dosage of aspirin may not be as critical in vivo as postulated on the basis of in vitro studies.

Clinical Trials with Dipyridamole and Aspirin

No trial evaluating dipyridamole alone has been undertaken, but its combination with aspirin has been tested. The rationale for combined treatment with dipyridamole and aspirin is based on a possible synergistic effect (aspirin inhibits production of the platelet-aggregating substance, thromboxane A_2, and dipyridamole enhances the action of prostacyclin, an inhibitor of platelet aggregation).[38]

The Persantine-Aspirin Reinfarction Study 1 (PARIS 1)

This study compared the effect of a combined treatment of dipyridamole and aspirin with that of aspirin alone or placebo on mortality and morbidity in patients with previous myocardial infarction.[39] In this double-blind trial conducted at 20 clinical centers in the United States and England, 2026 patients aged 30 to 74 years, of whom 1759 (87 percent) were men, were randomly allocated to one of the following treatments given three times daily: dipyridamole, 75 mg, and aspirin, 324 mg; aspirin, 324 mg, and one placebo tablet; two placebo tablets. There were 810 patients allocated to each of the two active treatment groups, and 406 to the placebo group. Patients were entered into the trial any time from 8 weeks to as long as 5 years after a myocardial infarction documented by ECG changes and enzyme elevations and were followed for an average of 44 months. The primary endpoints evaluated were total mortality, coronary mortality, and coronary incidence (coronary death or definite but nonfatal myocardial infarction). Of the total 2026 patients, 1666 completed the trial. Another 224 patients were reported deceased. The remaining 136 patients withdrew from the study; of these one was known to have died, 128 were known to be alive, and the fate of 7 was unknown at the time the results were reported.

Total mortality was 16 percent and 18 percent lower in the dipyridamole/aspirin and aspirin groups, respectively, than in the placebo group. Three quarters of the deaths were coronary in nature. There were 24 percent and 21 percent fewer coronary deaths in the dipyridamole/aspirin and aspirin groups, respectively, than in the placebo group. Coronary incidence was reduced by 25 percent and 24 percent in these groups. The aspirin group had the highest incidence of sudden coronary death, with 5.6 percent of the group's patients dying within 1 hour after the onset of symptoms. On the other hand, the aspirin group showed the lowest incidence of nonsudden coronary death—2.5 percent, compared with 5.7 percent and 4.0 percent in the placebo and dipyridamole/aspirin groups, respectively. None of the above differences was statistically significant at a Z value greater than 2.6, the critical value chosen for the study. However, significant differences in coronary incidence between the dipyridamole/aspirin and placebo groups were found after 4, 8, 12, 16, 20, and 24 months of treatment.

Patients enrolled in the study within 6 months after myocardial infarction had fewer deaths in the active treatment groups, a reduction of 44 percent in the combination group and 51 percent in the aspirin group. However, the number of patients enlisted so soon after myocardial infarction was limited (179 in the dipyridamole/aspirin group, 173 in the aspirin group, and 95 in the placebo group).

Both active treatment groups showed a reduction in incidence of definite nonfatal MI, angina pectoris requiring hospitalization, and stroke; however, both showed a higher incidence

Table 1. Cumulative annual mortality (%) by drug group in AMIS and PARIS

	Placebo	Aspirin	Dipyridamole/Aspirin
AMIS	8.8	9.6	
PARIS	11.4	9.0	9.4

of acute coronary insufficiency than the placebo group. The largest difference occurred for congestive heart failure; both active treatments showed a lower incidence than the placebo group, but neither difference was statistically significant.

COMMENT. While this study did not show a statistically significant benefit from treatment with aspirin alone or in combination with dipyridamole, nevertheless, in contrast with the results of the Aspirin Myocardial Infarction Study (AMIS), it does suggest an appreciable reduction in fatal coronary events and in combined fatal and nonfatal coronary episodes (coronary incidence). Furthermore, this beneficial effect could more readily be demonstrated among those patients who entered the trial within 6 months of their qualifying myocardial infarction, that is, during a period of increased mortality risk (early post-recovery period). In this respect, the findings in the aspirin group of PARIS 1 are reminiscent of the observations previously reported in the Elwood studies[29,30] and in the German-Austrian multicenter trial.[33,34]

Whether the addition of dipyridamole to aspirin in the dosages employed provided any additional benefit over that claimed for aspirin alone is not answered by this trial. Though some of the clinical endpoints appeared to favor the combination therapy, others favored aspirin alone.

Although PARIS 1 and AMIS had an essentially common protocol and were undertaken at the same time, their results appear to be dissimilar and have been interpreted differently. Perhaps this discrepancy relates to a major difference in the size of the placebo group relative to the test groups. In PARIS 1 there were only 400 placebo patients, compared with 800 patients in each of the active drug compartments. In essence, PARIS 1 was designed to take advantage of the large placebo compartment of 2257 patients in AMIS, on the assumption that the PARIS 1 and AMIS placebo results would be similar, and for this reason only a small placebo compartment would be necessary. However, as seen in Table 1, this supposition proved to be incorrect.

In effect, then, the benefits ascribed to aspirin and the combination therapy in PARIS 1 may just as well be related to a spuriously high mortality observed in the small placebo compartment of PARIS 1 as to any positive effect of the active drugs being tested. If the mortalities in the aspirin and dipyridamole/aspirin compartments of PARIS 1 are compared with that of the large placebo compartment of AMIS, which involved patients of a similar type studied at the same time, no difference is apparent.

The small placebo compartment in PARIS 1 also creates problems in interpretation of the differences in results for those patients who entered the trial within 6 months of their qualifying infarction and those who entered later. Because only approximately 20 percent entered less than 6 months after infarction, the benefit claimed is based on a study of only 95 placebo patients and 173 and 179 aspirin and dipyridamole/aspirin patients, respectively, and is related more to the soft endpoints (coronary events requiring hospitalization) than to the hard endpoint (mortality).

Persantine-Aspirin Reinfarction Study 2 (PARIS 2)

Because of the marked reduction in total and coronary deaths in patients entering the PARIS 1 trial within 6 months after infarction and treated with aspirin and dipyridamole, another large-scale study is being undertaken by the same investigators in patients within 4 months after myocardial infarction. This study will compare the combination treatment with placebo only and may provide an answer to the question of efficacy raised in PARIS 1.

Clinical Trials with Sulfinpyrazone

Sulfinpyrazone, a uricosuric agent used since the 1950s for the treatment of gout, was first reported to have platelet-regulating action in 1965.[40] In the ensuing decade, its effects were studied in the prevention of arteriovenous shunt thrombosis,[41] recurrent venous thrombosis,[42] and thromboembolism in patients with prosthetic cardiac valves.[43] In 1975, in a double-blind, placebo-controlled study of 291 elderly male patients, sulfinpyrazone was reported to significantly reduce mortality from vascular causes in a subgroup of 166 atherosclerotic patients.[44]

Anturane Reinfarction Trial

In 1975 a large-scale, double-blind study was undertaken of the effects of sulfinpyrazone on cardiac mortality in patients with a recent myocardial infarction.[45,46] The study, conducted over a 3-year period at 26 clinical centers in the United States and Canada, and designated the Anturane Reinfarction Trial, compared sulfinpyrazone, 800 mg daily (200 mg four times per day), with placebo for an average period of 16 months. Patients were enrolled in the study 25 to 35 days after the occurrence of a documented myocardial infarction.

In contrast with previous, "intent to treat" trials, the Anturane Reinfarction Trial was designed as a "clinical efficacy" study. This was considered possible without influencing bias for the following reasons: (1) sulfinpyrazone could not be differentiated from the placebo by either patient or physician on the basis of taste, color, or appearance; (2) sulfinpyrazone would produce no unique symptoms or signs that would allow it to be identified either by patient or physician; (3) all laboratory determinations were carried out in a central laboratory and, in addition, uric acid determinations were blanked out from any laboratory assays conducted on trial patients at the respective participating institutions; (4) all criteria for analyzability were set forth clearly in the protocol and operations manual before the trial was initiated; (5) the accuracy of the data collected was reviewed both during the trial and retrospectively during several audits carried out at different levels by independent groups with expertise in the conduct of such audits; and (6) all decisions were made on a blind basis without knowledge of drug assignment, and all such decisions were reviewed at three independent levels.

Therefore, it was deemed feasible to establish beforehand that the primary analysis would be only of cardiac deaths among eligible patients with analyzable events, according to clearly defined criteria for eligibility and analyzability established before the inception of the trial. Thus, prior to the start of the trial, special criteria were established for the classifications of death as "sudden death," "myocardial infarction," or "other cardiac" deaths. "Sudden death" was an unexpected, unobserved death or one that occurred within 60 minutes of the onset of symptoms. "Myocardial infarction" had to be documented at autopsy or by clinical evidence of pain, electrocardiographic findings, and by elevation of a serum enzyme (serum glutamic oxaloacetic transaminase, lactic dehydrogenase, or creatinine phosphokinase) to twice the normal level. The "other cardiac" category included congestive heart failure, arrhythmia, or cardiogenic shock.

All deaths in eligible patients were further classified as analyzable or nonanalyzable. A death was considered nonanalyzable if it occurred within 7 days after the initiation or more than 7 days following the termination of therapy or in a patient who did not comply with instructions, or if it could be attributed directly to surgery without association with a nonfatal event occurring during treatment. Analyzable deaths formed a basis for the primary analysis of the efficacy of sulfinpyrazone.

Of the original 1629 patients entered into the study, 1143 (73 percent) completed the protocol as planned and were included in the primary analysis. Of the remainder, 415 withdrew prematurely for various medical and nonmedical reasons, and 71 were excluded from analysis by the study's policy committee because they were judged, on a blind basis, not to meet the protocol criteria.

All 106 analyzable deaths reported in the study were cardiovascular in nature—105 were cardiac (the primary endpoint), and one was cerebrovascular. At 24 months, the observed reduction in cardiac mortality from sulfinpyrazone treatment was approximately 32 percent ($p = 0.058$). Over half of the deaths were sudden cardiac deaths, and the reduction in this category was mainly responsible for the overall reduction. There were 37 sudden deaths in the placebo group versus 22 in the sulfinpyrazone-treated group, a reduction of 43 percent ($p = 0.041$). This advantage occurred during the first 6 months of treatment when the rate of analyzable sudden deaths was 7 percent in the placebo group versus 1.8 percent in the sulfinpyrazone-treated group, a highly significant reduction of 74 percent ($p = 0.003$). Thereafter, however, the rates of sudden death were comparable for the two groups (2.0 percent with placebo versus 2.3 percent with sulfinpyrazone treatment).

The reduction in sudden deaths, when nonanalyzable sudden deaths were included, was 68 percent at 6 months for the sulfinpyrazone-treated group. By this time, the majority of sudden deaths had already occurred. For the entire 24-month observation period, the reduction rate was 41 percent.

Sulfinpyrazone had no effect upon analyzable deaths from myocardial infarction, there being 18 such deaths in the placebo group and 17 in the sulfinpyrazone group after 24 months.

In reporting these findings, the investigators noted that the first 6 months after myocardial infarction are a period of high risk (particularly from sudden death) directly related to the previous myocardial infarction, and it is during this period (early post-recovery period) that sulfinpyrazone exerts its effect. They also note that though the study was undertaken because of the known effects of sulfinpyrazone upon platelet function, the fact that sulfinpyrazone was effective in reducing sudden cardiac deaths but not deaths from myocardial infarction suggests that another, yet to be elucidated, mechanism of action exists.

Anturane Reinfarction Italian Study (ARIS)

A trial similar in design to the Anturane Reinfarction Trial and designated the Anturane Reinfarction Italian Study (ARIS) has been completed, but the results have not yet been reported.

This study was designed for a population of 650 patients of both sexes to be followed for a period of at least one year and differed from the larger American counterpart in several respects.[47] The daily dosage of 800 mg of sulfinpyrazone was given in two doses of 400 mg per day instead of four 200 mg doses. Moreover, patients were enrolled into the study a week or two earlier after their qualifying infarction—10 to 20 days. In addition to fatal reinfarction and sudden cardiac death, nonfatal myocardial infarction served as an endpoint for the study.

General Comment on Studies with Sulfinpyrazone

A great deal of publicity has been given to sulfinpyrazone, because the Anturane Reinfarction Trial is the only study that has claimed a major benefit for an agent in reducing cardiac mortality following an acute myocardial infarction, and this by virtue of a striking reduction in sudden death during the first 6 months (high-risk early post-recovery period) following discharge of the patient from the hospital. This claim was made possible because of the unique features of trial design as a "clinical efficacy" study; by avoiding the various dilution factors inherent in "intent to treat" trials, this study allowed a quantitative assessment of the actual effect of the drug in compliant patients. In addition, because of the early and narrow entry window (25 to 35 days after the qualifying infarction), the trial studied the effect of this drug on the natural history of mortality among recent survivors of an infarct both by period and by cause.

Considering the negative results of the Aspirin Myocardial Infarction Study (AMIS) and the inconclusive results of the Persantine-Aspirin Reinfarction Study (PARIS 1), it is not surprising that the trial has come under considerable criticism. In addition, the US Food and Drug Administration has raised serious questions as to the classification of certain of the deaths (sudden, myocardial infarction, other cardiac) within each treatment group.[48] An independent classification of the deaths by an outside independent panel of cardiologists recently convened for this purpose has confirmed that a significant reduction in total cardiac and sudden death mortality occurred during the first 6 months following trial entry.[49]

The observed reduction in cardiac mortality during the early post-recovery period in the Anturane Reinfarction Trial is not dissimilar to the beneficial trends ascribed to aspirin during this same period in both Elwood studies,[29,30] in the German-Austrian multicenter trial,[33,34] and for those patients receiving the combination of aspirin and dipyridamole in PARIS 1 who were entered within the first 6 months of their qualifying infarction.[39]

The claim that sulfinpyrazone reduces the incidence of sudden death and not fatal myocardial infarction has stimulated research on other actions of this drug which could account for this finding. Because most sudden deaths are due to the appearance of a lethal ventricular arrhythmia, the effect of this drug on experimentally induced ventricular arrhythmias arising from an ischemic myocardium in animals has been under study, and already a number of interesting observations have been made.[50-52] Inasmuch as an observation of a similar action by aspirin was reported previously,[53] an effect of these agents on prostaglandin pathways other than platelets may be involved in any possible beneficial therapeutic effect.

The striking results of the Anturane Reinfarction Trial require confirmation. Consequently, great interest can be attached to the results of the Italian study. Unfortunately, the size of this trial (approximately 650 patients) is probably too small to yield statistically significant differences even if the effects are similar to those described in the Anturane Reinfarction Trial. Therefore, the importance of this study probably will relate more to whether the various period and cause mortality rates are or are not influenced in a fashion similar to that described in the North American study.

CONCLUDING COMMENT

The investigation of the use of platelet-acting drugs as antithrombotic agents in the prevention of acute arterial vascular occlusions has opened a new and exciting chapter in medical therapeutics. Though a reasonably clear picture of their usefulness for certain selected clinical situations, such as the prevention of stroke and death in male patients with transient ischemic attacks, and for the prevention of thromboembolism from prosthetic valves has emerged, their value in reducing mortality following an acute myocardial infarction is, at present, less well established despite the preponderance of evidence supporting this conclusion. Theoretically the matter could be settled through additional trials, but it is unlikely that this will be accomplished. Considering the current widespread use of beta blockers in the post-infarct patient, and the beneficial effect in reducing mortality during the early high-risk period that has been attributed to these agents in several trials,[11,54-57] the opportunity to resolve this question is now markedly limited. Under the circumstances, physicians will probably have to decide on their own and on the basis of the present evidence as to whether there is virtue to their use, particularly during the early high-mortality period following an acute myocardial infarction.

REFERENCES

1. CRAVEN, LL: *Experiences with aspirin (acetylsalicyclic acid) in the nonspecific prophylaxis of coronary thrombosis.* Miss Valley Med J 75:38, 1953.

2. COBB, S, ANDERSON, F, AND BAUER, W: *Length of life and cause of death in rheumatoid arthritis.* N Engl J Med 249:553, 1953.

3. BOSTON COLLABORATIVE DRUG SURVEILLANCE GROUP: *Regular aspirin intake and acute myocardial infarction.* Br Med J 1:440, 1974.

4. BOSTON COLLABORATIVE DRUG SURVEILLANCE PROGRAM: *Regular aspirin use and myocardial infarction.* Br Med J 2:1057, 1976.

5. HAMMOND, EC, and GARFINKEL, L: *Aspirin and coronary heart disease: Findings of a prospective study.* Br Med J 2:269, 1975.

6. THE CORONARY DRUG PROJECT RESEARCH GROUP: *Aspirin in coronary heart disease.* J Chron Dis 29:625, 1976.

7. VERSTRAETE, M: *Registry of prospective clinical trials. Fourth report.* Thromb Haemost 43:176, 1980.

8. GENT, M, AND SACKETT DL: *The qualification and disqualification of patients and events in long-term cardiovascular clinical trials.* Thromb Haemost 41:123, 1979.

9. SACKETT, DL, AND GENT, M: *Controversy in counting and attributing events in clinical trials.* N Engl J Med 301:1410, 1979.

10. THE CANADIAN COOPERATIVE STUDY GROUP: *A randomized trial of aspirin and sulfinpyrazone in threatened stroke.* N Engl J Med 299:53, 1978.

11. THE NORWEGIAN MULTICENTER STUDY GROUP: *Timolol-induced reduction in mortality and reinfarction in patients surviving acute myocardial infarction.* N Engl J Med 304:801, 1981.

12. SHERRY, S: *The Anturane Reinfarction Trial.* Circulation 62(Suppl 5):73, 1980.

13. ZUMOFF, B, HART, H, AND HELLMAN, H: *Considerations of mortality in certain chronic diseases.* Ann Intern Med 63:595, 1966.

14. BEARD, OW, HIPP, HR, ROBINS, M, ET AL: *Initial myocardial infarction among 503 veterans. Five-year survival.* Am J Med 28:871, 1960.

15. COOPERATIVE STUDY: *Death rate among 795 patients in their first year after myocardial infarction.* JAMA 197:184, 1966.

16. HELMERS, C, LUNDMAN, T, MASSING, R, ET AL: *Mortality pattern among initial survivors of acute myocardial infarction using a life-table technique.* Acta Med Scand 200:469, 1976.

17. MADSEN, EB, SVENDSEN, TL, RASMUSSEN, S, ET AL: *Prognostic factors in acute myocardial infarction occurring within the first five days of ECG monitoring.* Dan Med Bull 25:155, 1978.

18. PELL, S, AND D'ALONZO, CA: *Immediate mortality and five-year survival of employed men with a first myocardial infarction.* N Engl J Med 270:916, 1964.

19. WEINBLATT, E, SHAPIRO, S, FRANK, CW, ET AL: *Prognosis of men after first myocardial infarction: Mortality and first recurrence in relation to selected parameters.* Am J Public Health 58:1329, 1968.

20. IBRAHIM, MA, SACKETT, DL, AND WINKELSTEIN, W, JR: *Acute myocardial infarction: Magnitude of the problem.* In SHERRY, S, BRINKHOUS, KM, GENTON, E, ET AL (EDS): *Thrombosis.* National Academy of Sciences, Washington, DC, 1969, p 106.

21. MOSS, AJ, DECAMILLA, J, AND DAVIS, H: *Factors associated with cardiac death in the post-hospital phase of myocardial infarction.* In KULBERTUS, HE, AND WELLENS, HJJ (EDS): *Sudden Death. Vol. IV. Developments in Cardiovascular Medicine.* Martinus Nijhoff, The Hague, Netherlands, 1980, p 237.

22. CANNOM, DS, LEVY, W, AND COHEN, LS: *The short- and long-term prognosis of patients with transmural and non-transmural myocardial infarction.* Am J Med 61:452, 1976.

23. HELMERS, C, AND LUNDMAN, T: *Sudden coronary death after acute myocardial infarction.* Adv Cardiol 25:176, 1978.

24. BIGGER, JT, JR, HELLER, CA, WENGER, TL, ET AL: *Risk stratification after acute myocardial infarction.* Am J Cardiol 42:202, 1978.

25. THIROUX, P: *Prevention des accidents aigus apres infarctus du myocarde par les beta-bloquants.* In *Proceedings of Colloquimon "Prevention des accidents aigus apres infarctus du myocarde." September 22, 1979, Nice, France.* Ciba-Geigy, France, 1980.

26. SCHULZE, RA, JR, STRAUSS, HW, AND PITTS, B: *Sudden death in the year following myocardial infarction. Relation to ventricular premature contractions in the late hospital phase and left ventricular ejection fraction.* Am J Med 62:192, 1977.

27. LURIA, MH, KNOKE, JD, MARGOLIS, RM, ET AL: *Acute myocardial infarction: Prognosis after recovery.* Ann Intern Med 85:561, 1976.

28. MOSS, AJ, DECAMILLA, J, AND DAVIS, H: *Potential for mortality reduction in the early posthospital period.* Am J Cardiol 39:816, 1977.

29. ELWOOD, PC, COCHRANE, AL, BURR, ML, ET AL: *A randomized controlled trial of acetylsalicylic acid in the secondary prevention of mortality from myocardial infarction.* Br Med J 1:436, 1974.

30. ELWOOD, PC, AND SWEETNAM, PM: *Aspirin and secondary mortality after myocardial infarction.* Lancet 2:1313, 1979.

31. THE CANADIAN COOPERATIVE STUDY GROUP: *A randomized trial of aspirin and sulfinpyrazone in threatened stroke*. N Engl J Med 299:53, 1978.

32. KELTON, JE, HIRSH, J, CARTER, CJ, ET AL: *Sex differences in the antithrombotic effects of aspirin*. Blood 52:1073, 1978.

33. BREDDIN, K, UBERLA, K, AND WALTER, E: *German-Austrian multicenter two years prospective study on the prevention of secondary myocardial infarction by ASA in comparison to phenprocoumon and placebo*. Sixth International Congress of Thrombosis and Haemostasis. Thromb Haemost 38:168, 1977.

34. BREDDIN, K, LOEW, D, LECHNER, K, ET AL: *Secondary prevention of myocardial infarction: Comparison of acetylsalicylic acid, phenprocoumon and placebo*. Thromb Haemost 40:225, 1979.

35. ASPIRIN MYOCARDIAL INFARCTION STUDY RESEARCH GROUP: *A randomized controlled trial of aspirin in persons recovered from myocardial infarction*. JAMA 243:661, 1980.

36. VERSTRAETE, M: *Registry of prospective clinical trials. Third report*. Thromb Haemost 39:759, 1978.

37. GENT, M: Personal communication, 1980.

38. MONCADA, S, AND KORBUT, R: *Dipyridamole and other phosphodiesterase inhibitors act as antithrombotic agents by potentiating endogenous prostacyclin*. Lancet 1:1286, 1978.

39. THE PERSANTINE-ASPIRIN REINFARCTION STUDY RESEARCH GROUP: *Persantine and aspirin in coronary heart disease*. Circulation 62:449, 1980.

40. SMYTHE, HA, OGRYZLO, MA, MURPHY, EA, ET AL: *The effect of sulfinpyrazone (Anturan) on platelet economy and blood coagulation in man*. Canad M A J 92:818, 1965.

41. KAEGI, A, PINEO, GF, SHIMIZU, A, ET AL: *Arteriovenous shunt thrombosis*. N Engl J Med 290:304, 1974.

42. STEELE, PP, WEILY, HS, AND GENTON, E: *Platelet survival and adhesiveness in recurrent venous thrombosis*. N Engl J Med 288:1148, 1973.

43. STEELE, P, WEILY, H, DAVIES, H, ET AL: *Platelet survival time following aortic valve replacement*. Circulation 51:358, 1975.

44. BLAKELY, JA, AND GENT, M: *Platelets, drugs and longevity in a geriatric population*. In HIRSH, J, CADE, JF, GALLUS, AS, ET AL (EDS): *Platelets, Drugs and Thrombosis*. S. Karger, Basel, 1975, p 284.

45. THE ANTURANE REINFARCTION TRIAL RESEARCH GROUP: *Sulfinpyrazone in the prevention of cardiac death after myocardial infarction*. N Engl J Med 298:289, 1978.

46. THE ANTURANE REINFARCTION TRIAL RESEARCH GROUP: *Sulfinpyrazone in the prevention of sudden death after myocardial infarction*. N Engl J Med 302:250, 1980.

47. POLLI, EE, AND CORTELLARO, M: *Anturane Reinfarction Italian Study Research Group* (Letter). N Engl J Med, 298:1258, 1978.

48. TEMPLE, R, AND PLEDGER, GW: *The FDA's critique of the Anturane Reinfarction Trial*. N Engl J Med 303:1488, 1980.

49. ANTURANE REINFARCTION TRIAL POLICY COMMITTEE: *Anturane Reinfarction Trial: Re-evaluation of outcome*. N Engl J Med 306:1005, 1982.

50. KELLIHER, GJ, DIX, RK, JURKIEWICZ, N, ET AL: *Effects of sulfinpyrazone on arrhythmia and death following coronary occlusion in cats*. In McGREGOR, M, MUSTARD, JF, OLIVER, M, ET AL (EDS): *Cardiovascular Actions of Sulfinpyrazone: Basic and Clinical Research*. Symposia Specialists, Miami, 1980, p 193.

51. MOSCHOS, CB, ESCOBINAS, AJ, AND JORGENSEN, DB: *Effects of sulfinpyrazone on ischemic myocardium*. In McGREGOR, M, MUSTARD, JF, OLIVER, M, ET AL (EDS): *Cardiovascular Actions of Sulfinpyrazone: Basic and Clinical Research*. Symposia Specialists, Miami, 1980, p 175.

52. POVALSKI, HJ, OLSON, R, KOPIA, S, ET AL: *Comparative effects of sulfinpyrazone and aspirin in the coronary occlusion-reperfusion dog model*. In McGREGOR, M, MUSTARD, JF, OLIVER, M, ET AL (EDS): *Cardiovascular Actions of Sulfinpyrazone: Basic and Clinical Research*. Symposia Specialists, Miami, 1980, p 153.

53. NOSCHOS, C, HAIDER, B, DeLaCRUZ, C, JR, ET AL: *Antiarrhythmic effects of aspirin during nonthrombotic coronary occlusion*. Circulation 57:681, 1978.

54. AHLMARK, G, AND SAETRE, H: *Long-term treatment with beta-blockers after myocardial infarction*. Europ J Clin Pharmacol 10:77, 1976.

55. VEDIN, A, WILHEMSSON, C, AND WERKO, L: *Chronic alprenolol treatment of patients with acute myocardial infarction after discharge from hospital*. Acta Med Scand (Suppl)575:7, 1975.

56. GREEN, KG, CHAMBERLAIN, DA, FULTON, RM, ET AL: *Reduction in mortality after myocardial infarction with long-term beta-adrenoceptor blockade*. Multicentre international study: supplementary report. Br Med J 2:419, 1977.

57. ANDERSEN, MP, FREDERIKSEN, J, JURGENSEN, HJ, ET AL: *Effect of alprenolol on mortality among patients with definite or suspected myocardial infarction*. Lancet 2:865, 1979.

189

Acute Myocardial Infarction—Coronary Thrombosis and Salvage of the Ischemic Myocardium*

Peter R. Maroko, M.D., Lair G. T. Ribeiro, M.D., and Sheldon Goldberg, M.D.

New developments in the treatment of patients with myocardial infarction have been achieved in all phases of the disease, that is, the pre-hospital, in-hospital, and post-hospital phases.

Many patients with acute myocardial infarctions die before reaching the hospital.[1] Much progress has been achieved in recent years by making treatment available to patients before they reach the hospital. The advent of mobile coronary care units, ambulances with physicians or paramedics trained in cardiovascular emergencies, and improved public education about emergency measures for acute myocardial infarction, including cardiopulmonary resuscitation, have been responsible for saving many lives.[2]

In hospitalized patients with acute myocardial infarction, the two main causes of death are arrhythmias and left ventricular failure, as manifested in its extreme form by cardiogenic shock and pulmonary edema. The establishment of coronary care units, electrocardiographic monitoring, and new antiarrhythmic drugs has improved dramatically the prognosis of patients with life-threatening arrhythmias. The treatment of severe left ventricular failure and its prevention continues to be a major clinical challenge.

In the post-hospital phase of treatment the main goal is to prevent future ischemic episodes that may progress to reinfarction or that may manifest themselves as life-threatening arrhythmias. The finding that several beta-adrenergic blocking agents such as timolol,[3] alprenolol,[4] atenolol,[5] metoprolol,[6] and propranolol[7-9] reduce significantly the rate of reinfarction and death of cardiac origin is the most remarkable advance in the treatment of this phase thus far.

Salvage of the acutely injured myocardium during the first hours of an acute myocardial infarction is a therapeutic approach to the minimization of left ventricular failure during the in-hospital phase. This approach will be presented in this chapter.

The rationale for reducing the ultimate size of myocardial infarctions is based mainly on the observation that there is a close correlation between the amount of myocardial damage and left ventricular failure.[10,11] The total noncontractile area resulting from either one single infarction or the sum of successive infarctions will determine subsequent left ventricular performance. Therefore it is to be expected that salvage of myocardial tissue immediately after each episode of an infarction will result in a larger contractile mass, better left ventricular function, and better prognosis. In addition to this expected amelioration in mechanical heart function, it has been shown that infarct size may be an important determinant of the occurrence of ventricular arrhythmias.[12]

*This work was partially supported by a grant from the W. W. Smith Charitable Trust.

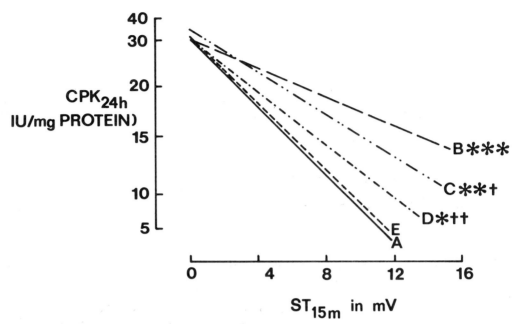

Figure 1. The relationship between ST segment elevation 15 minutes after coronary artery occlusion (ST_{15m}) and log creatine phosphokinase values of specimens obtained from same sites 24 hours later (CPK_{24h}). Group A (occlusion alone) (————): log CPK = $(-0.064 \pm 0.007)ST_{15m} + 1.48 \pm 0.02$; 12 dogs, r = -0.72 ± 0.04. Group B (hyaluronidase given 20 minutes after occlusion) (— — —): log CPK = $(-0.025 \pm 0.003)ST_{15m} + (1.48 \pm 0.02)$; 12 dogs, r = 0.72 ± 0.04. Group C (hyaluronidase given 3 hours after occlusion) (- · · · · · ·): log CPK = $(-0.037 \pm 0.05)ST_{15m} + (1.53 \pm 0.01)$; 8 dogs, r = -0.85 ± 0.02. Group D (hyaluronidase given 6 hours after occlusion) (- · · · · -): log CPK = $(-0.044 \pm 0.003)ST_{15m} + (1.49 \pm 0.001)$; 8 dogs, r = -0.78 ± 0.03. Group E (hyaluronidase given 9 hours after occlusion) (- - - -): log CPK = $(-0.06 \pm 0.006)ST_{15m} = (1.50 \pm 0.02)$; 6 dogs, r = -0.86 ± 0.006. Note that for any ST_{15m}, hyaluronidase given 20 minutes, 3 hours, or 6 hours after occlusion results in significantly greater myocardial CPK activity; in contrast, hyaluronidase given 9 hours after occlusion has no such effect. (* = $p < 0.05$, ** = $p < 0.025$, *** = $p < 0.0005$ in comparison to control; † = $p < 0.025$, †† = $p < 0.0005$ in comparison to hyaluronidase at 20 minutes.)

Myocardial infarction usually results from a complete interruption, or at least a severe reduction, in blood flow to a region of the myocardium. The reduction may reach so critical a level as to induce progressive myocardial damage per se or may be somewhat less severe but accompanied by other factors that worsen the balance between myocardial oxygen supply and demand, resulting in the same chain of histopathologic events leading to necrosis. In both instances, myocardial cells will progress to necrosis. This process, however, is not instantaneous but occurs over a period of several hours[13,14] (Fig. 1). At first the cells are injured only minimally, but with time this injury increases in severity and finally reaches a phase in which it is so intense that it cannot be reversed and will progress inexorably to necrosis. The exact moment that the reversibly injured myocardium becomes irreversibly injured during this process is not well determined, but it is known that it can be influenced by factors that determine the balance between oxygen supply and demand in each particular zone of the ischemic myocardium. Thus, if there is more coronary collateral blood flow to one region of the infarcting myocardium than to another, the cells in the region with greater collateral flow will survive longer and will remain longer in the reversible phase of injury than the cells in the region with less collateral flow. The period in which the cells are still reversibly injured is the time when a given therapy that can re-establish the balance between oxygen supply and demand, or at least tilt the imbalance in a favorable direction, can be effective.

In 1969, we demonstrated that myocardial infarction is a dynamic process and that the ultimate size of the myocardial infarction can be altered by many interventions administered early after coronary artery occlusion when myocardial injury is still in the reversible phase.[15,16]

The ultimate size of a myocardial infarction can be reduced by decreasing myocardial oxygen demand, by increasing oxygen supply to the infarcting zone, or by other miscellaneous mechanisms of action. The latter methods include stabilization of cell membranes, as in the case of glucocorticoids,[17] lidocaine,[18] and S1249;[18] reduction in the autophagic inflammatory type reaction, as in the case of aprotinin,[19] glucocorticoids,[17] and cobra-venom factor;[20] administration of hyaluronidase, which may act by reducing edema and facilitating penetration of nutrients and the washout of noxious catabolites;[21-24] the administration of nicotinic acid and other compounds that inhibit free fatty acids;[25] the reduction of edema by increasing osmolarity with mannitol;[26] and the administration of prostacyclins[27] or tilting the balance between thromboxane and prostacyclin toward prostacyclin,[28] which may decrease the inflammatory process.

The decrease in ultimate infarct size by a reduction in myocardial oxygen consumption can be achieved with beta-adrenergic blocking agents[15,16,29] or bradycardia,[16] and because beta-adrenergic blocking agents reduce heart rate, their beneficial effects in most circumstances will be additive (Fig. 2). However, it should be emphasized that the effect of a beta-adrenergic blocking agent is not due solely to its bradycardic action, although bradycardia parallels its other effects and may be used as an index of its effectiveness. Thus, for example, in the case of propranolol, over two thirds of its effect of decreasing myocardial injury, as measured spectrophotometrically by intramyocardial P_{CO_2}, was not due to a fall in heart rate, as was demonstrated in experiments in which the heart rate was maintained constant with electrical pacing.[30]

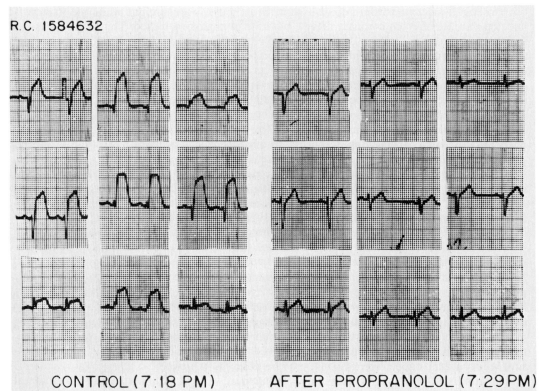

R.C. 1584632

CONTROL (7:18 PM)   AFTER PROPRANOLOL (7:29 PM)

Figure 2. The effect of propranolol on the reduction of ST segment elevation in a patient. The nine leads depicted are from the V_1, V_3, and V_5 positions and the corresponding sites one intercostal space above and below the standard positions.

193

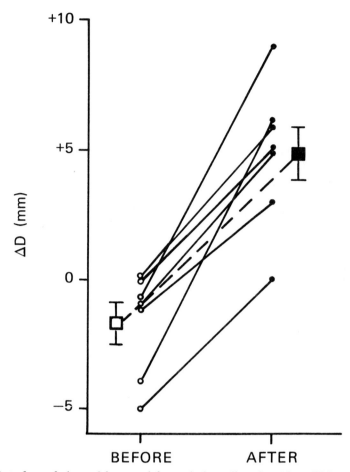

Figure 4. The effect of reperfusion at 3 hours on left ventricular wall motion. ΔD = EDD − ESD, where EDD = distance between beads at end-diastole and ESD = distance between beads at end-systole. Before *(open symbols):* 3 hours after occlusion and just before reperfusion. After *(closed symbols):* 30 minutes after reperfusion. Squares and bars indicate means and SEM.

are generally found in stenosed coronary arteries, although more rarely the underlying coronary artery appears normal angiographically.

Many investigations have been carried out to examine the effects of coronary artery reperfusion on infarct size. It has been shown that when the blood flow is re-established within the first 3 hours, a portion of the myocardial tissue is salvaged[44,45] and regional function is improved[45] (Fig. 4). Moreover, this procedure was accompanied also by reduced mortality in the conscious dog model.[57] However, re-establishment of blood flow through a previously occluded coronary artery presents some specific pathologic problems. One is the "no-reflow phenomenon," which is the consequence of vascular damage not permitting the re-established blood flow in the large coronary to reach the capillary level.[58,59] The "no-reflow phenomenon" and irreversible myocardial damage were recently quantified.[60] It was demonstrated that even after 3 hours of ischemia, 40 percent of the area of hypoperfusion (that is, the zone destined to necrose) could be salvaged by reperfusion. The other 60 percent of that hypoperfused zone necrosed; two thirds of this necrosed zone suffered the "no-flow phenomenon," and the other one third presumably had irreversible damage not directly due to the "no-reflow phenomenon." Thus, the re-establishment of blood flow is not enough to salvage the hypoperfused myocardium and is closely dependent on the duration of ischemia, because the latter is the main determinant of the extent of irreversible myocardial damage and the "no-reflow phenomenon." Another possible complication of reperfusion is hemorrhage, which has been observed in dogs[57,61-63] and baboons. Although hemorrhage is less frequent in patients after reperfusion, its frequency is not yet well determined and its potential detrimental effects not examined. In experimental animals, this hemorrhage can be diminished by propranolol,[62] barbiturate anesthesia,[62] and methoxy-verapamil, a calcium antagonist.[63]

Several of the beneficial interventions that were investigated in experimental animals were tried in humans. Although the analysis of the results in patients is much more difficult owing to the limitations in the techniques of measuring the effects of interventions on infarct size, the proteiform coronary architecture, and the pleiomorphic evolution of the disease, many studies concluded that various of the aforementioned interventions can decrease infarct size, reduce morbidity (heart failure and arrhythmias), or reduce mortality. These include studies of hyaluronidase[22,23,64-66] (Fig. 5), nitroglycerin,[47-53] glucose-insulin-potassium,[67] and beta-adrenergic blocking agents.[3-9,29,36] In the latter category, the metoprolol study[6] showed that the administration of this drug within 12 hours of the commencement of the infarction resulted in less myocardial tissue damage, less ventricular fibrillation, less heart failure, and smaller mortality.

To re-establish coronary flow by thrombolysis, two strategies have been suggested: (1) intravenous administration of thrombolytic agents, which was shown to improve significantly the prognosis in patients with moderately severe myocardial infarctions[68] and which was reported to be effective in reopening the occluded coronaries in a high percentage of patients,[69] and (2) intracoronary administration of the thrombolytic agent. Following the pioneering studies of Rentrop,[70] this technique is being examined in many centers.[71-76] The overall experience, which is still very recent, indicates that intracoronary thrombolysis, in experienced hands, is a safe technique that permits the re-establishment of anterograde coronary flow in

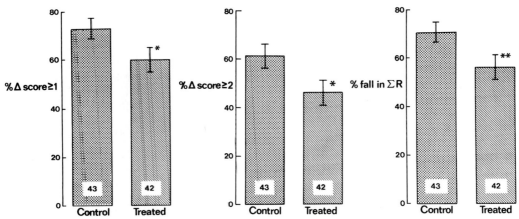

Figure 5. Changes in scores for ST segment elevation in hyaluronidase-treated and control groups. *Left panels* show the percentage of precordial sites with ST segment elevations ≥ 0.15 mV on the admission electrocardiogram with changes in QRS score of 1 or more in the tracing recorded on the seventh day. Numbers in the columns represent the numbers of patients in each group. Bars represent ± 1 SEM. The 43 control patients had 635 sites with ST segment elevations and the 42 hyaluronidase-treated patients had 591 sites. Note that the control patients had significantly more sites in which the QRS morphology changed than had the hyaluronidase-treated patients (* = $p < 0.05$). *Center panels* show the percentage of precordial sites with ST segment elevation ≥ 0.15 mV on the admission electrocardiogram with changes in the QRS score of 2 or more in the tracing recorded on the seventh day. In the 43 control patients the total number of vulnerable sites was 575, and in the hyaluronidase-treated patients it was 494. *Right panels* show the percentage fall in total R-wave voltage (ΣR) in the sites with ST segment elevations ≥ 0.15 on the initial electrocardiogram. Note that the controls had a significantly greater fall in ΣR-wave voltage than the hyaluronidase-treated patients (* = $p < 0.05$, ** $p < 0.01$).

approximately 80 to 90 percent of patients who had thrombotic occlusion (which is approximately 80 to 85 percent of the patients with acute transmural myocardial infarction).

The consequences of successful thrombolysis are not yet well established. The improvement in left ventricular function as generally assessed by left ventricular ejection fraction is rather small (for example, 51 to 54 percent[70]) and of doubtful biologic importance. However, it was suggested that ventricular function will improve further after several days or weeks and that the lack of immediate return of contractility is not an index of lack of final recuperation.[77] Moreover, it is possible that global function is not the most sensitive index of regional function, which is the one that should improve primarily. The evolution of regional function after thrombolysis is, however, also not very encouraging because in some patients it returns partially to normal and in others the effect is not obvious. The possibility of delayed beneficial effects, that is, "stunned myocardium," should be again considered. The electrocardiographic signs of necrosis, that is, fall in the R wave voltage and appearance of a Q wave, have a biphasic behavior. They fall to the same degree after thrombolysis as without it, but within a week there is an increase of voltage of the R waves. This "regrowth of the R wave phenomenon" probably corresponds to the repair of the myocardial cells.[78] Because creatine kinase and other enzymes are released more promptly and in greater amounts per unit of necrosed myocardium after reperfusion, this index of myocardial necrosis cannot be used.[79] Thus, although most parameters indicate that patients may improve following thrombolysis, the effects in many patients are not striking. It is possible that when other interventions that may reduce the extent of the "no-reflow zone" and of hemorrhage are added to thrombolysis, the favorable effects will be markedly improved.

In summary, the extent of myocardial infarction after an acute coronary artery occlusion can be minimized by many favorable interventions in experimental models. The initial results in patients confirm the experimental results. It is possible that the most effective manner to reduce ultimate infarct size in patients will be a combination of interventions that re-establish an effective blood flow to the infarcting myocardium by thrombolysis while at the same time insuring the integrity of the ischemic capillaries and the viability of the myocytes by other interventions.

REFERENCES

1. PANTRIDGE, JF, AND GEDDES, JS: *A mobile intensive care unit in the management of myocardial infarction.* Lancet 2:271, 1967.

2. COBB, LA, WERNER, JA, AND TROBAUGH, GB: *Sudden cardiac death.* Mod Concepts Cardiovasc Dis 49:31, 1980.

3. THE NORWEGIAN MULTICENTER STUDY GROUP: *Timolol-induced reduction in mortality and reinfarction in patients surviving acute myocardial infarction.* N Engl J Med 304:801, 1981.

4. ANDERSEN, MP, FREDERIKSEN, J, JURGENSEN, HJ, ET AL: *Effect of alprenolol on mortality among patients with definite or suspected acute myocardial infarction.* Lancet 2:865, 1979.

5. YUSUF, S, RAMSDALE, D, PETO, R, ET AL.: *Early intravenous atenolol treatment in suspected acute myocardial infarction: Preliminary report of a randomized trial.* Lancet 2:273, 1980.

6. HJALMARSON, A, HERLITZ, J, MALEK, I, ET AL: *Effect on mortality of metoprolol in acute myocardial infarction.* Lancet 2:823, 1981.

7. BETA-BLOCKER HEART ATTACK TRIAL RESEARCH GROUP: *A randomized trial of propranolol in patients with acute myocardial infarction.* JAMA 247:1707, 1982.

8. BETA-BLOCKER HEART ATTACK STUDY GROUP: *The beta-blocker heart attack trial.* JAMA 246:2073, 1981.

9. HANSTEEN, V, MOINICHEN, E, LORENTSEN, E, ET AL: *One year's treatment with propranolol after myocardial infarction: Preliminary report of Norwegian multicentre trial.* Br Med J 284:155, 1982.

10. PAGE, DL, CAULFIELD, JB, KASTOR, JA, ET AL: *Myocardial changes associated with cardiogenic shock.* N Engl J Med 285:133, 1971.

11. YASUDA, I, BINGHAM, JB, MAROKO, PR, ET AL: *Early strenuous exercise on ventricular function following acute myocardial infarction.* Circulation 60:II-236, 1979.

12. ROBERTS, R, HUSAIN, A, AND AMBOX, D, ET AL: *Relation between infarct size and ventricular arrhythmia.* Br Heart J 37:1169, 1975.

13. HILLIS, LD, FISHBEIN, MC, BRAUNWALD, E, ET AL: *The influence of the time interval between coronary artery occlusion and the administration of hyaluronidase on salvage of ischemic myocardium.* Circ Res 41:26, 1977.

14. FISHBEIN, MC, HARE, CA, GISSEN, SA, ET AL: *Identification and quantification of histochemical border zones during the evolution of myocardial infarction in the rat.* Cardiovasc Res 14:41, 1980.

15. MAROKO, PR, BRAUNWALD, E, COVELL, JW, ET AL: *Factors influencing the severity of myocardial ischemia following experimental coronary occlusion.* Circulation 40:III-140, 1969.

16. MAROKO, PR, KJEKSHUS, JK, SOBEL, BE, ET AL: *Factors influencing infarct size following coronary artery occlusions.* Circulation 43:67, 1971.

17. LIBBY, P, MAROKO, PR, BLOOR, CM, ET AL: *Reduction of experimental myocardial infarct size by corticosteroid administration.* J Clin Invest 52:599, 1973.

18. MAROKO, PR, CHEUNG, W-m, AND FARIA, DB: *Comparison of the effects on the extent of myocardial ischemic damage of lidocaine and of S1249.* Circulation 62:IV-243, 1980.

19. DIAZ, PE, FISHBEIN, MC, DAVIS, MA, ET AL: *Effect of the kallikrein inhibitor aprotinin on myocardial ischemic injury following coronary artery occlusion in the dog.* Am J Cardiol 40:541, 1977.

20. MAROKO, PR, CARPENTER, CB, CHIARIELLO, M, ET AL: *Reduction by cobra venom factor of myocardial necrosis following coronary artery occlusion.* J Clin Invest 61:661, 1978.

21. MAROKO, PR, LIBBY, P, BLOOR, CM, ET AL: *Reduction by hyaluronidase of myocardial necrosis following coronary artery occlusion.* Circulation 46:430, 1972.

22. MAROKO, PR, DAVIDSON, DM, LIBBY, P, ET AL: *Effects of hyaluronidase administration on myocardial ischemic injury in acute infarction. A preliminary study in 24 patients.* Ann Intern Med 82:516, 1975.

23. MAROKO, PR, HILLIS, LD, MULLER, JE, ET AL: *Favorable effects of hyaluronidase on electrocardiographic evidence of necrosis in patients with acute myocardial infarction.* N Engl J Med 296:893, 1977.

24. MAROKO, PR: *Effect of hyaluronidase on infarct size.* In LEFER, AM, KELBTER, GJ, AND ROVETTO, MS (EDS): *Pathophysiology and Therapeutics of Myocardial Ischemia.* Spectrum, New York, 1977.

25. KJEKSHUS, JK, AND MJOS, OD: *Effect of inhibition of lipolysis on infarct size after experimental coronary artery occlusion.* J Clin Invest 52:1770, 1973.

26. POWELL, WJ, JR, DIBONA, DR, FLORES, J, ET AL: *Effects of hyperosmotic mannitol in reducing ischemic cell swelling and minimizing myocardial necrosis.* Circulation 53:I-45, 1976.

27. FARIA, DB, CHEUNG, W-m, HASTIE, R, ET AL: *Effect of prostacyclin on infarct size—analysis of discrepancies.* Circulation 64:IV-280, 1981.

28. JUGDUTT, BI, HUTCHINS, GM, BULKLEY, BH, ET AL: *Infarct size reduction by prostacyclin after coronary occlusion in conscious dogs.* Clin Res 27:177A, 1979.

29. GOLD, HK, LEINBACH, RC, AND MAROKO, PR: *Propranolol-induced reduction of signs of ischemic injury during acute myocardial infarction.* Am J Cardiol 38:689, 1976.

30. HILLIS, LD, KHURI, SF, BRAUNWALD, E, ET AL: *The role of propranolol's negative chronotropic effect on protection of the ischemic myocardium.* Pharmacology 19:202, 1979.

31. RUDE, RE, KLONER, RA, MAROKO, PR, ET AL: *Effects of amrinone on experimental acute myocardial ischemic injury.* Cardiovasc Res 14:419, 1980.

32. WATANABE, T, COVELL, JW, MAROKO, PR, ET AL: *Effects of increased arterial pressure and positive inotropic agents on the severity of myocardial ischemia in the acutely depressed heart.* Am J Cardiol 30:371, 1972.

33. MAROKO, PR, BRAUNWALD, E, AND ROSS, J, JR: *The metabolic costs of positive inotropic agents.* In CORDAY, E, AND SWAN, HJC (EDS): *Myocardial Infarction.* Williams & Wilkins, Baltimore, 1973.

34. COVELL, JW, SONNENBLICK, EH, ROSS, J, JR, ET AL: *Studies of Digitalis XVI. Effect on myocardial oxygen consumption.* J Clin Invest 45:1535, 1966.

35. JENTZER, JH, LEJEMTEL, TH, SONNENBLICK, EH, ET AL: *Beneficial effect of amrinone on myocardial oxygen consumption during acute left ventricular failure in dogs.* Am J Cardiol 48:75, 1981.

36. GOLD, HK, LEINBACH, RD, MAROKO, PR, ET AL: *Reduction of injury during acute myocardial infarction: Dependence on coronary anatomy.* Circulation 55 and 56:III-66, 1977.

37. GOLD, HK, LEINBACH, RD, AND MAROKO, PR: *Regional beta blockade with intra-coronary propranolol.* Circulation 54:II-173, 1976.

38. REIMER, KA, LOWE, JE, AND JENNINGS, RB: *Effect of the calcium antagonist verapamil on necrosis following temporary coronary artery occlusion in dogs.* Circulation 55:581, 1977.

39. SMITH, HJ, SINGH, BN, NISBET, HD, ET AL: *Effects of verapamil on infarct size following experimental coronary occlusion.* Cardiovasc Res 9:569, 1975.

40. HENRY, PD, SHUCHLEIB, R, BORDA, LJ, ET AL: *Effects of nifedipine on myocardial perfusion and ischemic injury in dogs.* Circ Res 43:372, 1978.

41. ZALEWSKI, A, FARIA, DB, CHEUNG, W-m, ET AL: *Comparison of the effectiveness of various calcium antagonists in protecting acutely ischemic myocardium.* Clin Res 30:232, 1982.

42. HIRSHFELD, JW, JR, BORER, JS, GOLDSTEIN, RE, ET AL: *Reduction in severity and extent of myocardial infarction when nitroglycerin and methoxamine are administered during coronary occlusion.* Circulation 49:291, 1974.

43. SMITH, ER, REDWOOD, DR, MCCARRON, WE, ET AL: *Coronary artery occlusion in the conscious dog. Effects of alterations in arterial pressure produced by nitroglycerin, hemorrhage, and alpha-adrenergic agonists on the degree of myocardial ischemia.* Circulation 47:51, 1973.

44. MAROKO, PR, LIBBY, P, GINKS, WR, ET AL: *Coronary artery reperfusion I: Early effects on local myocardial function and the extent of myocardial necrosis.* J Clin Invest 51:2710, 1972.

45. GINKS, WR, SYBERS, HD, MAROKO, PR, ET AL: *Coronary artery reperfusion II: Reduction of myocardial infarct size at one week after the coronary occlusion.* J Clin Invest 51:2717, 1972.

46. REDWOOD, DR, SMITH, ER, AND EPSTEIN, SE: *Coronary artery occlusion in the conscious dog; effects of alterations in heart rate and arterial pressure on the degree of myocardial ischemia.* Circulation 46:323, 1972.

47. BORER, JS, REDWOOD, DR, LEVITT, B, ET AL: *Reduction in myocardial ischemia with nitroglycerin or nitroglycerin plus phenylephrine administered during acute myocardial infarction.* N Engl J Med 293:1008, 1975.

48. COME, PC, FLAHERTY, JT, BAIRD, MG, ET AL: *Reversal by phenylephrine of the beneficial effects of intravenous nitroglycerin in patients with acute myocardial infarction.* N Engl J Med 293:1003, 1975.

49. FLAHERTY, JT, REIN, PR, KELLY, DT, ET AL: *Intravenous nitroglycerin in acute myocardial infarction.* Circulation 51:132, 1975.

50. CHIARIELLO, M, GOLD, HK, LEINBACH, RD, ET AL: *Comparison between the effects of nitroprusside and nitroglycerin on ischemic injury during acute myocardial infarction.* Circulation 54:766, 1976.

51. DERRIDA, JP, SAL, R, AND CHICHE, P: *Nitroglycerin infusion in acute myocardial infarction.* N Engl J Med 297:336, 1977.

52. BUSSMAN, WD, PASSEK, D, SEIDEL, W, ET AL: *Reduction of CK and CK-MB indexes of infarct size by intravenous nitroglycerin.* Circulation 63:615, 1981.

53. EPSTEIN, SE, KENT, KM, GOLDSTEIN, RD, ET AL: *Reduction of ischemic injury by nitroglycerin during acute myocardial infarction.* N Engl J Med 292:29, 1975.

54. RADVANY, P, DAVIS, MA, MULLER, JE, ET AL: *Effects of minoxidil on coronary collateral flow and acute myocardial injury following experimental coronary artery occlusion.* Cardiovasc Res 12:120, 1978.

55. CHIARIELLO, M, RIBEIRO, LGT, DAVIS, MA, ET AL: *Reverse coronary steal induced by coronary vasoconstriction following coronary artery occlusion in dogs.* Circulation 56:809, 1977.

56. DEWOOD, MA, SPORES, J, NOTSKE, R, ET AL: *Prevalence of total coronary occlusion during the early hours of transmural myocardial infarction.* N Engl J Med 303:897, 1980.

57. BAUGHMAN, KL, MAROKO, PR, AND VATNER, SF: *Effects of coronary artery reperfusion on myocardial infarct size and survival in conscious dogs.* Circulation 63:317, 1981.

58. KLONER, RA, GANOTE, CE, AND JENNINGS, RB: *The "no-reflow" phenomenon after temporary coronary occlusion in the dog.* J Clin Invest 54:1496, 1974.

59. SCHAPER, W, AND PASYK, S: *Influence of collateral flow on the ischemic tolerance of the heart following acute and subacute coronary occlusion.* Circulation 53:57, 1976.

60. CHEUNG, W-m, KJEKSHUS, H, RIBEIRO, LGT, ET AL: *Quantification of "no-reflow phenomenon" by dual autoradiography after different times of occlusion and its relationship to necrosis.* Am J Cardiol 49:1047, 1982.

61. BRESNAHAN, GF, ROBERTS, R, SHELL, WE, ET AL: *Deleterious effects due to hemorrhage after myocardial reperfusion.* Am J Cardiol 33:82, 1974.

62. DIAZ, PE, VATNER, SF, AND MAROKO, PR: *Factors determining the appearance of hemorrhage following coronary artery reperfusion.* Circulation 54:II-69, 1976.

63. ENDO, T, RIBEIRO, LGT, CHEUNG, W-m, ET AL: *Reduction in hemorrhage and the extent of necrosis by methoxy-verapamil in dogs with coronary artery reperfusion.* Circulation 64:IV-98, 1981.

64. SALTISSI, S, ROBINSON, PS, COLTART, DS, ET AL: *Effects of early administration of a highly purified hyaluronidase preparation (GL enzyme) on myocardial infarct size.* Lancet 1:867, 1982.

65. FLINT, EJ, DEGIOVANNI, J, CADIGAN, PJ, ET AL: *Effect of GL enzyme (a highly purified form of hyaluronidase) on mortality after myocardial infarction.* Lancet 1:871, 1982.

66. HENDERSON, A, CAMPBELL, RWF, AND JULIAN, DG: *Effect of a highly purified hyaluronidase preparation (GL enzyme) on electrocardiographic changes in acute myocardial infarction.* Lancet 1:874, 1982.

67. ROGERS, WJ, SEGALL, PH, MCDANIEL, HG, ET AL: *Prospective randomized trial of glucose-insulin-potassium in acute myocardial infarction.* Am J Cardiol 43:801, 1979.

68. EUROPEAN COOPERATIVE STUDY GROUP FOR STREPTOKINASE THERAPY IN ACUTE MYOCARDIAL INFARCTION: *Streptokinase in acute myocardial infarction.* N Engl J Med 301:797, 1979.

69. SHRODER, R, BIAMINO, G, VON LEITNER, ER, ET AL: *Intravenous short time thrombolysis in acute myocardial infarction.* Circulation 64:IV-10, 1981.

70. RENTROP, P, BLANKS, H, KARSCH, KR, ET AL: *Selective intracoronary thrombolysis in acute myocardial infarction and unstable angina pectoris.* Circulation 63:307, 1961.

71. MATHEY, DG, KOOK, KH, TILSNER, V, ET AL: *Nonsurgical coronary artery recanalization in acute transmural myocardial infarction.* Circulation 63:849, 1981.

72. GANZ, W, BUCHBINDER, N, MARCUS, H, ET AL: *Intracoronary thrombolysis in evolving myocardial infarction.* Am Heart J 101:4, 1981.

73. LEINBACH, RC, AND GOLD, HK: *Regional streptokinase in myocardial infarction.* Circulation 63:498, 1981.

74. GOLDBERG, S, MAROKO, PR, AND ENGEL, TR: *Editorial: Intracoronary streptokinase therapy in patients with acute myocardial infarctions.* Ann Intern Med 96:115, 1982.

75. GOLDBERG, S, URBAN, PL, GREENSPON, AJ, ET AL: *Combination therapy for evolving myocardial infarction: Intracoronary thrombolysis and percutaneous transluminal angioplasty.* Am J Med 72:994, 1982.

76. MARKIS, JE, MALAGOLD, M, PARKER, JA, ET AL: *Myocardial salvage after intracoronary thrombolysis with streptokinase in acute myocardial infarction.* N Engl J Med 305:777, 1981.

77. KLONER, RA, DEBOER, LWV, DARSEE, JR, ET AL: *Persistent myocardial abnormalities following brief periods of temporary coronary occlusion not associated with necrosis.* Circulation 62:III-80, 1980.

78. GOLDBERG, S, GREENSPON, AJ, URBAN, PL, ET AL: *Reperfusion arrhythmias: A marker of intracoronary thrombolysis during acute myocardial infarction.* Clin Res 30:189A, 1982.

79. VATNER, SF, BAIG, H, MANDERS, WT, ET AL: *Effects of coronary artery reperfusion on myocardial infarct size calculated from creatine kinase.* J Clin Invest 61:1048, 1978.

Reduction of Infarct Size with Thrombolytic Agents

Paul Urban, M.D., Herman K. Gold, M.D., and Sheldon Goldberg, M.D.

In 1912, Herrick attributed acute myocardial infarction to coronary thrombosis.[1] Subsequently, some investigators believed coronary thrombosis was the result of myocardial necrosis rather than the immediate cause of the infarct. As outlined in a previous chapter in this book,[2] the history of ideas concerning coronary thrombosis and myocardial infarction reflects the background of scientists examining these phenomena. Two critical observations have brought us to a new threshold of therapeutic intervention in evolving myocardial infarction. The first observation was the angiographic demonstration by DeWood and coworkers[3] that acute transmural myocardial infarction is associated with complete coronary occlusion in 87 percent of patients studied within the first 4 hours of myocardial infarction. These occlusions are commonly due to coronary thrombi in the large epicardial coronary arteries. In DeWood's study, total coronary occlusion was observed in 110 of 126 patients evaluated within 4 hours of the onset of symptoms. The percentage decreased substantially to 65 percent (37 of 57 cases) when patients were catheterized 12 to 24 hours after the onset of symptoms (Fig. 1). These findings suggest that complete interruption of coronary blood flow and subsequent spontaneous recanalization are frequent features of evolving myocardial infarction. The second critical observation was Rentrop's finding that coronary thrombi could be lysed by direct administration of lytic enzymes into the affected coronary artery.[4] Because the morbidity and mortality of acute myocardial infarction are related to the amount of tissue necrosis,[5] the concept of restoring antegrade coronary blood flow by intracoronary thrombolysis, and thereby salvaging myocardial cells, has enormous appeal.

PHYSIOLOGIC CONSIDERATIONS DURING ACUTE MYOCARDIAL INFARCTION

Re-establishing coronary blood flow during acute myocardial infarction is completely different from improving coronary blood flow in patients with chronic ischemic heart disease, as is done by coronary bypass surgery. The latter therapy increases myocardial blood flow by bypassing critically narrowed regions of the epicardial coronary arteries. Although in chronic ischemic disease the target myocardium is hypoperfused, it is not in imminent danger of necrosis. The goal of intracoronary thrombolysis is not only to re-establish blood flow through the occluded artery but also to salvage myocardial cells destined to undergo necrosis. Thus, it is not sufficient to demonstrate mere opening of the occluded coronary artery with intracoronary thrombolysis; rather, smaller infarcts and more viable contracting myocardium are important endpoints by which this therapy will be judged.

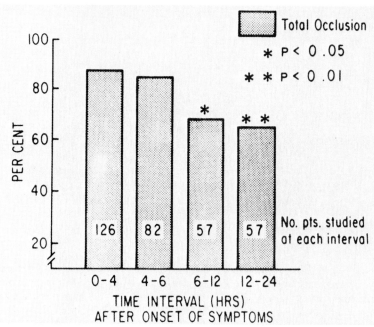

Figure 1. Incidence of complete coronary occlusion during the early hours of myocardial infarction. From DeWood et al, N Engl J Med 303:897, 1980.

Myocardial cells acutely deprived of coronary blood flow become ischemic and will progress to necrosis, depending on the degree of hypoperfusion and the time elapsed from occlusion. Cells in the periphery of the hypoperfused zone, where there is less reduction of blood flow than in the center, will undergo necrosis more slowly than cells in the center, where perfusion may be totally absent.[6,7] Myocardial cells completely deprived of blood flow may show signs of irreversible damage within half an hour, whereas myocardium with some residual flow through collateral channels may resist necrosis for several hours. These time-dependent phenomena suggest that if coronary blood flow is acutely interrupted, some myocardial necrosis will inevitably occur unless intervention is almost immediate. Although myocardial necrosis cannot be totally prevented in the clinical setting, a considerable portion of myocardium can be salvaged by prompt treatment.

The extent of myocardial necrosis can be reduced by decreasing oxygen demand and/or by increasing myocardial oxygen supply.[8,9] For example, beta-blocking agents may reduce infarct size after coronary occlusion by decreasing myocardial oxygen demand,[10–12] whereas intra-aortic balloon counterpulsation has the dual capability to decrease myocardial demand by reducing afterload and to increase coronary collateral blood flow by augmenting diastolic coronary perfusion pressure.[13] Nitroglycerin can increase coronary collateral flow and thereby reduce infarct size.[14–18] Agents with other mechanisms of myocardial salvage, such as calcium antagonists[19,20] and hyaluronidase,[21] also have shown promise in limiting infarct size. However, the beneficial effect of these latter agents used alone has not been clinically striking.

Reperfusion of myocardium made acutely ischemic by interruption of blood flow can be accomplished either by coronary bypass surgery[22–25] or by intracoronary thrombolysis. Maroko[26] and Ginks[27] and their colleagues showed that infarct size was reduced and local myocardial function improved by reperfusion undertaken as long as 3 hours after experimental coronary artery occlusion. More recently, Baughman and associates[28] studied the effects of coronary reperfusion on infarct size and survival in conscious dogs. Reperfusion after either 1 or 3 hours produced a beneficial effect on survival. In addition, infarct size at 1 week (measured by gross pathology and myocardial creatine kinase depletion) was smaller in the reperfused dogs. All experimental studies agree that after approximately 20 minutes the most severely ischemic myocardial cells inevitably progress to necrosis and that later reperfusion will not save all jeopardized cells. Re-establishment of flow within hours of coronary occlusion will salvage the more peripheral regions in the myocardium rendered ischemic by flow interruption. Thus, the ultimate improvement in ventricular function is dependent on collateral flow to the peripheral zone and on the time elapsed from occlusion to reperfusion. Because one could seldom achieve intracoronary thrombolysis clinically within 20 minutes of onset of coronary occlusion, evidence of some myocardial necrosis would be expected even with dramatically improved ventricular function. Therefore, myocardial infarction cannot be completely prevented, but a significant amount of myocardium can be salvaged.

CLINICAL STUDIES WITH INTRACORONARY THROMBOLYSIS

Rentrop and coworkers[29] reported that 22 of 29 acutely occluded coronary arteries were successfully opened by intracoronary thrombolysis using streptokinase. Chest pain was relieved and ST segment elevation reduced in the majority of patients. Left ventricular function was improved in the 14 patients in whom contrast ventriculography was performed. Ejection fractions were 50.5 ± 12 percent before and 54.6 ± 9 percent immediately after ICT (p less than 0.05). Mathey and associates[30] reported similar results. Using intracoronary streptokinase plus plasminogen within 3 hours of onset of symptoms, they were able to achieve reflow in 30 of 41 patients with acute myocardial infarction. Though chest pain and ST segment responses were favorable, new Q waves or R wave loss occurred in 24 of the 30 patients. Left ventricular ejection fractions improved from 37 ± 5 percent in the control phase to 47 ± 4 percent (p less than 0.0025) predischarge (Fig. 2). Reduto and colleagues[31] achieved

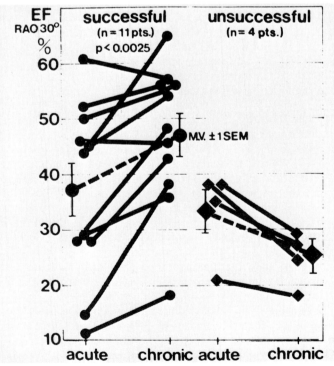

Figure 2. Control and predischarge ejection fractions in patients undergoing intracoronary thrombolysis. (From Mathey et al,[30] with permission of the American Heart Association, Inc.)

similar results by reperfusing 18 of 26 acutely occluded coronary arteries. They performed intracoronary thrombolysis up to 18 hours after onset of chest pain. In the latter study, a delay of 10 days to 2 weeks occurred before left ventricular ejection fraction improved. Ejection fractions measured by radionuclide angiography before and immediately after successful intracoronary thrombolysis were 44 $\pm$ 15 percent and 46 $\pm$ 14 percent respectively (ns). However, ejection fractions measured at a mean time of 10 days improved significantly to 55 $\pm$ 7 percent (p = 0.007). In patients who had unsuccessful attempts at thrombolysis and also in a group of patients with acute myocardial infarction treated with standard therapy, left ventricular function did not improve even at 10 days. Six patients with acute myocardial infarction had severe stenosis, but not total occlusion, of the involved coronary artery. These patients showed no improvement of the stenosis with the intracoronary nitroglycerin and streptokinase, and early and late left ventricular function was unchanged.

The aforementioned studies used standard cardiac catheterization techniques, and reflow was established in approximately 75 percent of cases. To increase the concentration of thrombolytic agents directly at the site of thrombus, Ganz and coworkers[32,33] modified the procedure by using subselective catheterization, that is, a small catheter was introduced through a standard coronary catheter and positioned adjacent to the thrombus. Using this technique, reflow was achieved in 34 of 36 (94 percent) patients. Regional left ventricular wall abnormalities improved at late (10 to 14 day) followup.

Further evidence for myocardial salvage comes from studies examining myocardial cell viability by nuclear imaging and electrocardiographic techniques. Markis and associates[34] assessed the efficacy of intracoronary thrombolysis by the use of intracoronary thallium-201.[34] Nine patients with acute myocardial infarctions underwent cardiac catheterization 2.3 to 4.3 hours after the onset of symptoms. Intracoronary thallium was injected before and after streptokinase-induced thrombolysis. The scintiscans in seven of nine patients showed a definite improvement in thallium uptake in the distribution of the recanalized coronary artery. The distribution of injected thallium-201 depends not only on delivery of this tracer by the coronary circulation but also on extraction of thallium-201 by the myocardium. Since viable myocardial cells with intact membranes are required for thallium-201 extraction, this study suggests that thrombolysis can salvage jeopardized myocardium.

Studies examining electrocardiographic changes associated with thrombolytic therapy also suggest infarct size reduction. Goldberg and Greenspon[35] found that arrhythmias occurred precisely at the time of restoration of antegrade coronary flow in the majority of patients undergoing thrombolytic therapy. The arrhythmia most often noted was accelerated idioventricular rhythm during left and right coronary artery reperfusion, with marked slowing of rate and atrioventricular block when right coronary arteries were recanalized. Because accelerated idioventricular rhythm is most likely due to increased automaticity and because irreversibly damaged myocardial cells are unlikely to show an enhanced rate of depolarization, these findings suggest that reperfusion arrhythmia in the setting of intracoronary thrombolysis is a marker of coronary reflow and may be an electrophysiologic indicator of myocardial salvage. Blanke[36] and Goldberg[37] and their colleagues also reported that reflow was associated with rapid control of injury current (ST segment elevation) and late decline in Q waves and regrowth of R waves.

Several illustrative cases show the therapeutic potential of intracoronary thrombolysis and also demonstrate important clinical considerations regarding management of patients treated with this therapy.

PATIENT A. A 73-year-old man developed unstable angina. During a typical attack there was T wave inversion in the precordial leads (Fig. 3A). During a severe episode of chest pain, a repeat electrocardiogram showed ST segment elevation in the precordial leads (Fig. 3B). The pain and electrocardiographic changes were unrelieved by nitroglycerin. After informed consent was obtained, the patient was taken to the cardiac catheterization laboratory where left ventriculography revealed anterior wall dyskinesis (Fig. 3C), corresponding to the electrocardiographic injury zone. An angiogram of the right coronary artery revealed a high-grade, fixed stenosis. Angiography of the left coronary artery showed total occlusion of the left anterior descending coronary artery (Fig. 3D) and fixed lesions of the circumflex artery. Intracoronary nitroglycerin failed to restore flow. Intracoronary streptokinase was then administered, and after 40 minutes there was restoration of antegrade flow in the left anterior descending artery with a residual high-grade stenosis (Fig. 3E). Concomitant with reflow, chest pain was relieved and ST segment elevation decreased. However, immediately after the procedure, new Q waves developed (Fig. 3F). A post-therapy ventriculogram demonstrated improved anterior wall motion (Fig. 3G). An ECG taken one week after thrombolytic therapy showed loss of Q wave and regrowth of R wave (Fig. 3H). However, 18 days later the patient developed severe unstable angina, requiring emergency coronary artery bypass surgery. The post-surgical course was uneventful, and the patient was angina-free one year later.

PATIENT B. A 63-year-old man was hospitalized with severe chest pain, and the electro-cardiogram revealed an acute anterior myocardial infarction (Fig. 4A). A percutaneous intra-aortic balloon pump was inserted. The ventriculogram showed anterior dyskinesis. The right coronary arteriogram was normal. The left coronary angiogram showed total occlusion of the left anterior descending coronary artery (Fig. 4B). Intracoronary nitroglycerin had no effect, but intracoronary streptokinase infusion 3 hours after onset of symptoms resulted in resto-ration of antegrade flow (Fig. 4C) with a residual high-grade left anterior descending artery stenosis. Reflow was accompanied by accelerated idioventricular rhythm (Fig. 4D). Following intracoronary thrombolysis, chest pain was relieved and ST segment elevation subsided (Fig. 4E). Evidence for improved left ventricular function is demonstrated by echocardiograms performed before and after intracoronary thrombolysis (Figs. 4F,G). The left ventricular ejection fraction measured by contrast ventriculography improved from 26 to 38 percent. The patient was returned to the coronary care unit and treated with aspirin and dipyridamole. Eleven days later he sustained a recurrent anterior infarction, and efforts at repeat throm-bolysis were unsuccessful.

PATIENT C. A 50-year-old woman sustained an acute inferior myocardial infarction. A percutaneous intra-aortic balloon pump was inserted. Ventriculography showed inferior wall akinesis. The left coronary artery was normal. The right coronary artery was totally occluded (Fig. 5A). Intracoronary streptokinase resulted in restoration of antegrade right coronary artery flow and a residual high-grade stenosis remained (Fig. 5B). Chest pain and ST segment elevations subsided. Two days later, after discontinuation of heparin therapy, there was recur-rence of chest pain and ST segment elevation. Repeat angiography showed reocclusion of the right coronary artery. The patient was again treated with intracoronary thrombolysis (dou-bling the dose of streptokinase), and the artery was reopened. Six hours later, percutaneous transluminal coronary angioplasty using a Gruntzig balloon catheter (Fig. 5C) was per-formed, with reduction of the high-grade lesion to a luminal irregularity (Fig. 5D). The patient made an uneventful recovery without recurrence of symptoms, and followup angiog-raphy 3 months later showed continued vessel patency.

These illustrative cases demonstrate the potential for myocardial salvage by intracoronary thrombolysis. There was improvement in ventricular function as demonstrated by contrast ventriculography and/or echocardiography. In addition, the electrocardiographic findings of control of injury current, appearance of reperfusion arrhythmia, and regrowth of R wave lend further support for reduction of infarct size. However, recurrent ischemic events, including unstable angina and reinfarction, are frequent. In an effort to optimize therapy, Gold and coworkers studied the course of patients after attempted intracoronary thrombolysis.[38] Intra-coronary streptokinase was given to 40 patients with acute transmural myocardial infarction. Twenty-eight (70 percent) had reflow which was stable enough to control myocardial injury. Late reocclusion was seen in five cases at intervals ranging from 6 days to 11 months. All in-hospital occlusions occurred in patients with underlying coronary artery stenoses of 70 percent or more. The most consistent association was with inadequate anticoagulation. In three cases,

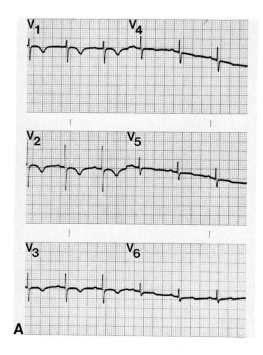

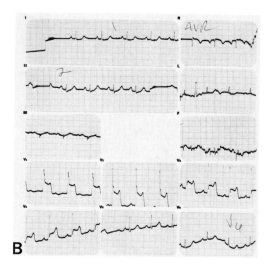

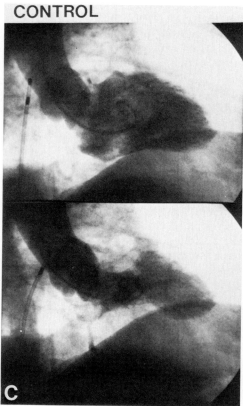

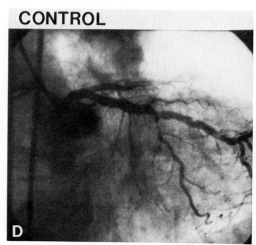

Figure 3. *A*, Electrocardiogram from patient A shows T wave changes during an anginal attack. *B*, The ECG during prolonged chest pain shows precordial ST segment elevation. *C*, Left ventriculography in the RAO projection during pain and ST segment elevation revealed anterior wall dyskinesis. *D*, Left coronary angiography in the RAO projection performed during pain and ST segment elevation. There is total occlusion of the left anterior descending coronary artery.

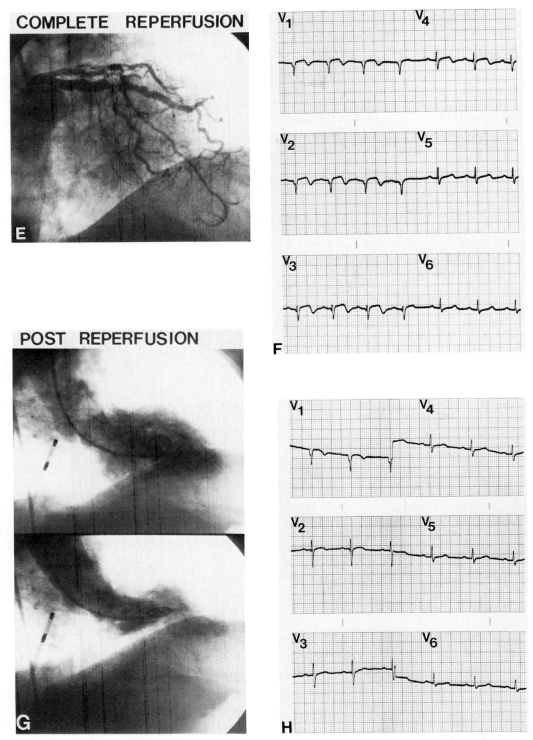

Figure 3. *E*, Following intracoronary streptokinase infusion, there is restoration of left anterior descending artery flow. A high-grade, fixed lesion remains at the site of prior total occlusion. Pain and ST segment elevation subsided. *F*, The ECG obtained immediately following streptokinase infusion disclosed reduction in ST segment elevation, but new Q waves developed. *G*, Ventriculography after reflow shows improvement in anterior wall motion. Ejection fraction increased from 0.51 to 0.59. *H*, The ECG taken one week after reflow reveals loss of Q waves and regrowth of R waves, further suggesting myocardial salvage. (From Goldberg, et al,[37] with permission of the American Heart Association, Inc.)

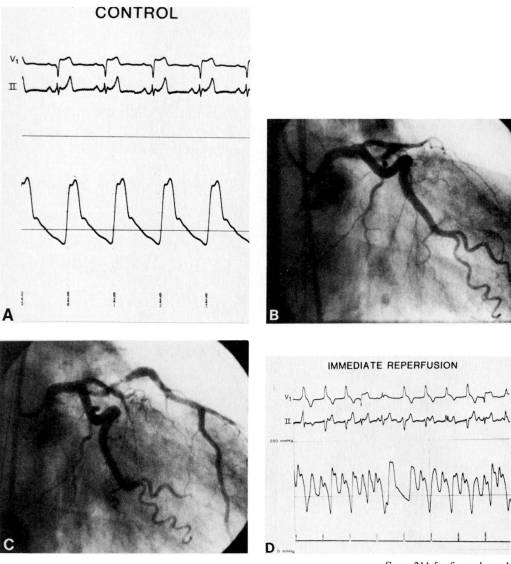

CONTROL

IMMEDIATE REPERFUSION

See p 211 for figure legend.

heparin or warfarin had been discontinued because of bleeding complications, and two patients were taking only aspirin. The factors influencing reocclusion in these patients are shown in Table 1. The clinical manifestations of late reocclusion ranged from no symptoms to reinfarction, shock, and sudden death (Table 2). Percutaneous transluminal angioplasty at the time of intracoronary thrombolysis was performed in 7 patients with 6 successes. Bypass surgery was performed after successful intracoronary thrombolysis in eight. Followup revealed recurrent ischemia or cardiac death in approximately half of the patients treated with intracoronary thrombolysis alone, but only in 1 patient with successful thrombolysis combined with percutaneous transluminal coronary angioplasty or bypass surgery.

LATE REPERFUSION

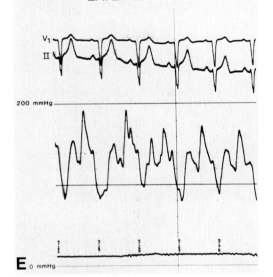

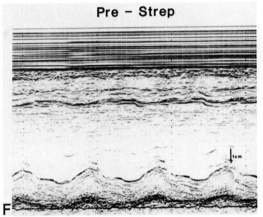

Pre – Strep

Post – Strep

Figure 4. *A,* The ECG and pressure tracing during acute myocardial infarction in patient B. Q waves are already present in V_1, and there is marked ST segment elevation. *B,* The left coronary angiogram reveals total occlusion of the left anterior descending coronary artery. *C,* The left coronary angiogram after intracoronary streptokinase infusion discloses restoration of antegrade flow in the left anterior descending coronary artery. However, a high-grade proximal lesion remains at the site of prior occlusion. *D,* The ECG obtained precisely at the time of reflow shows accelerated idioventricular rhythm. *E,* The ECG obtained after the procedure discloses subsidence of ST segment elevation and persistence of Q waves. *F,* Pre-thrombolysis echocardiogram reveals septal akinesis. *G,* Post-thrombolysis echocardiogram: Septal motion is dramatically improved. (From Goldberg, et al,[37] with permission of the American Heart Association, Inc.)

Table 1. Factors influencing late reocclusion

Pt	Time of reocclusion	Dose SK (U)	Residual stenosis (%)	Plaque ulcer**	Wall motion*	Anticoagulation
1	15 days	150,000	90	0	+	Interrupted day 13
2	6 days	160,000	85	+	+	Interrupted day 2
3	13 days	300,000	70	+	+	Interrupted day 5
4	2 months	110,000	50	+	+	ASA
5	11 months	250,000	50	0	0	ASA

*Wall motion = + when akinesis involves 75% of zone at risk.
**Plaque ulcer present = +.
Pt = patient, SK = streptokinase, ASA = aspirin
(From Gold et al,[38] with permission of the American Heart Association, Inc.)

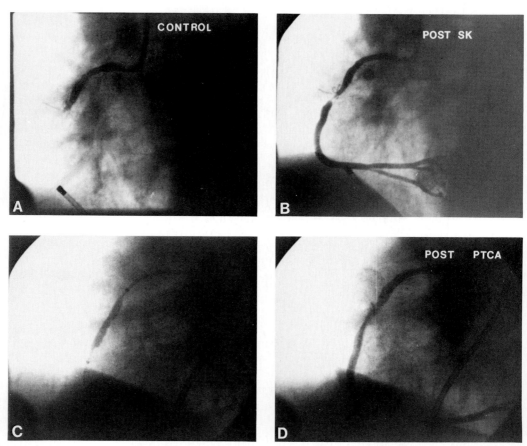

Figure 5. *A*, Right coronary angiogram of patient C shows total occlusion of the vessel. *B*, Following intracoronary streptokinase, reflow occurs and a high-grade stenosis remains in the mid portion of the vessel. *C*, Inflated Gruntzig balloon. Note the indentation of the balloon by the lesion. *D*, The post-angioplasty angiogram shows marked improvement in luminal diameter of the right coronary artery. (From Goldberg, et al,[44] with permission.)

Table 2. Clinical manifestations of late coronary reocclusion

Pt	Location of lesion	Time after reflow	Clinical signs
1	LAD	15 days	Sudden death*
2	RCA	6 days	Reinfarction, shock
3	RCA	13 days	None
4	RCA	2 months	Angina
5	RCA	11 months	Reinfarction

*Reocclusion confirmed at postmortem examination.
LAD = left anterior descending coronary artery.
Pt = patient.
RCA = right coronary artery.
(From Gold et al,[38] with permission of the American Heart Association, Inc.)

IMPLICATIONS AND FUTURE DIRECTIONS

The studies described in this chapter indicate that intracoronary thrombolysis establishes reflow in approximately 70 to 90 percent of patients with acute myocardial infarction. There is preliminary evidence of infarct size reduction studied by electrocardiographic, scintigraphic, and ventriculographic techniques. It is encouraging that the clinical course of patients with evolving myocardial infarction was not generally complicated either by the cardiac catheterization studies or by the thrombolytic therapy, and preliminary nonrandomized studies suggest a reduced in-hospital mortality.[39] Nonetheless, there are potential complications that should not be overlooked, such as occurrence of hazardous arrhythmia or coronary artery dissection or perforation. The possibility of myocardial hemorrhage after reperfusion should also be considered; this complication, which is common in experimental animals,[40] has also been reported in patients who died after successful intracoronary thrombolysis.[41]

The optimal technique for thrombolytic therapy needs clarification. Is subselective catheterization necessary, as recommended by Ganz? An exciting recent report by Schroder and associates showed that administration of *intravenous* streptokinase resulted in reflow in 80 percent of patients with evolving infarction.[42] Moreover, reduced mortality was shown in patients with acute myocardial infarction who received intravenous streptokinase therapy in a large multicenter trial.[43] There are other critical, unanswered questions regarding this treatment. For example, after how may hours of coronary occlusion will reperfusion reduce infarct size enough to be clinically relevant? What is the effect on mortality both in-hospital and long-term? Should adjunctive therapy with agents that protect ischemic myocardium be used? What is the role of regional or systemic nitrates, beta blockers, calcium blockers, and intra-aortic balloon counterpulsation? Finally, what is the best therapy after intracoronary thrombolysis—coronary artery bypass surgery or percutaneous transluminal coronary angioplasty?[44] And how soon after thrombolysis should the latter procedures be performed? Coronary recanalization is promising and may have enormous clinical benefit. At this time, carefully designed multicenter randomized trials are in order.

REFERENCES

1. HERRICK, JB: *Clinical features of sudden obstruction of the coronary arteries.* JAMA 59:2015, 1912.

2. BREST, AN, AND GOLDBERG, S: *Coronary thrombosis: Historical aspects.* In GOLDBERG, S: *Coronary Artery Spasm and Thrombosis.* Cardiovascular Clinics Series, vol 14, number 1. FA Davis, Philadelphia, 1983.

3. DeWOOD MA, SPORES, J, NOTSKE, R, ET AL: *Prevalence of total coronary occlusion during the early hours of transmural myocardial infarction.* N Engl J Med 303:897, 1980.

4. RENTROP, P, BLANKE, H, KOSTERING, K, ET AL: *Acute myocardial infarction: Intracoronary application of nitroglycerin and streptokinase in combination with transluminal recanalization.* Clin Cardiol 2:354, 1979.

5. CAULFIELD, JB, LEINBACH, R, AND GOLD, H: *The relationship of myocardial infarct size and prognosis.* Circulation 53(Suppl 1):1, 1976.

6. FISHBEIN, MC, HARE, CA, GISSENSA, A, ET AL: *Identification and quantification of histochemical border zones during the evolution of myocardial infarction in the rat.* Cardiovasc Res 14:41, 1980.

7. REIMER, KA, LOWE, JE, RASMUSSEN, MM, ET AL: *The wave front phenomenon of ischemic cell death.* Circulation 56:786, 1976.

8. MAROKO, PR, KJEKSHUS, JK, SOBEL, BE, ET AL: *Factors influencing infarct size following experimental coronary artery occlusions.* Circulation 43:67, 1971.

9. MAROKO, PR, AND BRAUNWALD, E: *Effects of metabolic and pharmacologic interventions on myocardial infarct size following coronary occlusion.* Circulation 53(Suppl 1):1,1976.

10. MIURA, M, THOMAS, R, GANZ, W, ET AL: *The effect of delay in propranolol administration on reduction of myocardial infarct size after experimental coronary artery occlusion in dogs.* Circulation 58:1148, 1979.

11. GOLD, HK, LEINBACH, RC, AND MAROKO, PR: *Propranolol-induced reduction of signs of ischemic injury during acute myocardial infarction.* Am J Cardiol 38:689, 1976.

12. SINGH, BN, AND BURNAM, MH: *The role of beta-adrenergic blocking drugs in early myocardial infarction.* Cardiovasc Rev Report 1:281, 1980.

13. ROBERTS, AJ, ALONSO, DR, COMBES, JR, ET AL: *Role of delayed intraaortic balloon pumping in treatment of experimental myocardial infarction.* Am J Cardiol 41:1202, 1978.

14. EPSTEIN, SE, KENT, KM, GOLDSTEIN, RE, ET AL: *Reduction of ischemic injury by nitroglycerin during acute myocardial infarction.* N Engl J Med 292:29, 1975.

15. COME, PC, FLAHERTY, JT, BAIRD, MG, ET AL: *Reversal by phenylephrine of the beneficial effects of intravenous nitroglycerin in patients with acute myocardial infarction.* N Engl J Med 293:1003, 1975.

16. CHIARIELLO, M, GOLD, HK, LEINBACH, RC, ET AL: *Comparison between the effects of nitroprusside and nitroglycerin on ischemic injury during acute myocardial infarction.* Circulation 54:766, 1976.

17. BUSSMAN, WD, PASSEK, D, SEIDEL, W, ET AL: *Reduction of CK and CK-MB indexes of infarct size by intravenous nitroglycerin.* Circulation 63:615, 1981.

18. JUDGUTT, BI, BECKER, LC, HUTCHINS, GM, ET AL: *Effect of intravenous nitroglycerin on collateral blood flow and infarct size in the conscious dog.* Circulation 63:17, 1981.

19. REIMER, KA, LOWE, JE, AND JENNINGS, RB: *Effect of the calcium antagonist verapamil on necrosis following temporary coronary artery occlusion in dogs.* Circulation 55:581, 1977.

20. HENRY, PD, SHUCHLEIB, R, BORDA, LJ, ET AL: *Effects of nifedipine on myocardial perfusion and ischemic injury in dogs.* Circ Res 43:372, 1978.

21. MAROKO, PR, HILLIS, LD, MULLER, JE, ET AL: *Favorable effects of hyaluronidase on electrocardiographic evidence of necrosis in patients with acute myocardial infarction.* N Engl J Med 296:898, 1977.

22. BERG, R, KENDALL, RW, DUVOISIN, GE, ET AL: *Acute myocardial infarction: A surgical emergency.* J Thorac Cardiovasc Surg 70:432, 1975.

23. DEWOOD, MA, SPORES, J, NOTSKE, RN, ET AL: *Medical and surgical management of myocardial infarction.* Am J Cardiol 44:1356, 1979.

24. PHILLIPS, SJ, KONGTAHWORN, C, ZEFF, RH, ET AL: *Emergency coronary artery revascularization; A possible therapy for acute myocardial infarction.* Circulation 60:241, 1979.

25. MULLER, JE, ANTMAN, E, GREEN, LH, ET AL: *Salvage of acutely ischemic myocardium by emergency coronary artery bypass grafting.* Clin Cardiol 3:276, 1980.

26. MAROKO, PR, LIBBY, P, GINKS, WR, ET AL: *Coronary artery reperfusion I; Early effects on local myocardial function and the extent of myocardial necrosis.* J Clin Invest 51:2710, 1972.

27. GINKS, WR, SYBERS, HD, MAROKO, PR, ET AL.: *Coronary artery reperfusion II: Reduction of myocardial infarct size at one week after coronary occlusion.* J Clin Invest 51:2727, 1972.

28. BAUGHMAN, KL, MAROKO, PR, AND VATNER, SF: *Effects of coronary artery perfusion on myocardial infarct size and survival in conscious dogs.* Circulation 63:317, 1981.

29. RENTROP, P, BLANKE, H, KARSCH, KR, ET AL: *Selective intracoronary thrombolysis in acute myocardial infarction and unstable angina pectoris.* Circulation 63:307, 1981.

30. MATHEY, DG, KUCK, KH, TILSNER, V, ET AL: *Nonsurgical coronary artery recanalization in acute transmural myocardial infarction.* Circulation 63:489, 1981.

31. REDUTO, LA, SMALLING, RW, FREUND, GC, ET AL: *Intracoronary infusion of streptokinase in patients with acute myocardial infarction: Effects of reperfusion on left ventricular performance.* Am J Cardiol 48:403, 1981.

32. GANZ, W, BUCHBINDER, N, MARCUS, H, ET AL: *Intracoronary thrombolysis in evolving myocardial infarction.* Am Heart J 101:4, 1981.

33. GANZ, W: *Intracoronary thrombolysis in evolving myocardial infarction.* Ann Intern Med 95:500, 1981.

34. MARKIS, JE, MALAGOLD, M, PARKER, JA, ET AL: *Myocardial salvage after intracoronary thrombolysis with streptokinase in acute myocardial infarction.* N Engl J Med 305:777, 1981.

35. GOLDBERG, S, GREENSPON, A, URBAN P, ET AL: *Reperfusion arrhythmia: A marker of restoration of antegrade flow during intracoronary thrombolysis in acute myocardial infarction.* Am Heart J 105:26, 1983.

36. BLANKE, H, KARSCH, KR, SCHLIUTER, G, ET AL: *Preservation of R waves after acute LAD occlusion by streptokinase reperfusion.* Circulation 64:45, 1981.

37. GOLDBERG, S, GREENSPON, A, URBAN, P, ET AL: *Limitation of infarct size with thrombolytic agents: Electrocardiographic indices.* Circulation (Suppl) (In press).

38. GOLD, HK, LEINBACH, RC, PALACIOS, IF, ET AL: *Coronary reocclusion after selective administration of streptokinase.* Circulation (Suppl) (In press).

39. WEINSTEIN, J, SONNENBLICK, EH, COWLEY, MJ, ET AL: *Improved left ventricular function and reduced hospital mortality following intracoronary thrombolysis in myocardial infarction with diminished ejection fraction.* Am J Cardiol 49:961, 1982.

40. BRESNAHAN, GF, ROBERTS, R, SHELL, WE, ET AL: *Deleterious effects due to hemorrhage after myocardial reperfusion.* Am J Cardiol 33:82, 1974.

41. Mathey, DG, Kloppel, G, and Kuch, KH: *Transmural hemorrhagic infarction following intracoronary streptokinase: Clinical, angiographic and autopsy findings.* Circulation 64:4, 1981.

42. Schroder, R, Biamino, G, and Von Leitner, ER: *Intravenous short time thrombolysis in acute myocardial infarction.* Circulation 64:4, 1981.

43. European Cooperative Study Group for Streptokinase Treatment in Acute Myocardial Infarction: *Streptokinase in acute myocardial infarction.* N Engl J Med 301:797, 1979.

44. Goldberg, S, Urban, PL, Greenspon, AJ, et al: *Combination therapy for evolving myocardial infarction: Intracoronary thrombolysis and percutaneous transluminal angioplasty.* Am J Med 72:994, 1982.

Index

An *italic* numeral indicates a figure.
A "t" indicates a table.

DATE DUE

AUG 3 1 '99			

338

DEMCO 13829810